A COMPREHENSIVE GUIDE TO DAOIST NEI GONG

by the same author

Heavenly Streams
Meridian Theory in Nei Gong
Damo Mitchell
ISBN 978 1 84819 116 7
eISBN 978 0 85701 092 6

The Four Dragons
Clearing the Meridians and Awakening the Spine in Nei Gong
Damo Mitchell
Foreword by Dr Ole Saether
ISBN 978 1 84819 226 3
eISBN 978 0 85701 173 2

Daoist Nei Gong for Women
The Art of the Lotus and the Moon
Roni Edlund and Damo Mitchell
ISBN 978 1 84819 297 3
eISBN 978 0 85701 247 0

The Yellow Monkey Emperor's Classic of Chinese Medicine
Damo Mitchell and Spencer Hill
Artwork by Spencer Hill
ISBN 978 1 84819 286 7

Daoist Nei Gong
The Philosophical Art of Change
Damo Mitchell
ISBN 978 1 84819 065 8
eISBN 978 0 85701 033 9

Daoist Reflections from Scholar Sage
Damo Mitchell and his students
ISBN 978 1 84819 321 5
eISBN 978 0 85701 274 6

White Moon on the Mountain Peak
The Alchemical Firing Process of Nei Dan
Damo Mitchell
Foreword by Jason Gregory
ISBN 978 1 84819 256 0
eISBN 978 0 85701 203 6

A Comprehensive Guide to

DAOIST NEI GONG

DAMO MITCHELL

Foreword by Paul Mitchell

SINGING DRAGON
LONDON AND PHILADELPHIA

First published in 2018
by Singing Dragon
an imprint of Jessica Kingsley Publishers
73 Collier Street
London N1 9BE, UK
and
400 Market Street, Suite 400
Philadelphia, PA 19106, USA

www.singingdragon.com

Library of Congress Cataloging in Publication Data
A CIP catalog record for this book is available from the Library of Congress

British Library Cataloguing in Publication Data
A CIP catalogue record for this book is available from the British Library

ISBN 978 1 84819 410 6
eISBN 978 0 85701 372 9

Printed and bound in Great Britain

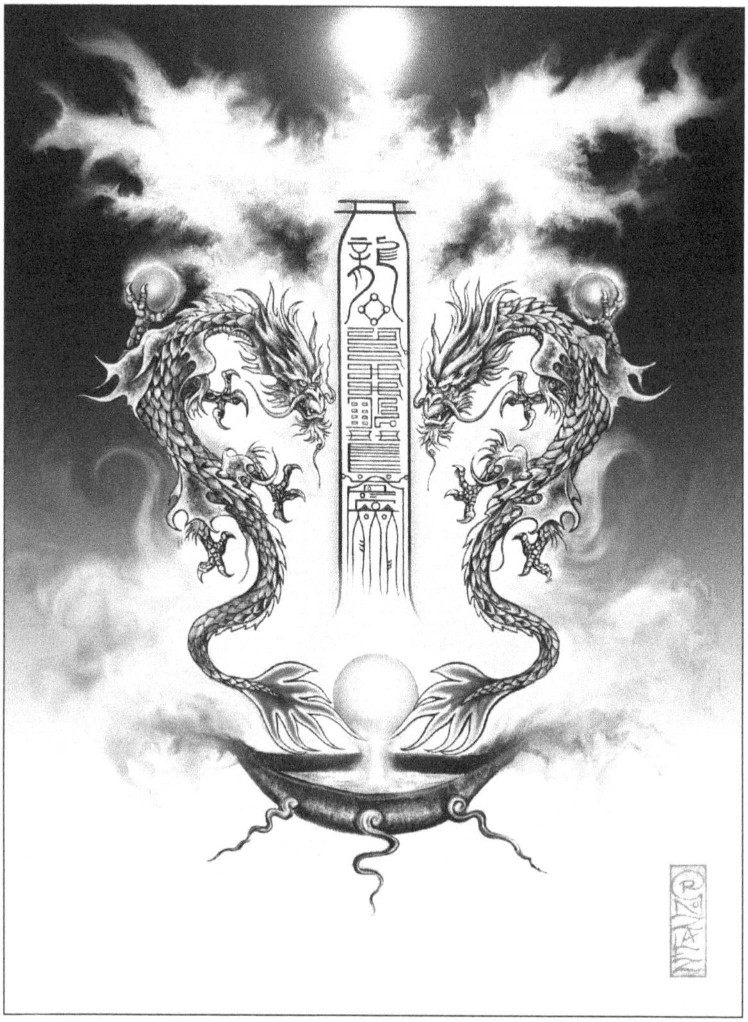

Contents

Foreword

Paul Mitchell

I, with a large degree of fatherly pride, was extremely pleased to be asked by my talented oldest son to write the foreword for his latest book.

It has been several decades since I, with high hopes for his future, began to train him in the Martial Arts of Asi. I did not, at this time, realise how this would begin a lifelong quest of discovery for him and consequently lead to a deep and profound understanding of a vast array of topics ranging from both external and internal martial arts through to Nei Gong, meditation and Chinese medicine.

It has been several years since Damo's first book on the Nei Gong process, and although it was certainly a ground-breaking piece of writing, his studies and understanding of this method of human development have greatly magnified and evolved. His new book most certainly reflects this evolution within him. In my opinion, my eldest son's greatest ability is his grounded approach to life, and this I feel sets him apart from others that profess to know and subsequently write upon and teach the Daoist arts. In some ways, I feel that maybe his generous nature causes him to make, what is all said and done, generally considered to be 'inner door' information readily available to the general public. However, I am myself no stranger to the teaching of these arts, having become a student of my son upon the realisation that his knowledge likely rivalled all but the most elite within the Daoist world. This has taught me that, for those that have not completed the correct groundwork, this 'inner door' information is of little use. The groundwork or indeed the building of a good foundation for a person's internal process is both essential for their future development as well as being a test of their character. For this reason, my concerns regarding the making public of the many revelations contained within this book have been dispelled. It is certainly true that in this modern time of instant gratification and love of shallow pursuits there is a very real danger that the health benefits, skills and personal development made possible through the processes intricately described within this book will all but disappear; this would be a crying shame. The watering down of classical systems, in order to fit in with people's lives, is a common occurrence in this time, and I know that my son feels a heavy burden of responsibility regarding the correct transmission of these arts in order to preserve them for future generations.

The material covered in this piece of work is certainly extensive. It takes the reader through relatively simple Qi Gong principles through standing practices and Daoist philosophy into energetic realms that are beyond the reach of all but the very resilient of us. Although I myself have studied these ways for many years, I discovered within this book many a facet previously untouched by my mind. As I stated earlier, I could not have known the journey that our humble beginnings within the martial arts would set in motion, but with hindsight there has been, in my opinion, nothing random about it. This piece of written work is in my opinion a simple extension of all that has gone before and is the culmination and encapsulation of my son's teaching up to this point. It is often true that what I would refer to as a 'journey person' (and, to my mind, my son is certainly one of those) will find it necessary to almost crystallise their accumulated knowledge at a given point in time and, beyond some personal practices that are between his teachers and himself, this book is just that. It is in my experience a rare thing for a teacher to put in black and white in an open and honest manner just what it is they are attempting to transmit through their teaching, and even rarer for them to write down for all to see how they do it. This again, in my opinion, speaks volumes about Damo's personal attainment within the arts, and therefore his openness and willingness to share his knowledge with all those fine souls that are willing to listen and make the necessary effort.

My son's previous books outlined the processes necessary in order to move a person through Dao Yin training in order to purge themselves of internal pathogens into Qi Gong exercises in order to regulate and rebalance themselves, and then into the deeper aspects of using these movements as tools in order to go far deeper into the realms of Nei Gong. This work has gone deeper still into this process and also includes many previously unmentioned aspects, including maybe one of the first written, certainly in English, explanations of the connective tissues or the 'Huang'. This is surely an important read for all who study body work, from gymnasts through to exponents of Taijiquan, back through to all those who profess to practise Nei Gong. I know it has long been a concern of my son that some people embark upon a Nei Gong practice without the background knowledge or work and without the guidance of an authentic teacher, and this can often cause them to harm themselves. For this reason, he has also included a section of possible dangers and methods for avoiding them.

I personally cannot state strongly enough that before one embarks upon a deep study of any internal system they must first find a good teacher. I know that, as the author's father, it is likely or even inevitable that I carry some degree of positive bias when it comes to this written piece, but I like to think that my many years working upon myself have given me the ability to separate my emotions from my ability to be objective. I found this book to not only be informative beyond most of what I have read on similar subjects but also exceptionally readable; a rare thing indeed in my experience. I think that this book will be a vitally important addition to anybody's collection if they intend to progress within the Daoist arts.

Paul Mitchell
Somerset, UK, January 2018

Preface

Back in 2011, the publishing house Singing Dragon released my first professional book on the subject of Nei Gong. The book was a simple overview of the internal process inherent within the Daoist arts. My aim was to shed some light on some of the more intricate aspects of internal training as well as to put forth the idea that Daoism was a fairly linear path, at least in the context of practices such as Qi Gong or the internal martial arts. The underlying ethos of most Eastern traditions is that there is a very strong relationship between our actions and the results that these actions generate; this is known as the rule of cause and effect. Within a practice such as Qi Gong, we establish the cause through what we do and then we allow the effect to arise as a result of this cause. The effect is not forced in any way, we don't struggle or strive for it, we simply establish the causes and allow this to take us where we wish to go. In the case of Qi Gong, the cause is generally the result of the principles we are adhering to combined with the exercises we are practising. The result is the change that this may have upon our health, well-being and the efficiency of the way in which our mind and body function. As we continue to practise in this way, we are led along a path of transformation that takes place within us; this path is what we call Nei Gong.

Qi Gong exercises can be practised in isolation from an internal path of development, and can simply be treated as a form of gentle exercise. On the other hand, if we understand the wider picture of Daoism and alchemical change, then we can begin to see these exercises as tools; now our focus can switch from practising Qi Gong exercises simply for their own sake, to using them as a way to develop ourselves internally through the Nei Gong process. Of course, neither of these two ways of practice is more correct than the other, they are simply different approaches. This book, however, adopts the view that Qi Gong exercises are tools that we use to lead us along the path of Dao.

You will see that though there is a great deal of information contained within this book, there is only a very small percentage of the book dedicated to moving Qi Gong practices. Instead, the majority of the book looks at the principles of practice and how they can affect the mind and body. This is because I would imagine the majority of people reading this book to already have a Qi Gong practice of their own. Though many people may know a series of Qi Gong exercises, fewer are aware of the internal processes that may be initiated through the practice of these exercises. To help make it clear, I have outlined the process that I have been moving through; this is also the process that I guide my students into as well. Though not all systems of practice will follow this same path, there are likely to be some similarities as well as some differences. Recognising these can be helpful as it can shed light on your own practice.

I started my journey into the Eastern arts when I was four years old. This journey began with martial arts training, and though I knew little of what I was doing at that age, I was establishing the base for what would turn out to be a lifelong fascination with these arts. I continued in my training until I turned fourteen and encountered the internal arts of China; initially this was the practice of Taijiquan from within the Yang family tradition but, with time, this study expanded into Qi Gong, meditation, medicine and Nei Gong. I was consumed with a passion for my studies and quickly sought out as many high-level teachers as I could here in the West. This satisfied me for a short while but then I began to look further afield and so headed into China and South-East Asia.

Over the years I have spent a great deal of my life seeking out those who can help me move deeper into these practices; sometimes my searching proved fruitful and at other times I was led down dead ends by teachers who proclaimed to know more than they actually did. This is all a part of the journey that myself and so many others have been on. Whilst these dead ends can also provide us with a valuable life lesson, it would have been nice to get the time back that I spent pursuing practices that would essentially lead me nowhere. I often wished that I had access to more information on the nature of the journey itself as well as detailed explanations of what I was to look for as signs of progress; this kind of information is often very difficult to come by within the internal arts community. For this reason, I have put together this book, to try to provide some of the guidance that I would have liked to have had access to much earlier on in my personal development.

I have tried to give an overview of the Nei Gong process with a heavy emphasis upon the important principles and practices at each stage as well as spending time underlining the key elements of the training that many people struggle with understanding. I have tried to include clear signs of when you are starting to attain Gong (an embodied quality or skill associated with your practice) at each stage in the training along with pitfalls and possible errors that you may make. It is my hope that some of this information will prove at least a little helpful to those who are embarking on their journey into the internal arts.

You will notice that I spend a fair amount of time looking at the body and how to work with it on a physical level. This is of paramount importance to me: the 'workshop' where all of your work will take place is your body. If the workshop is not properly prepared then the work you produce will be of a poor quality. For this reason, I have given a detailed description of the sinew-changing practices of the internal arts in order to help demonstrate just how the body should be developed. Despite the Sinew-Changing Classic, the text from which almost all Qi Gong teachings regarding the transformation of the body are derived, being a key component contained within all of the internal arts, especially arts such as Qi Gong, it is often poorly understood and applied.

Another key factor that you will notice from my writings is that I rarely talk of using the imagination. Visualisation and generated mental imagery are not a part of the system I teach. Instead, various qualities of mental abiding are developed along with a connection to the somatic experience of the practice. It is an important quality of Qi Gong practice that we learn to relax, expand and absorb the mind into our practice. This can only happen when the mind is free from action. The mind cannot be free from action if it is generating visual experiences or engaging with your imagination; in this way, the process of mental release and visualisation are in direct conflict with one another.

I am still very much a student myself on this path; I am exploring and practising and have no delusion that I am anything other than scratching the surface of these arts. For this reason, I can only present to you what I have been taught, what I have experienced and how I understand these arts according to my current position. I ask, therefore, that you don't take anything written in this book as gospel. To take everything you are told 100 per cent on faith is never a healthy way to approach life, but neither should we be closed off to new information. The best approach to studying any art like this is to listen to what we are told, consider it, try it out and then see what conclusions we come by through this practice. An open and explorative mind is the healthiest mind we can have when engaging with a practice such as Nei Gong.

Just a quick note now about text usage. Throughout this book I have used the Pinyin system of Romanisation for the majority of Chinese words. Please note that much of the theory in this book differs greatly from Western science.

The classical Chinese approach to understanding the organs of the body, for example, is based around the function of their energetic system rather than their physical anatomy. To distinguish the two understandings from each other I have used capitalisation to indicate the Chinese understanding of the term. 'Heart', for example, refers to the classical Chinese understanding of the organ, whilst 'heart' refers to the physical organ as understood within contemporary Western biological sciences.

Also, I have had a lot of correspondence from native Chinese speakers who have been reading my books. This, combined with an increase in Chinese students, means that it is now wise to put the Chinese characters next to each Pinyin term used. In order to not 'overcrowd' the text I have included the Chinese character the first time each Pinyin term is used. The exception to this is if it seemed relevant to include the Chinese character on another occasion such as when listing Pinyin terms. As well as this, there is a full glossary of Chinese terminology at the end of this book.

I hope the book is helpful to some of you reading this and I wish you all the best in your own development.

Damo Mitchell
Portugal, January 2018

Acknowledgements

As with all writing projects of this kind, there are always a number of people involved. I would like to express my thanks to all those who helped me in various ways when I was putting this text together; without you, my task would have been a whole lot more difficult!

First, thanks must go to those who taught me these arts; there has been a variety of masters and teachers around the world, both here in the West and abroad in Asia. Over the past thirty years or so of practice, I have had the chance to be led into these practices and shown the way to proceed along my practice and Ming. Much gratitude and recognition of debts I can never even come close to paying back for all you have shared with me.

Second, thank you to my students around the world; it is a pleasure to teach you guys, and without the school, I would not have had the need nor experience required to analyse the Nei Gong process enough to put it into a written format.

Many thanks to my father for being my first teacher and for writing the Foreword for this book. Thank you for starting me out on this journey and then continuing to travel it with me.

Much gratitude to Roni, my beautiful wife, for putting up with me and the mess whilst I wrote this book and for assisting with reading sections of the text; I love you dearly and could not hope for a better life or training partner.

Many thanks to Jana 'fan of squids' Reidenbach for tirelessly working her way through the book when it was in its earliest draft and helping with such thorough corrections and suggestions. You made the book sound a lot more professional.

Cheers to my student and friend Jason Smith for working on the diagrams that fill the book. They make things very clear and you did a neater job than I would have done.

Xuelian 'Julie' Qin was as generous as ever with her assistance with the Chinese characters in the book. Thank you for helping me out with that darn confusing language, Chinese.

Thanks to Spencer Hill and Joe Andrews for their help with the line drawings that appear in the book. Especially well done to Spencer for reproducing the Hun and Po deities from such badly reproduced classical sources.

Much gratitude to the students who appeared in the photos of this book: Tom Burrows, Roni (once again), Susan Casserfelt, Ramut Rodriguez and Jason (again).

Thanks to Rob Aspell for his help with the Chinese medicine sections of the book. Thanks to Ramut Gonzalez for the fancy Dragon, Ding and Fu image on the inside cover. Great work.

As always, thank you to the good folk of Singing Dragon and Jessica Kingsley herself for helping to bring this book to life and for always doing an excellent job with regard to the final product.

Last, but not least, thank you to Oscar Idelji-Tehrani for making those adjustments of simplified to traditional Chinese characters for me in the glossary as well as throughout the main text.

To anybody else who was involved who I forgot to mention: I am truly sorry, just let me know next time I see you and I shall apologise profusely...

Chapter 1

QI GONG, NEI GONG AND QI

Throughout history, numerous spiritual traditions have each developed their own understanding of human life. Though the models may be different, the basis of all of their teachings is that we comprise much more than just our physical body. Animating the vessel of our form is a spirit, an intangible soul. Connecting the mind and body together, there is generally an intangible, unseen force that is seen as 'flowing' around the body. In each tradition, this understanding of how we exist on different levels was then used to inform systems of practice. Some are based on forms of meditation, some on moving exercises, and others on stretching and conditioning the body in various ways. Though their eventual outcomes may differ, there is always the shared view that in order to elevate the spirit, we must first learn to understand and work with the various elements that make up our existence.

Easily one of the most widespread esoteric 'models' of human existence today is that of the ancient Chinese. To place an exact historical date upon the start of Chinese internal development is impossible. Exercises and spiritual teachings are understood to originate way back in the early days of Chinese history with shamanic characters known simply as the Wu (巫). It is likely that the Wu developed their understandings through a combination of experience and spiritual insight. My personal teachers explained to me that the Wu served as medicine men, tribal guides and magicians of sorts. What is for certain is that the ancient methods of this time evolved and developed throughout history to become exercises such as Dao Yin (導引) and Qi Gong (氣功). Today, Qi Gong exercises are practised in parks around the world as well as in community centres and village halls in many places here in the West. In the majority of cases, these exercises are practised for medical purposes, the view being that if a person can regulate their Qi (氣), then it will help bring the body closer to a state of good health. In this way, what we are seeing is an amalgamation of exercise with Chinese medicine theory.

Other forms of Qi Gong include practices aimed at strengthening the body for martial purposes, systems developed to help a person gain spiritual elevation, and even religious systems aimed at connecting a person to deities and gods. Qi Gong as a practice has evolved and diversified into hundreds of different forms, though the core principles behind each practice remain the same.

Qi Gong is an interesting practice. It is often compared to a mix of Yogic asana and meditation, but this is only partially true. As with the movements we commonly associate with Yoga, there is a certain degree of working with and changing the body, though this is where the similarities end. Whilst Yoga works to stretch and open up the body, Qi Gong aims to divide the body into parts and reshape it from the inside out. In order to compare Qi Gong to meditation, we must understand that meditation takes many forms, but in the majority of cases is aimed at working solely with the practitioner's consciousness. In Qi Gong practice, we aim to develop a very particular mindset that does indeed share qualities with the mindset of meditation, but the route to getting there is very different indeed. Rather than going directly to consciousness-based exercises, we instead work with the tangibility of the body first before progressing into the subtler realms of the mind.

Though Qi Gong exercises are fairly well known now, less well understood is the process of Nei Gong (内功). Nei Gong means 'internal skill'; if we take the term literally, it is referring to a very specific series of changes that the body can go through if trained in the correct manner. Nei Gong does not have any specific 'exercises' as such. It is simply a process that is laid out in a very clear and surprisingly linear manner. Movement through the Nei Gong process is the inherent aim within most classical schools of Qi Gong, whereby the Qi Gong exercises themselves are simply seen as 'tools' that are used to facilitate this process.

For those wishing to practise Qi Gong exercises solely for the (more than acceptable) aim of relaxation or as a form of health exercise, there is no need for study of the Nei Gong process. It is a long and complex path that only the most dedicated of students should really concern themselves with.

What Does Nei Gong Entail?

The big question that many newcomers to Nei Gong may ask is 'What exactly does Nei Gong training entail?' When first encountering teachings on the subject of Nei Gong, it can be a little overwhelming. There is a great deal of philosophy involved, volumes of alchemical writings and almost impenetrable terminology which can initially seem very off-putting. The good news, though, is that Chinese arts always tend to be the same: the theory is initially very complex, but the actual practice involved is fairly straightforward. The theory is there to help shape the mind in the right way and guide us through the processes of change we will inevitably go through, but ultimately, it is our engagement with the practice that will yield the results.

We can divide Nei Gong training into three main aspects – standing exercises, moving exercises, and seated practice. There are then further adjunct practices, but these three broad categorisations make up the majority of our work. Standing exercises are the starting point of the tradition. These are aimed at developing certain fundamental skills such as 'sinking the Qi' and 'locating the lower Dan Tian (丹田)'. From here, there is a general progression into moving and, finally, seated practice. Moving exercises help to circulate Qi through the body, and seated exercises are used for the more intricate aspects of the process. At first, when learning these arts, you will switch between the three types of exercises according to what you are practising, but with time you should find that you gravitate more towards seated work; at this stage of the training, your standing and moving exercises will become less and less important.

What is most important to recognise is that we have a clear distinction between two terms. These terms are 'Nei Gong' and 'Qi Gong'. Essentially, Nei Gong is the process of change we should be aiming to move through, whilst Qi Gong exercises are the tools we use to move through this process. This means that for the majority of our training, we will be studying Qi Gong and using these exercises on a daily basis. In the background to all of this, we should be developing an understanding of the Nei Gong process and our placement along the spectrum of this path. This will enable us to understand exactly where we are and when we need to move on to the next stage of our training.

Who Should Not Train?

Though Nei Gong is no more dangerous than any other internal practice (as long as it is trained according to the guidelines) there are a few groups of people who really should not undertake the practices in this book.

First, people under the age of 18 should not practise Nei Gong of any sort. Other internal practices such as Taijiquan are fine to study but Nei Gong itself is a bad idea. Throughout childhood and the early teens, there are many shifts taking place within a person's energetic matrix as well as within the elemental makeup of their mind. It takes until the late teens or early adulthood for a person's Xing to enter into some kind of settled state and for the emotions to move into a more stable place. If a younger person engages with Nei Gong, then they are essentially adding another variable, a potent one at that, into a rapidly changing set of conditions. It is wiser to wait until a person is at a more stable age before they start to study an art that can lead to such powerful internal changes.

Second, women who are pregnant or who think they may be pregnant should not practise Nei Gong at all. The Qi and Shen within a pregnant woman are already undergoing all sorts of alchemical changes; these will unfold as they are supposed to. It could be problematic if a woman then has a process of change taking place at the same time that is a result of her practice. Allow the energies within the body to move as they are supposed to and stick with gentle stretching and breathing exercises during pregnancy; there should be no Dan Tian-focused work at all.

Those with a recognised, chronic mental illness should not practise Nei Gong, as the chance of developing Qi Gong deviation-type sickness is increased greatly within those with psychiatric imbalance. This is especially true in the case of mental disorders that swing between extreme highs and lows or for those medicated with anti-psychotic medication.

People with severe heart disorders should be cautious with their approach to the practice of Nei Gong. Whilst correct practice of the system will be fine, it is easy to make an error and send the Qi of the heart into a hyperactive state. Whilst this is rare, it could be problematic for those with pre-existing heart problems. If you are unsure of how your heart condition could be affected by Qi Gong training, then consult with a skilled Chinese medical practitioner as well as with your teacher. Generally, as an aside on problems with the heart, practitioners of Nei Gong run the risk of disturbing their heart rhythm if they practise whilst extremely stressed, practise whilst chronically exhausted, drink too much coffee alongside their practice, cannot sink their Qi properly, or use too strong a level of mental focus. Generally, if people have problems with their heart during practice, it is due to one of these factors.

People who regularly use recreational drugs, especially hallucinogenic drugs, should not practise Nei Gong, as this can lead to severe problems developing within the Shen. As well as this, you should never practise whilst intoxicated in any way.

> Those with cancer should notify their teacher of their condition and work carefully with them to ensure that they progress in a safe fashion. The only form of cancer that really should not be combined with Nei Gong is cancer that is present within the lymphatic system. This is because the increased flow of Qi through the body also influences the lymphatic system and there is the risk of spreading the condition at a faster rate.

Fa versus Gong

Within the practice of Qi Gong, we can divide the process of learning into two main stages. The first is the stage of learning the Fa (法) and the second is the attaining of Gong (功). Fa can be translated as 'the method' or 'technique'. This is what all students begin with when they start any practice. The method must be developed over a period of time until it is good enough to be considered a skill. The point of a 'method' is that it is designed to achieve a particular goal, and so we use said method until this goal is reached. Within the internal arts, once a method has been practised for long enough that it achieves its goal, it can be said to have transformed into a 'Gong'. Gong is commonly translated as 'skill' or 'work', when in actual fact, if we look at the way the term 'Gong' is used within arts such as Qi Gong, it would be better to translate it as a 'quality'. In short, a practitioner of the internal arts learns how to develop and use Fa until they attain Gong.

This fact is often misunderstood within contemporary internal arts practice, whereby many modern people think they have achieved a high level once they can do the technique correctly; in actuality they are still stuck at the stage of Fa. An example would be a person who learns a set of Qi Gong exercises that are intricate and complex, perhaps a set such as the Dragon Dao Yin or the Five Animal Frolics. They spend all of their practice time making sure that each movement is as neat as possible, that the movements flow, and that from the outside it looks relaxed and beautiful. What has been missed here is that the point of exercises such as this is to achieve a very specific goal; each part of the exercise has been meticulously developed over a long period of time to affect the inside of the body or mind in a very specific manner. By focusing on the 'technique' to the detriment of the 'result', through a lack of awareness of this fact, they have stopped themselves from ever reaching a state of Gong. This is a common error I term 'overfocusing on the tools'.

To achieve Gong takes a long time and lots of repetition. I disagree with the common traditional mindset that even with a lack of understanding, a person will still reach mastery if they repeat what they are doing enough times. This may work for a small number of people, but in the majority of cases, having a deeper understanding of what they are doing will help a person more efficiently develop towards a higher level of skill. In this way, theory will 'shape the Yi (意)'. This is a concept I will return to when we discuss 'regulation of the mind'.

If we apply this understanding of the term 'Gong' to our practice, we can see that even the names for what we are doing imply reaching a certain level of expertise. So, to understand Qi Gong now as a practice, we can see that it should be translated as 'practising with our Qi until we reach Gong'. A practice such as Nei Gong should be translated more fully as 'working with our internal environment until we reach Gong'. In this way, the names of what we are doing serve to tell us where we are aiming for rather than what we are doing.

Daoism and the Arts

Daoism is a tradition that most likely evolved out of the esoteric practices of the Wu people. It is considered to be China's primary internal tradition since the other two primary traditions of China include Confucianism, which is primarily concerned with 'external' methods of cultivation in the form of philosophical guidance, and Buddhism, which originated in Nepal before being exported to China at a later date. Daoism was really consolidated as a tradition with the teachings of the legendary figure Laozi (老子) and his pivotal text, the Dao De Jing (道德經). Scholars debate whether or not Laozi was a real person or if he was used as a figurehead for the collected wisdom of a number of people. Whatever the truth, Daoism as a tradition was formalised at this time, over 2,500 years ago. There is further disagreement as to whether Daoism was ever a philosophical tradition devoid of a religious aspect. Some state that it was always a religion with hierarchal structures and a pantheon of gods. Others claim that it was instead a practical 'method-based' system of practice that later evolved into a religion when it merged with religious Buddhist beliefs. The truth of the matter is that it is rather irrelevant since nowadays there is definitely a divide between the two schools of thought. Some practise a very ritual- and worship-based form of Daoism which takes a similar format to other organised religions, whilst others either practise the 'methods' of Daoism, or apply its philosophical teachings to their lives. I am personally from the 'method-based' form of Daoism and have little interest in its religious expression.

It would be disingenuous to the other spiritual traditions of China to say that Qi Gong was purely from Daoist roots; instead, we can say that Daoism had a major influence upon Qi Gong's development, and certainly much of the terminology and philosophy of the practice is taken directly from Daoist sources. You will see, as the book continues, that many Daoist and even shamanic concepts underpin everything that we do in our practice.

If we are to take the three most important concepts of Qi Gong that were derived from Daoism, these would undoubtedly be Yin Yang (陰陽) theory, the concept of Heaven and Earth, and the principle of Wei Wu Wei (為無為). The first two concepts will be explored in more detail later, but for now we will begin with Wei Wu Wei.

Wei Wu Wei

Note that when I use this term in full, I write 'Wei Wu Wei' instead of simply 'Wu Wei' as it is usually seen. The use of 'Wei Wu Wei' is specifically important to Qi Gong practice, as it concerns the transference from 'Fa' to 'Gong' that was discussed above. Wei Wu Wei can be translated as 'doing, non-doing' or rather 'doing until we reach the stage of non-doing'. This concept is important within our practice because it dictates how long we do each exercise or method within our system as well as why we do it. Everything in life is about 'cause and effect'; the internal arts are no different. The original 'doing', the 'Fa', is practised until the correct quality, or Gong, is achieved. Then we allow the quality we have achieved to unfold on its own within us. Once the correct effect is achieved, there is no need for 'doing' any more. Now we have reached the level of applying Wu Wei to our practice.

Think of an example like this: I have an exercise designed to draw Qi into the region of the lower abdomen. This method involves a series of breathing methods and arm movements combined with mental exercises. I learn the method and then practise it for a long time. This is the stage of having learnt Fa and now using Fa to generate the correct 'cause' within the body. I practise for a year or so, and now the Qi begins to move to a high degree into my lower abdomen. It starts to become so natural for the body to do this that I no longer need the external movements nor breathing methods. Instead, I can simply sit and let my mind become aware of the process. The simple act of being aware strengthens the process, and so now I no longer need to 'do' anything. The 'cause' has established the desired 'effect'. I have now reached the state of 'non-doing' or Wu Wei. Remaining with the process that is now unfolding will start to lead me towards Gong, an inherent quality built into my body, until it is a natural and continuous process. All that is required is steady observance with the mind.

It is for this reason that there is a traditional rule within Qi Gong communities that beginners should practise 90 per cent moving exercises and 10 per cent static exercises. This is because the need for Wei or Fa is much greater. In contrast to this, advanced practitioners should move towards 90 per cent static practice and only 10 per cent moving exercises. They are static a lot more of the time, as they are simply being aware of the 'cause and effect' they have successfully established within themselves. The stage of Wu Wei is more important to them in their movement towards Gong. Wu Wei is considered a more desirable stage, as there is less room for human error, but we must go through Wei first.

Two potential pitfalls for Qi Gong practice revolve around poor application of this concept. If a person tries to apply Wu Wei too early, then they are essentially observing a 'cause and effect' relationship that has not been set up. The result will be that very little happens. On the other hand, if a practitioner continues with the stage of 'doing' for too long, past the stage of having already attained the desired result, they will actually slow their progress. Daoists call this 'over-sharpening the knife until it becomes blunt'. It is because of these pitfalls that one important role of a teacher was to tell a student when it was time to move on with what they were doing. Teachers should understand the clear signs of when their students have attained the desired result and so should move into the next stage of their development. Without this knowledge and guidance, we are essentially working in the dark. In the past, I have had teachers who knew the methods but not the signs of when to move on; the result was that I did not practise in a very efficient manner, and so my progress was slowed. I then had teachers later who knew the signs and knew exactly when I had done enough work to move on. I experienced a clear increase in efficiency in what I was doing when I moved into working under their instruction. Often, knowledge of the signs of progress have been lost or forgotten, so throughout this book I have tried to include clear, tangible signs that you should be able to recognise to understand exactly where you are in your development and when to move on.

Increasing the Efficiency of the Body

If we are to look at the main reasons why people practise Qi Gong exercises, it generally either comes down to looking for a way to relax or else to improve their health. Of course, there are many other reasons why people practise arts like this, but I am just focusing on the two largest groups. These are good reasons to study an art like Qi Gong, but they are certainly only a part of the practice and not the be all and end all of the training. Basically, relaxation of the mind and body in Qi Gong practice is required so that we can 'enter the gate' of the practice. In this case, relaxation is not a goal as such but rather a 'way in' to the practice. The second reason why most people practise, to attain good health, is more in line with many of the other positive side-effects of training Qi Gong. The reason for this is that it is based upon making the mind and body function more efficiently. Now, that might sound glaringly obvious, but it is worth repeating and keeping in mind, because many people I have met in the Qi Gong world seem to miss this fact. Qi Gong training is designed, as a practice, to make your mind and body function more efficiently. The actual process of 'change' that helps this efficiency to grow is called the Nei Gong process. Different systems have their own aims and each can take people to a different level of 'efficiency', depending upon how effective the system is, but in essence, this is all they are doing. Even the masters who show skills that look almost supernatural are only working at a higher level of efficiency than the majority of people. The capability is there within people, it is just getting the body to function in the correct manner and at the right level that can be elusive. If we look at the stages involved in increasing the efficiency of the body's functioning, we can see that, in most cases, they follow the basic series of steps outlined in Figure 1.1. These stages begin with working on what most people would consider as 'improving health' and then progress onto deeper stages.

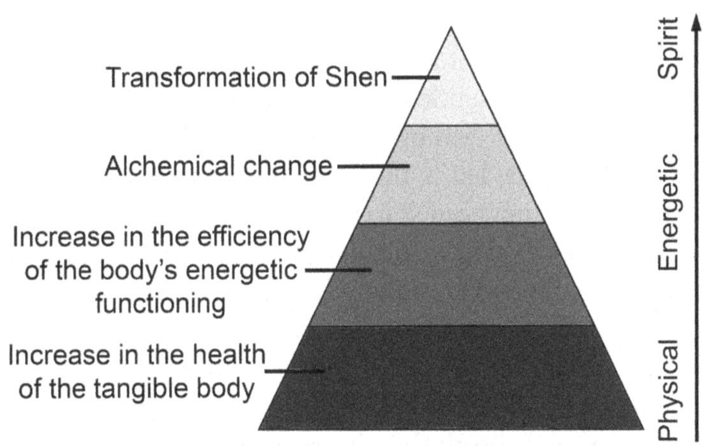

Figure 1.1: The Stages of Increasing the Body's Efficiency

At the base of the pyramid structure is an 'increase in the health of the tangible body'. This happens as a result of the increase in efficiency of the body's functioning. These changes take place in everything from the way that we use our body to move around, sit, stand and carry out actions on a daily basis, through to how the internal organs function and relate to one another. The connection of mind to body means that even at this level, as the body changes, so does the functioning of the mind. It is always more difficult to focus and relax your mind when the body is in a state of dis-ease.

Beyond this change to the body's physical functioning, we then have an 'increase in the efficiency of the body's energetic functioning'. Note that here, in the first chapter of the book, I use the term 'energy' to refer to the circulations and actions of the body's Qi. In truth, I find the term 'energy' a little non-specific and sometimes unhelpful when approaching an art like Qi Gong. Further on, I shall define the term more exactly and clarify what I mean by 'circulations of Qi'. For now though, it is enough to understand that sitting 'behind' the tangible body's form is a more subtle level of functioning that we need to learn how to work with and improve the efficiency of if we wish to move deeper into our practice. This stage works cyclically with the previous stage. The more we increase the efficiency of the body's functioning on an energetic level, we also help the body's physical state and vice versa.

The third stage of improving the efficiency of the body's functioning is through 'alchemical' change. The term 'alchemical' is referring to the manner in which the three treasures of Jing (精), Qi (氣) and Shen (神) relate to one another. This is a complex aspect of the internal arts to which a great deal of time and thought was given by classical Daoist teachers. A large percentage of the classical texts that have been passed down through the generations to the modern day spend a lot of time trying to decipher the mysteries of these three aspects of our subtle body. To be perfectly honest, this stage of attainment takes a great deal of time and effort. For those interested in simply reducing their stress levels, there is no need to commit to the amount of hours and inner scrutiny needed to touch upon this aspect of the arts.

Beyond this stage of training, there begins work on 'energetic density'. This is important for intermediate-to-advanced practitioners so that they may soften the quality of their mind with regard to how it interacts with the body. Essentially, the mind can be thought of as having a 'shape' of sorts. In order to move towards the deeper aspects of Qi Gong and Nei Gong, we must be able to fully absorb the 'shape' of the mind into the body. For this to happen, there has to be a series of 'anchors' established within the body. These anchors then root the mind into our being, even when we are in a passive state. Though not as complex as it can sound, it takes time to achieve this kind of level in your practice, and many Qi Gong practitioners never reach this important stage, simply because they don't have the correct information. We will discuss this in great detail further into the book.

The final two stages of increasing the efficiency of how we function are to do with the Shen and its elevated form, the Ling (靈). These stages correspond with the advanced stages of moving beyond work with the body into pure 'consciousness development'. At this level, the training is more akin to Nei Dan (内丹) or 'internal alchemy' than it is to Qi Gong.

A Linear Path

Of course, this description is just a rough outline of the various stages of development we are going through, the different levels of human existence that are worked on as we progress. Each stage of work involves various exercises, processes and stages that we should be aware of. It often surprises people just how 'linear' a process all of this is when you understand the 'roadmap' of how we develop within the arts. More fitting with the contemporary 'alternative arts' scene would be to describe everything as being non-linear or to simply say, 'There is no journey, we are already there!', but in actual fact, the path of Nei Gong, and indeed Daoism, must be walked. This is hinted at in one common translation for Daoism which is 'the way' or 'the path'. If we look at the Chinese character for 'Dao', we can even see that it shows a wild-haired shamanic-looking character walking along a path. Figure 1.2 shows the character and how it is constructed.

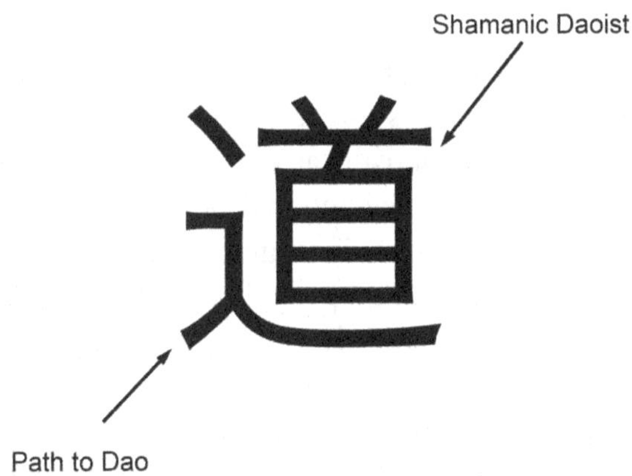

Figure 1.2: Dao

This character can be seen to the right. The character is showing us that in order to reach Dao, we should 'walk along the path'. A path is a linear route through a practice that starts at A and leads you through to B. If we then look at any of the internal arts, we can see that true transmission of the methods involves following a systematic path of progression that takes you through a series of developmental stages. If we do not have these developmental steps, then we will, at some stage, become 'lost' in our practice and, as the Daoists would say, will 'stray from the path'.

Curiously, the basis of Daoism is that we have to adhere to a tradition and then, at the correct time (the term 'correct' here is very important!), we must step away from the tradition and instead simply allow Dao to unfold within us. This is highlighted within the line 'Dao Ke Dao Fei Chang Dao (道可道非常道)' or 'The Dao that can be followed is not the true and unmoving Dao.' This implies that although the 'path' of Dao must be walked, at the right stage in our practice we must forget the path and let our prior work lead us towards the next stage in our development.

The basis of understanding when to 'leave the path' is looking at what the path does. The systematic internal training of the Daoist arts works to regulate the body, energetic matrix and consciousness in such a way that when we relax and allow ourselves to merge with Dao, we are in the right condition to do so. If we try to 'simply be with Dao' before this, then we will have little hope. The quality of our Jing, Qi and Shen is not right. Instead, we prepare the body, the vessel, through systematic practice until such time as everything is as it should be. Practice leads us into a specific state of being, and then we allow the fruits of our labour to unfold within us of their own accord. This is known as the balance between Wei (doing) and Wu Wei (non-doing). Getting this balance right is of paramount importance and is the reason for the usefulness of traditional training within an internal system.

Many Qi Gong systems do not really have a step-by-step nature to the way that they are taught. This is fine for those who wish to relax and move their bodies gently, but it is not really an efficient way to study for those who really want to go deep into their internal practice. Every classical system of practice from an authentic root is taught in a step-by-step manner, with each stage in the practice building upon what came before. The student first works towards developing the body in the right way, then the energetic system, and finally the mind. Though there is, of course, some crossover between these stages of development, we generally work in this manner.

For each stage of development, there are defined exercises to practise and expected results. The 'landmarks' show us when to move on, and this is where the role of the teacher comes in. The teacher must help the student develop along the 'path' as effectively as they can.

Mastering control of the efficiency of the body requires first mastering control of our Qi, hence the name of the practice – Qi Gong. Beyond this, we must master the control and development of our internal environment; this is alluded to in the name of the process of our development – Nei Gong. If we actually look at the stages of 'efficiency increasing' within Figure 1.1, we can see that it starts with the physical body, moves into the energetic realm, and then finally leads into direct work with the mind and spirit. This is the classical order for work within the Daoist arts. It ensures that a solid foundation is built in the tangible before exploration of the subtle is undertaken: a vital principle to ensure we remain 'grounded' in our lives.

A Developing Process

The process of development that we go through whilst practising is important to understand. Whilst there is room for some flexibility within any given process, there is generally a main route that we should follow. In many Qi Gong schools, the 'process' is not laid out in a clear fashion, whilst the general tendency of schools calling themselves 'Nei Gong schools' is that they have a clear path of internal development. Though some will balk against having a linear path of progression to follow, I myself have always found it helpful. When meeting many Qi Gong practitioners for the first time, I tend to ask them where they are on their own path and where they are headed. What is the point of the exercises they are doing? Of course, this is only for those who wish to move deep into the arts. For those who wish to use their training to improve their health, it is not so necessary. In many cases, people find it difficult to answer, so the first mission is to go back to the process, 'the way', and ascertain what stages of development they are comfortable with. What 'Gong' have they achieved and what are they weak in? Once you have a clear idea of this, then it can create a massive shift in your practice. All of a sudden, you can start to ascertain what it is you are supposed to be focusing on in your training.

The basic Nei Gong process that I work with within my school is as follows:

1. Conditioning and preparing the physical body
2. Regulation of breath and mind
3. Beginning the stage of Jing to Qi
4. Awakening the energy system
5. Movement and governance of the Yang Qi
6. Attainment of internal vibration/life

7. Beginning the stage of Qi to Shen
8. The stage of Shen to Ling and Dao

I have written about this process previously in a very 'introductory' manner. In the book *Daoist Nei Gong: The Philosophical Art of Change*, published by Singing Dragon in 2011, I gave a brief introduction to the Nei Gong process and outlined some of the stages inherent at each step. In this book, I wish to go deeper into these stages and really take apart what happens at each part of the process, certainly for the foundation and intermediate stages of training. If we wish to understand each step along the way fully, we can subdivide them into the following parts:

1. Conditioning and preparing the physical body
    a. Stretch and strengthen the body in the correct manner
    b. Learn to 'hang the muscles' from the frame
    c. Learn how to align the body
    d. Learn how to maintain alignments whilst moving
    e. Learn to locate the lower Dan Tian in the correct fashion
    f. Control the placement of the centre of mass
    g. Learn to effectively move the centre of mass
2. Regulation of breath and mind
    a. Regulate the breath according to the 'keywords' of Qi Gong
    b. Understand the nature of 'passive' and 'active' breathing
    c. Connect breath to the process of release
    d. Understand the nature of mind
    e. Understand Daoist teachings on mind training
    f. Understand the 'shape' of the mind
    g. Application of Wei Wu Wei in practice
    h. The balance of focus and release
3. Beginning the stage of Jing to Qi
    a. Consolidation of Jing

   b. Retraining of Jing movement
   c. Understanding healthy patterns of Jing maintenance
   d. Control of the lower basin of the body
4. Awakening the energy system
   a. Dan Tian awakening
   b. Fire and Water governance
   c. Opening of the channels
   d. Microcosmic orbit
   e. Understanding the nature of Qi
   f. Purging, nourishing and regulating Qi
   g. Sinking the Qi in the correct manner
5. Movement and governance of the Yang Qi
   a. Understanding the nature of Fire and Water Qi
   b. Understanding the nature of Yin and Yang Qi
   c. Balancing and combining of Fire and Water
   d. Mixing of Fire and Water
   e. Generation of Yin and Yang
6. Attainment of internal vibration/life
   a. Conversion of mental activity to 'listening'
   b. Full absorption of consciousness into the body
   c. Application of the Sinew-Changing Classic to the practice
   d. Return to the consolidation of Dan Tian
   e. Building the 'gourd'
   f. Expanding the Qi
   g. Attainment of 'radiation'
7. Beginning the stage of Qi to Shen
   a. Stilling the mind

    b. Combining the five elements
    c. Finding the 'white moon on the mountain peak' (see Chapter 12)
8. The stage of Shen to Ling and Dao
    a. Advanced alchemical study
    b. Shen Gong and development of spirit (神功)

After an initial look at the background philosophy of the arts and a discussion of health according to Daoism and Qi Gong, I shall spend the rest of the book exploring these stages and what they mean.

What Is Qi?

It is clear to see that within any of these kinds of arts, no matter the system, the main concern is going to be finding and working with your Qi. There is no way around this term or the fact that an in-depth experiential study of Qi will be involved in your practice. I have had the misfortune to come across a couple of 'Qi Gong' schools that had completely dropped the term altogether and instead turned their practice into breathing exercises based on Western physiotherapy theory, but luckily, most systems have not gone down this route. Throwing out a term simply because you do not understand it or you feel that the ancient understandings were archaic is not a good idea. I have found time and time again that once I actually penetrated deeper into the arts, there were clear and specific definitions for every single term being used. You will often hear the phrase 'Qi as a term is impossible to define, as it is an abstract thing'; I do not believe this to be the case. Qi has a very specific set of meanings, it just depends upon what context the term is being used within. So, for example, the term 'Qi' appears in Chinese medicine, Qi Gong, martial arts and countless other Chinese practices. It is also used within general conversation where the 'Qi' of the weather may be discussed and so on. If we mistakenly assume that the term 'Qi' is the same within each of these contexts, then obviously we will suddenly have a very broad spectrum of definitions. Now, it is difficult for us to understand the term or give it a very specific definition; but if we look at each art in isolation, we can actually start to discover its meaning. This meaning is useful, as without a definition of Qi that we can work with, it will be hard to progress far into our practice.

The Qi of Chinese Medicine

Within Chinese medicine terminology, Qi is used in two main ways: first as an 'action' or 'function', and second as a very specific entity that flows through the channel system. We shall look at the definition of Qi within the channels separately since it is relevant to Qi Gong practice as well.

We can see the term 'Qi' being used as an 'action' within phrases such as 'the Qi of the Heart'. What is the 'Qi of the Heart'? Essentially, it is the functional activity of the Heart system. So, if the Heart has healthy Qi, then it means that it is performing its functions properly. 'Heart Qi Deficiency' essentially means that the Heart is not performing its 'actions' as well as it should, for whatever reason. In this way, Qi acts like a verb rather than a noun. When we discuss the various 'Qi' of the body in this way within Chinese medicine, we are discussing the various activities of the organ systems and how efficiently they are carrying out their functions.

The Qi of the Channels

This one is a bit more difficult to understand at first. It takes a fair amount of experiential understanding before you can really engage with what is taking place within the channel system of the body. To understand the 'Qi of the channels', we must first understand that Qi is born from Shen within classical Daoist thought. Essentially, this means that 'spirit' is the seed of life, and that Qi extends down through us as we are developing within the womb. The Jing or 'essence' that we are gifted gives birth to the physical body, whilst the Shen extends its influence through our body via the action of the Qi. This process is shown in Figure 1.3. This is how mind and body come together as we develop within the womb. Traditional Daoist terminology would call this the 'coming together of Yin and Yang' or the 'merging of Heaven and Earth'.

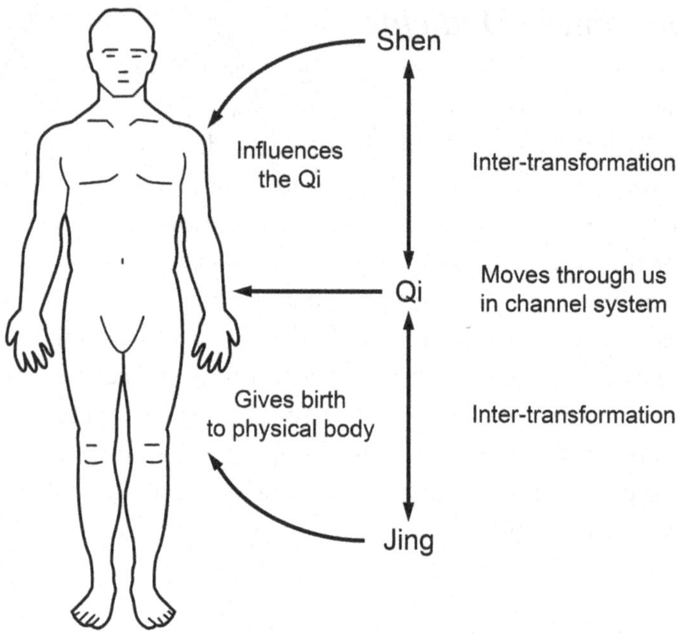

Figure 1.3: Mind and Body Forming

One classical name for the channel system is the 'hall of lights'. Many have been confused by this ancient name for the channels, but it is essentially because when you attain a certain level of ability within these arts, you can begin to visually perceive the inside of the body. The mind begins to view different layers of existence within your internal environment, and when you see the channel system for the first time, it appears like a large mass of silvery white threads that extend through the body. Sadly, the pathway of the channel system is nowhere near as neat and simple as shown in acupuncture textbooks. Instead, it is a huge tangle of complex pathways that reach every part of your body. The reason why the channels appear lit up is that the brain can perceive different energetic layers in different ways. When Shen or consciousness is perceived, it generally appears as a white light – the 'white light of illumination' that many traditions talk of. The channel system is lit up white, as it is an extension of the consciousness through the body. It is the way in which the spirit reaches through the body like so many tendrils to animate us and bring us life.

A second classical name for the channels refers to them as 'heavenly streams'. This is because they are like streams that extend through the body from Heaven which, in this case, is used as an analogy for consciousness. Consciousness is the 'mini Heaven' of our own internal environment.

It is primarily this aspect of Qi we are working with when we do any work to open or clear channel pathways within Qi Gong and Nei Gong practice. This is why so many of the stages of clearing or changing Qi also have a direct and often profound impact upon our state of mind. It is also the reason why so many of the points stimulated in acupuncture also have an impact upon our state of mind. By applying manual pressure or inserting small needles, we are accessing the extensions of the mind.

Note here that the term 'opening the channels' is vitally important to our training. We shall return to this at the relevant stage in this book and look at what it means to open a channel, how it is done, and how to focus on this in our practice.

Since this form of Qi is an extension of the mind, I often simplify this by letting beginning students mull over the definition of Qi as being a form of 'conscious information'. This definition has become useful as a teaching tool, as it gives me a simple working model that gets students in the correct mindset and pulls them away from the rather inadequate definition of Qi being 'energy'.

The Qi of Standing and Martial Arts

I have placed 'standing' and 'martial' arts into one category as, to me, they are essentially discussing the same process. Here, I am primarily talking about the Qi discussed within arts such as Taijiquan (太極拳) rather than external forms of combat. I will not go into a great amount of detail concerning the martial arts, as this is a book on Qi Gong and Nei Gong. I am only including information on 'martial Qi' so as to show that there are different uses of the term.

One of the greatest misunderstandings within the internal martial arts is made by those thinking that it is the 'Qi of the channels' that is important. Whilst it may well be the case that repeated practice of Taijiquan opens up the channels of the meridian system, this is not the aim. The term 'Qi' is used in a very different context here. The Qi of internal martial arts falls into two main types: Qi that is sunk, and Qi that is mobilised. The reason I place martial arts and the Qi of standing practices such as Zhan Zhuang (站樁) into one category is that the mechanism behind them both is essentially the same. Static Qi Gong forms, like Taijiquan, rely on being able to first 'sink' the Qi and then to 'mobilise' the Qi. The mobilisation arises as a direct result of the sinking. Quite simply, if you cannot 'sink the Qi', then the Qi will never mobilise effectively.

'Sinking the Qi' takes place in a series of stages. These stages are as follows:

1. Relaxing the contractive muscles
2. Sinking the mass actively through the body
3. Filling the lower abdomen
4. Expanding the lower abdominal region
5. Stretching the connective tissues of the body
6. Connecting the soft tissues into one unit
7. Stressing the soft tissues through increased release of mass
8. Generating expansive 'space' within the body

All of these stages take place sequentially, with each stage taking place as a direct result of the previous stage reaching a high enough level. As with all stages of development in the internal arts, it is the 'how' rather than the 'what' that is important. If the 'how' is not applied correctly, then the desired results will not be achieved. In this case of 'sinking the Qi', it is the second stage that, in my experience, people tend to make mistakes with. The keyword in the second stage of the above list is 'actively'. Sinking your mass actively means to drop your weight down to the ground through your body so that it has the effect of stretching all of the connective tissues on its way past. Most practitioners 'passively' sink: they drop their weight through to the ground with no effect upon their body. There is no stretching inside and so no engagement of the connective tissues. If this happens, then the 'Qi' cannot be sunk.

Once the tissues are stretched under the force of the weight actively dropping through the body, then this begins to lead you towards the stage of 'mobilising the Qi'. This means that the connective tissues can be used to a far greater degree than the contractive muscles. This is the basis for the internal martial arts as well as a key skill to come from static Qi Gong practices such as Zhan Zhuang. It is a tricky skill to get the hang of at first and one that almost certainly needs the guidance of an experienced teacher.

Types of Qi

If we look at the three broad categories of Qi discussed above, we can see that they are essentially three very different things. These 'types' of Qi are summarised in Table 1.1.

Table 1.1: Types of Qi

Use of the term 'Qi'	Meaning
Qi of Chinese medicine	The quality of an action or function
Qi of the channels	Extension of consciousness through the body
Qi of standing/martial arts	The reaction to sinking and changing the body

On top of these three broad categories, there are also other types of Qi and uses of the word, from a general level of vitality in a person, through to the strength of the auric field. The list could be much longer. The reason I have focused on the three uses of the term 'Qi' above is that I have found many practitioners to be mixing these up within their practice. If you do not have a clear idea of what sort of Qi we are discussing, then your practice is likely to become confused and so weakened.

The final aspect of Qi I really wish to concern you with here in the first chapter of the book is that of Yin and Yang Qi. These two terms come up time and time again within the arts, and for anybody practising either high-level Nei Gong training or internal alchemy, these two types of Qi will be of prime concern.

Essentially, Yin and Yang Qi are the two purest forms of Qi that the body can generate. In this case, we are essentially discussing the Qi that circulates within the channels – the extension of conscious awareness through the body. To open the channels and work with the Dan Tian at some of the more advanced stages of training, we need to learn how to produce the purest forms of Qi that we can. Within classical Daoist terminology, the pure forms of Qi were called Yin and Yang. The distorted versions of Qi within the body were generally known as Fire and Water. Thus it became of great importance to the Daoists to study how to transform Fire and Water back into Yin and Yang. This was a model for them of how to condition the mind and control the body in order to purify the quality of Qi that flowed within the channel system. On top of the above model, we then have a whole spectrum of Qi qualities that are not even pure enough to be called Fire and Water. This concept is shown in Figure 1.4. It shows the types of Qi that we generally experience and feel moving through the body during our practice.

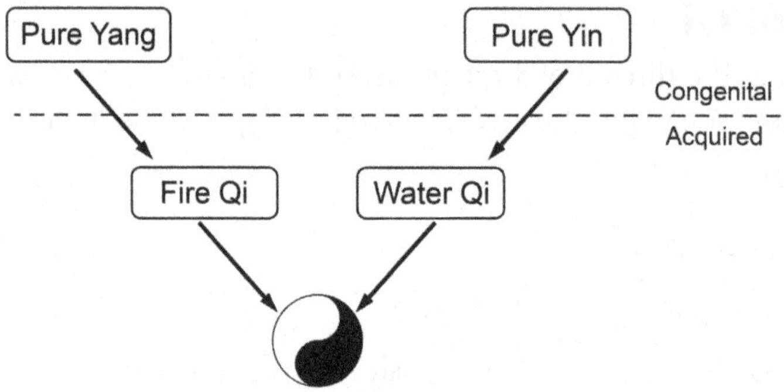

Figure 1.4: Yin, Yang, Fire, Water and the Spectrum of Qi

One of the key 'languages' that we have when learning how to work with Qi is that of our body's sensations – the language of feeling. Though it is a somewhat flawed sense function that is certainly not beyond the realms of delusion, it is the best way we have of knowing what form of Qi we are working within in the earliest stages of our training. Yin, Yang, Fire and Water will be returned to many times in this book, and we will look at them in great detail. For now, it is enough to know roughly what they feel like within the body when they are produced and experienced. Whilst each of us will process an internal experience in our own unique way, there are always certain experiences that are going to be shared.

Yang Qi (陽氣) feels like an electrical current that moves through the channels in a strangely fluid-like manner. It may sound strange to those who have never felt it for themselves, but 'liquid electricity' is how I would best describe it. Yin Qi (陰氣) feels like a strong form of magnetism that bends and stretches the insides of the body. When you generate enough Yin Qi it is as if your internal environment is being physically reformed under the control of a series of magnetic fields.

Yin and Yang Qi are quite advanced types of Qi to generate within the body; they are not usually experienced by practitioners for a long time; instead it is Fire, Water and everything in between that we encounter during the early and intermediate stages of our training. Fire Qi feels like a shaking or vibrating pathway that moves along the length of the channels. Most of the more 'impure' forms of Qi that we feel are also variations on this; for this reason, most of the Qi you are going to experience in the early stages of training are going to feel like vibrations and shaking taking place inside of your body. Water Qi is experienced as a kind of 'heaviness' within the body. It can feel like gravity suddenly got much stronger and started to pull down on your insides. In the majority of cases, it can feel like quite hard work to resist the effects of Water Qi building within you and, as we will discuss later, it can even pull you right down to the ground.

These feelings of being pulled by the more Yin forms of Qi and the vibratory lines of movement generated by the more Yang types of Qi are what we are going to be working with for a long time when we begin Qi Gong. The basic process is that we generate these types of Qi, these reactions and experiences, and we then purify the Qi as best we can so that we start to locate and generate pure Yin and Yang energies. From here, we then learn how to work with these two forces, make them work as one unit and combine them within the body. This is the premise of work inherent within the Nei Gong process.

A Note on Heat

For those of you who are new to these kinds of arts, I am sure by now you are already confused! It may seem that this first chapter is an unusual mix of information on experiences, feelings in the body, philosophy, and how to practise. The reason for this is that learning Qi Gong has to take all of these factors into account. It is a circular study, whereby a fair understanding of various pieces of the puzzle must be developed in order to grasp the bigger picture. This is what makes it such a challenging and fascinating subject.

The final 'experience' I should discuss here is the feeling of heat that many people develop in their practice right from the early stages. This heat can be an overall feeling of increased body temperature, localised heat in patches around the body, heat along the length of a channel, or heat building in the lower abdomen. The reason I want to focus on this sensation of heat is because it is very common and also because it is often misunderstood. In the majority of cases, heat is not Qi, though it is generated as a result of the movement of Qi. Heat is generally being generated due to resistance within the body. When Qi tries to move through a region of the body that is tight and not open enough, then the resistance starts to generate a sensation of heat. This is why, if a person is practising correctly, then sensations of heat should start to fade away. The experience should be temporary, as the channels open up more and the resistance is lessened.

This kind of heat is quite distinct from warmth resulting from increased circulation. Once you have the experience, you can clearly feel how they differ.

The Eight Experiences

It is important to understand that within Qi Gong practice, it is the Qi of the channels we are first going to work with and feel. This type of Qi is an extension of the mind down through the body, as shown in Figure 1.5. The connection between the Qi of the channel system and the mind is absolute. It is almost like an energetic version of the nervous system.

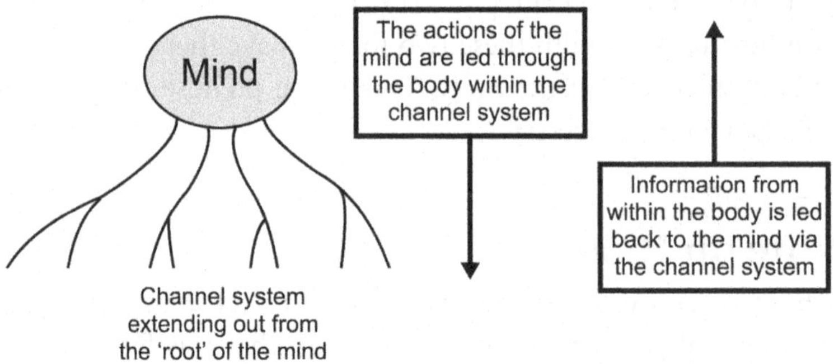

Figure 1.5: Extension of the Mind into Channels

This Qi moves through us as a form of vibrational information. This information can have an emotional quality to it, which is why, when we touch upon Qi, it can also begin to release trapped emotional experiences, as when this 'emotional Qi' leaves the body, it is normal for us to have brief emotional swings. This is because the mind is reading the information contained within our Qi and processing it as an experience for us. It is nothing to worry about and all quite normal. On top of these emotional experiences, we also have what the Chinese classically call the Ba Chu (八触) or 'eight experiences'. These experiences are generally listed as Diao (掉) or 'shaking', Yi (猗) or 'excitement', Leng (冷) or 'feeling cold', Re (熱) or 'feeling hot', Fu (浮) or 'feeling light', Chen (沈) or 'feeling as if sinking', Jian (堅) or 'feeling tight' and Ruan (軟) or 'feeling soft'.

All of the above are general reactions to the movement and effects of Qi. As the 'information' begins to move in the channels, it is sent back to the mind where it is processed as a tangible experience. It is these experiences we can use to navigate the path of Nei Gong. Whilst the experience itself is not the goal, it is a useful way for us to know what is taking place. If we look at the eight experiences individually, we can see that they correspond with the following:

- *Diao (shaking):* Feeling like you are shaking inside is due to the movement of the more Yang forms of Qi including Fire Qi.

- *Yi (excitement):* This indicates a hyperactivity of the inside of the body and sometimes the mind. It can leave you 'buzzing' for some time afterwards; this is a sign of the Qi moving at an increased rate.
- *Leng (feeling cold):* Feelings of cold are usually how the body processes a region of the body with a chronic deficiency of Qi, or else, if the cold feels as if it is moving along a channel, it is usually how you experience an energetic pathogen leaving the system.
- *Re (feeling hot):* This is the heat of resistance discussed above. A very common experience.
- *Fu (feeling light):* As Qi moves upwards in the body, it can be a little 'unrooting', which makes you feel light and as if you could float.
- *Chen (feeling as if sinking):* As the more Yin types of Qi, including Water Qi, are experienced, they can feel as if you are becoming heavier or being drawn down towards the ground.
- *Jian (feeling tight):* If Qi conducts strongly through a channel, then it can actually tighten the channel temporarily. This is because the connective tissues of the channel are reacting to the increased information of the Qi passing along their length.
- *Ruan (feeling soft):* As channels open and release tension from their length, it is normal for the body to suddenly feel as if it is softening or slackening to a certain degree.

Beginning a Practice

Traditionally, whatever the system of Qi Gong a person practised, they always had to begin in the same way: first they had to regulate the body's condition, then they had to regulate the breath, and finally they had to regulate the mind. These are the 'three regulations' of Qi Gong and the way that we ensure we are getting ourselves ready to move as deep as possible into our practice. Much of the rest of this book will be discussing the three regulations of internal practice as well as the underlying philosophy and wider process of Nei Gong.

It would be dishonest of any author not to point out at this stage that the most effective way to train Nei Gong, Qi Gong or any associated art form is to make contact with an experienced teacher and receive hands-on tuition. In this age of 'information sharing', 'online classes' and general 'ease of access' to theoretical information, it is wise to remember that these arts were always passed on as a kind of apprenticeship between teacher and dedicated student. Whilst there are many benefits to how easily we can access information now, there are also pitfalls. The sheer number of people learning solely from books and videos has meant that the arts are now more widespread, but they are also practised to a lower quality than they were in the past. For this reason, I would like to point out that I have written this book, and indeed several others, in order to provide supporting theoretical guidance to those either thinking of looking for a teacher, or who already study with one. Feel free to give the material in this book a try, but if you wish to progress past the earliest stages of practice, then you should seek out personal assistance.

The key to all of this work is the Wuji (無極) posture, which is discussed in Chapter 4. If you really want to make Nei Gong a part of your life, then a lot of time should be spent studying this standing exercise and making sure you have integrated all of its teachings into your body. You should have gone beyond Fa into the Gong of the exercise in order to have built a solid-enough foundation. Not spending long enough on the basics is an easy mistake to make. It is a tempting 'trap' of these arts to want to move too quickly; I know, I have made the same mistake myself many times in the past. Almost every time I hit a glass ceiling in my training and my development is stalled, it is due to something within the fundamentals of my practice being incorrect. I generally have to take a step back and re-check the basics to see where the issue lies.

The key to developing these arts is to understand that it is daily practice that really makes a difference. When starting out, it is my experience that the majority of people cannot maintain a daily practice. There are generally too many distractions, mental resistance and all number of other 'excuses' that the mind will come up with to prevent a person from knuckling down to developing a daily practice routine. It is for this reason that I would say this is the first and most important thing for new students to look at. These arts rely on consistency to really work. Intermittent practice with a constant personal battle against laziness will never really take you anywhere beyond the surface levels. One of the first things we must accept is that 'what we put in, we get back out', and so we must be realistic with what we can achieve in relation to how much effort we put in. I would suggest that newcomers to the arts should begin with a short daily practice of around thirty minutes. From here, you should work to expand up to an hour's session per day, and then from here, once a daily practice routine is established, it will naturally expand out into longer times.

Chapter 2

HEALTH AND PERSONAL EVOLUTION

Probably the most common reason for a person to begin studying Qi Gong or associated arts is to improve their health. Though there are many other reasons why Qi Gong exercises were developed, it is undeniable that the practice of Qi Gong was connected to medicine far back in history. Even one of the oldest-known records of internal exercises, the Dao Yin Tu (導引圖), discussed the use of Qi developmental training to help alleviate sickness; this chart is dated to approximately 160 BCE. The tradition of Daoism has long since had a close connection to the development of various medical practices such as acupuncture and herbal remedies.

In fact, it may be fair to say that the healing aspects of Qi Gong were emphasised for the general public, whereas for those said to be 'inside the door' – a term meaning that they had access to the full and complete teachings of a tradition – it was known that attaining good health was simply the beginning. A solid baseline of sound physical and mental health was required in order for a person to progress onto more advanced work aimed directly at elevating the spirit. In this way, the practices coming out of Daoism were often at odds with other spiritual traditions of the time which viewed the body as pretty much inconsequential. To the Daoists, the physical world and the spiritual world were inextricably linked and so one could not be cultivated without the other. The body was a vehicle through which to engage with the world, and also the 'workshop' where all of your practice was to be carried out. If the workshop was a mess, how would any effective work ever be completed?

Health According to Daoism

In line with modern Western definitions, health is viewed by the Daoists as a state of complete physical and emotional well-being. It is a state of being free from disease and, ultimately, it comes down to the efficiency of the body and mind's functioning. It was also understood by the Daoists that, unfortunately, attainment of this state was nigh on impossible. From the moment of conception, we are subject to imbalance of some sort, and this imbalance will continue to be a part of our existence until the moment we die. Only those said to have attained 'immortality' through means of cultivation are considered to be truly 'healthy' and so perhaps, compared to the Western definition, the Daoists set the bar fairly high!

That being said, there is a vast spectrum of levels of imbalance, and consequently, through practice, the Daoists did their best to develop their body and mind so that they functioned as efficiently as they could. This is where the absolute crux of understanding Nei Gong can be found: it all comes down to efficient functioning of the body and mind. As we train ourselves in a very specific manner, we first begin to change the quality of our health. This happens as a by-product, rather than a direct aim, of our practice. From here, as the efficiency of the body's functioning increases, we raise ourselves above the foundation of good health and move into the more 'super-normal' aspects of the training. Whereas the foundation of good health generally relies on what we have the innate capacity to manage, the stages beyond this can be life-changing, and many are surprised to see just what the human body and mind are capable of. Even when we see true masters emitting Qi from their body or governing the spirit around them with apparently supernatural ability, this is all simply an expression of how efficient they have made their body and mind's functioning. Essentially, you could argue that their skills are merely an expression of health – health taken to a very high level. It was classically said that Qi Gong exercises could take a person to a state of good health, but Nei Gong training was needed to take people beyond this foundation. Figure 2.1 shows the relationship of these practices to health and our personal development.

There is a trap to be aware of here, though. It may sound strange for me to say, but if we overfocus on our health through the training, then we actually hinder our ability to develop. I am aware that, by saying this, I am placing myself into a clear minority, especially since the vast majority of Qi Gong available to people falls under the 'medical' category. I have a very specific reason for making this statement, though, and from my experience of teaching hundreds of people around the world, I have seen this to be the case. Intention is everything. That which I overly 'intend' begins, after a while, to become a kind of attachment. All Eastern traditions make it very clear that attachments can be negative factors on your path to personal cultivation.

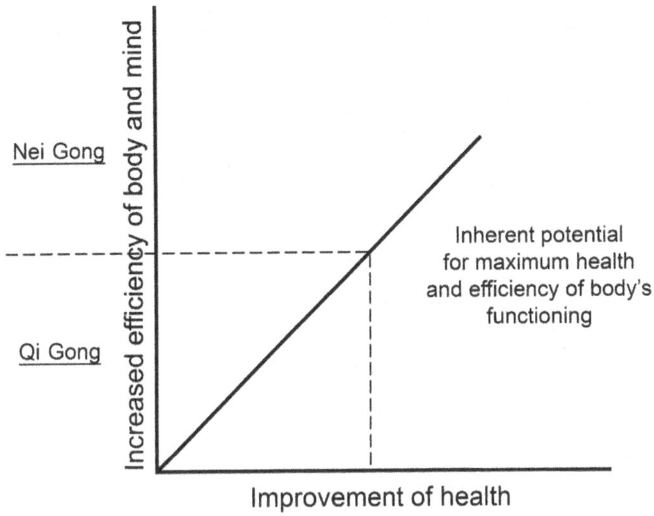

Figure 2.1: Health and Personal Development through Practice

I have seen this to be the case in students coming into the school to seek out freedom from a specific malady. For example, I may have a student come into the class who is looking for Qi Gong practice to help with their severe asthma, or perhaps their depression. They tell me very clearly from the start that this is the sole reason that they are in the class. They are also generally keen to find very specific exercises to help them with these conditions. Perhaps they want a specific exercise or movement they can work on to cure their asthma, or maybe they are seeking a 'depression exercise' to do each day. In almost all of these cases, I see minimal improvement in their condition. There may be a little change, but essentially, the root of the condition still remains within their body. Whilst they are practising, they are free from the influence of the condition, but when they stop their practice and return to everyday life, their condition comes back. This is because they are overly attached to the condition that they are suffering from. If, on the other hand, I have a student who comes into the class and is training simply because they find the arts interesting, I see them go through a whole process of transformation that takes care of many of these kinds of illnesses. By absorbing themselves into the practice and not seeking out any specific goal with regard to their health, they will improve their health as a by-product in the background of their training. It is for this reason that when students ask me for a specific exercise just for them and their condition, I rarely give it to them; I simply take them through the same process that the whole school goes through.

The Nine Palaces of Heart Health

The Daoists took a very rounded approach to health and developed the model of the nine palaces. These are nine aspects of a person's health that should be in balance to ensure that the person is moving towards a more beneficial state of being. These 'palaces' take into account a person's physical, emotional, even social health. As a model, it formed a large part of many Chinese medical systems, though contemporary Chinese medicine practice rarely includes it, and we can still see the model featuring heavily in many forms of practice such as Feng Shui (風水). The palaces are classically linked to compass directions as well as symbolic energies, as shown in Figure 2.2. For the purposes of understanding health, these associations are not so important, though, and I have simply included them here for interest.

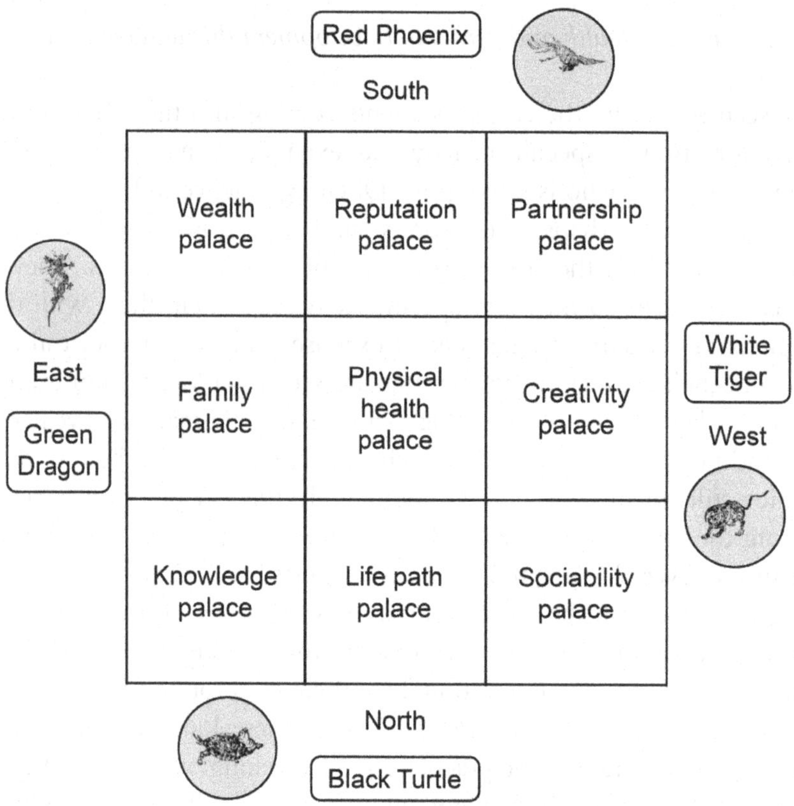

Figure 2.2: The Nine Palaces

The nine palaces are explored below in more detail. Each of these nine areas of health can be adjusted through practice and improving the efficiency of the body and mind.

The Physical Health Palace

This palace is the most important to the Daoists and thus it takes its position at the 'centre' of the compass directions. If the body is not functioning efficiently according to Chinese medical principles, then essentially none of the other palaces will ever be in order. At the same time, there is a reciprocal relationship here that means that the state of the other eight palaces will impact upon the central palace of physical health as well. Physical health in this sense includes not only the strength and vitality of the tissues and organs but also the efficient circulation of Qi and Blood.

The Knowledge Palace

It was considered important for a person to continue to develop their knowledge over the course of their lives. Life is about change and evolution. It is a sad state of affairs that many people in modern society are under the impression that all of their study should take place in their formative years; once they have left school or college, they have no more directed learning to do and instead they simply plod through life with no real aim to continue the development of their mind. This would be considered a sign of poor health according to this palace, and so it can lead to further psychological and physical imbalance developing.

Learning can either be intellectual, in the form of academic study, or it can take other forms, such as the study of Qi Gong or even reading a book, like you are right now. There are many ways to develop the mind and keep evolving your personal knowledge. Just be careful, though: the mind absorbs information at an incredible rate, and so whatever we 'give' our mind to feed on will have a direct influence upon how we develop. Think of how our mind may be affected if we absorb ourselves in tabloid newspapers and horror movies compared to deep study of a subject we are impassioned by.

The Family Palace

Family was long considered by the Chinese to be one of the most important aspects of an individual's life. Honouring ancestors is still clearly seen in Asian culture, and life generally revolves around family dos and events. Interestingly, there was traditionally seen to be a shared quality of health running through a family (clear to see when we think of genetics) as well as a shared Karmic nature of the cause-and-effect harmonics taking place through a genetic lineage. It was for this reason that how one family member acted was said to have an impact upon the rest of the family's lives. In many cases, this idea developed into an unhealthy societal obsession with not 'bringing shame' onto the family – something that became very restrictive. Children were even (and still are) sent off to the monasteries to bring credit to the family with the heavenly realm.

It was also seen as unhealthy to not have any relationship with your own family members, and I have certainly seen this to be the case. Within my own extended family, there are several rifts that have formed over the years between various relatives, and I can see the long-term impact this has upon those individuals' health. Whilst family relations can often be some of the most difficult to sustain, they are worth fostering due to the closeness that can only come from people with a genetic link.

The Wealth Palace

The Daoist approach to life has always been a fairly pragmatic one. Whilst obsession with money and personal gain is obviously detrimental to a person's development, not having enough in the way of resources can also be a real nuisance! It was understood that for a person to be able to focus on their inner development, they needed to be free from too much stress over having enough money. Now, this is where some common sense comes in; the practical needs of a monk living in retreat are quite different from those of a practitioner living in the middle of Tokyo or London, but essentially it comes down to the same issue. Do we have enough money for food, shelter, to provide for those who are dependent upon us, and also to have peace of mind? It has been stated to me quite clearly by several of my teachers at different times that, in order to really progress in these arts, I must find a way to be financially secure enough to not have stresses in this area. We only need to look at the negative impacts of stress on our health as well as where the main causes of stress in people's practical lives come from to see the sense in this idea.

With regard to the wealth palace and how it impacts upon a person's health, I can see three main areas which people need to look at: not having enough, striving for too much, and overly attaching to wealth. It is the relationship between these three that really needs to be looked at.

The Reputation Palace

This may initially seem like an odd inclusion to the nine palaces, but to the ancient Daoists, your reputation was seen as important to your health.

We live in a time where we are often told, 'Do not worry what others think of you,' and 'Don't be affected by others' thoughts,' but I rarely see this to be the case. We only have to take a short trip into the world of social media to see people declaring adamantly how much they don't care what others think of them, whilst at the same time it is clear to see the internal hurt that is motivating them to make such statements. In fact, it is often the case that whatever has hurt us is what drives us to do what we do; in the majority of cases, this hurt comes from other people and either what they have done to us or what they view us to be. This is what the Daoists were talking about when they discussed 'reputation'. It is almost inevitable that by placing ourselves into the view of others, we will draw negative attention. It is the human condition to find fault in others and, generally, they like to express these views as widely as possible! The cause-and-effect relationship that exists between all of us will inevitably mean that some of this negativity will have an impact upon our thoughts and actions, but all we can do is manage this as best as we can.

Within my practice of Chinese medicine, I have seen many cases of people's internal health being negatively impacted due to personal attacks on their 'reputation' by a person or group of people. This can be from family members, employees, the public or any number of other sources, but the outcome is the same. In many cases, this person will adamantly declare that they are not bothered by the attacks that they are receiving, but the state of their inner health generally tells a different story.

All we can do to manage this aspect of our health is to act with as much integrity and kindness as we can. Work towards generating as little enmity as you can in others and yet, at the same time, recognise that you can't keep everybody happy!

The Partnership Palace

The nature of human life is to live in partnership with another. Whether this is an innate biological need or a socially generated one is irrelevant; the end result is the same – we are conditioned to seek out another individual to share our life with. Now, saying this, I am aware that people will be disagreeing and thinking about those who are happy to be single and those who live in polyamorous relationships. I would argue that these people are the exceptions and not the norm.

In times past, the correct partner was so important for a person's health that choosing this partner was rarely left up to the people involved! Arranged marriages were based upon practical issues, finance, joining of family lines, and astrological readings to check for compatibility. In modern times this is rarely the case, but still, a wholesome and loving partnership with another person is generally considered the healthiest situation to be in. Sadly, many people live in unhappy relationships and this can be hugely detrimental to a person's health. To be loved and to give love in a healthy manner is an important aspect for the lives of most of us.

The Creativity Palace

Creativity is an expression of the Heart and its associated spirit, the Shen (神). If the Heart was not able to express itself, then this was said to be bad for your health. This creativity can be expressed through art, movement or countless other ways, but it must be expressed. If there is a lack of self-expression through creative means, then the spirit begins to weaken and so our health is damaged.

It is for this reason that Daoism also influenced and created many forms of art, from music and poetry through to calligraphy and martial arts. The ancient Daoists were working on an aspect of the self that can only become healthy through an expression of creativity. This often confuses my Chinese medical patients when they have come to me for advice after the treatment. They are expecting herbs, exercise or dietary suggestions, but instead I send them out to explore dance, painting, singing or something similar. No amount of herbs or other healthcare will be as helpful for certain spiritual conditions as immersing yourself into an expressive art form.

The Sociability Palace

Having a social outlet is a normal and healthy part of human life. Humans are essentially pack and communal animals. Living alone, completely isolated from the rest of our community, is rarely healthy; in fact, loneliness can be one of the biggest killers. This has been recognised by several charities and scientific studies in the West that now reach out to those living alone, especially the elderly, and help to provide them with company and support.

Daoism never advocated a monastic lifestyle. The addition of monks and isolation to the tradition came much later on in its development. Instead, Daoism advised a policy of 'one foot in and one foot out'. What was meant by this was that people should live amongst others and become a part of their community and yet, at other times, retreat into solitude to focus upon their personal cultivation. I have had a large number of teachers over the past three and a half decades of studying the Eastern arts. Contrary to what people might expect, many of the highest-level Daoist masters I have trained with did not live in the mountains; instead, they lived in busy Asian cities such as Beijing, Taipei and Kuala Lumpur. They generally held down jobs working closely with their community, whilst the people they interacted with rarely knew the level of attainment that they had reached in their development. In essence, they lived a 'social' life whilst remaining somewhat invisible with regard to their skills.

I should add here that it is common for people to train in an art like Nei Gong or meditation and reach a stage where they find it difficult to socialise with those who don't also practise. You will always see the signs of this developing as the practitioner starts to refer to non-practitioners as 'normal people' in a somewhat dismissive manner. I know, I have been here several times – it is an easy trap to fall into and one to recognise and pull yourself out of. These experiences of having difficulty connecting with others are because of changes inside, but it should be recognised that they are temporary shifts. Just wait, be patient with yourself, and things will change. You will, once again, at some stage find that socialising with people becomes pleasurable. Do not wear these temporary bouts of 'unsociability' like some kind of mark of achievement. If you do this, then they will stick. The attachment to this state will make it permanent, and you will find that life has a way of giving you what you are unintentionally asking for. It will not be long before you are indeed socially isolated, and that will do you no good whatsoever.

The Life Path Palace

The final palace is often called the 'career palace', but this is a somewhat limiting name for it. It implies a paid job that is useful to society in a conventional manner. Whilst this kind of career may be just right for the majority of people, there are many others who find that it does not suit them. Perhaps your calling is in overseas charity work, or art, dance, or any one of infinite possibilities. My own life path is based around preserving a very old Eastern tradition and helping enough people to understand it so that it survives the dumbing-down of spiritual arts that seems prevalent today. This life path gives me purpose and satisfaction; from these two qualities I derive joy. My previous 'life paths' of working on building sites or as a social worker did not bring me the same sense of fulfilment and, ultimately, were bad for my mental health!

Having the 'right' life path is important for people, and these life paths can also adjust with us as we develop internally. Oftentimes, people are too fixed with their path and unable to change direction when they need to. This almost always brings detriment to a person's health.

I see this issue most in people who are just at school-leaving age. They often enter into a kind of purgatory where they have no life path, no idea what this path should be, and then, on top of that, they are pressured into the wrong paths by well-meaning older people! The result is often depression or emotional flatness. It would be far healthier for them to get some kind of temporary work in order to help build up some finance and then head out into the world for several years, trying as many different things as they can to find out just what it is they are passionate about. When they find their passion, they will generally find their life path is somewhere in there. Retirement is so far away; there are plenty of years to spend working yet. Go and waste some time searching for your passion instead!

Figure 2.3 summarises the nature of the nine palaces as well as the effects that they have upon the overall quality of a person's health.

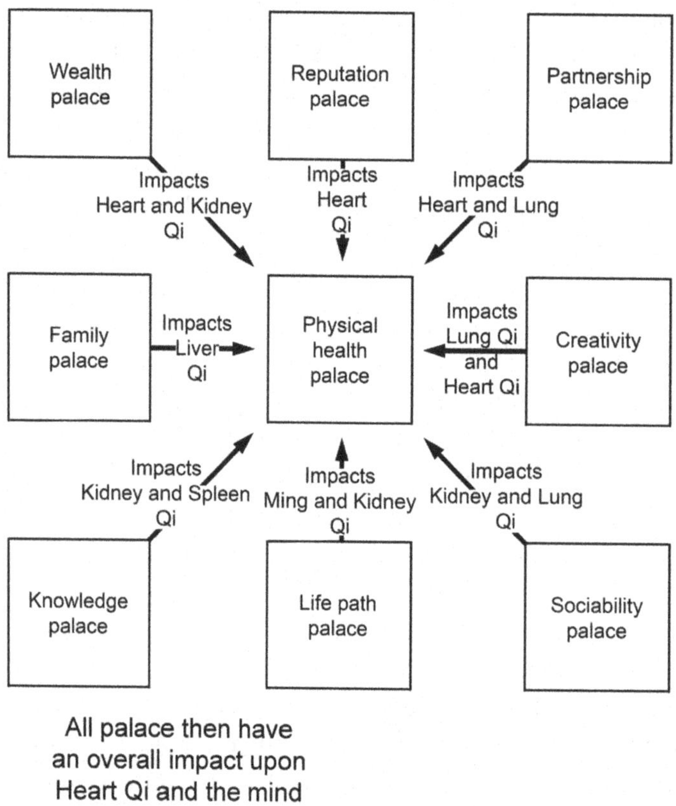

Figure 2.3: The Influence of the Nine Palaces on Health

Training as You Age

My own school is a fairly large organisation with many people from around the world studying these arts; we currently have around a 50/50 split of men and women, and there is a variety of ages, spreading from people in their early twenties through to fairly elderly students. Whilst it is great to have a spread of students from all sorts of backgrounds, it can be tricky teaching a large group, especially when it comes to the issue of age differences. We rather jokingly tell our students that younger people should train hard and older people should train properly!

What we mean by this is that people should train according to the inherent quality of their body and Qi. Younger students (generally) still have an abundance of active Yang energy within their systems and so they can stretch, strengthen and work the body to get it prepared not just for practice, but for life. It is a foolish person in their twenties who only looks after their Qi and does not consider the building of their physical body as well; they will certainly pay the price for this approach to practice when they are older.

As we move towards middle age, the ability of the physical body to rebuild and restructure is lessened; it can still take place, of course, but there should be a slower and more gradual approach to how the body is changed. A lot of internal work should be used as the basis for any physical development and certainly there should be little in the way of pushing the body; in no way should this group ever go to their limits as, instead of building their body up, they are essentially going to run the risk of breaking it down.

When people enter their twilight years, then almost all of the work that they undertake should involve the building of Qi and the regulation of Shen. The body should keep adapting purely as a result of energy work, deep relaxation methods and gentle restructuring of the body.

Essentially, the processes outlined in this book are fine for all ages, the only exception being much younger students who should ensure that they are building their physical body in the right way through exercises such as martial arts or other body movement-based training. This is what is meant by the phrase 'younger people should train hard and older people should train properly': the Yang of youth can be used to generate strength in the body, whilst the Yin of older age should be nurtured and used to transform the body and mind in a different way – a way, ultimately, more in keeping with the tenets of Daoism.

One of the major hurdles to this is societal programming regarding age. There is most certainly a 'cult of youth' within modern society and a kind of shame attached to the ageing process. This is both unhealthy and completely insane; ageing affects us all and the body goes through various energetic changes during this natural process. The activity of Yang and the stillness of Yin are equally important, they are energies that dominate our functioning at different stages in our life; this is both natural and healthy. Those who can learn how to harness the inherent energetic strength of their personal stage in life will develop in the most effective manner; those who ignore this factor and train in the wrong way will either slow down their process or cause lasting harm. The path to Dao is open to all as long as we understand our own internal rhythms and work with them.

The Nine Palaces and Nei Gong

Some of you may now be wondering what the section above on the nine palaces has to do with Nei Gong. When I first encountered these teachings, I felt the same. I was visiting with a teacher and expectantly waiting for instruction on how to build and circulate my Qi and was instead presented with a series of lectures on how I should approach life. Though initially uninterested in this seemingly irrelevant aspect to the training, I have come to understand it and see how integral this is to practice. Essentially, Nei Gong cannot be separated from the tradition from which it was born; this tradition is Daoism. Many have tried to divorce the arts from their 'mother philosophy', Westernise them or else strip out what is viewed as 'irrelevant', but this never works. The point of a tradition is not just to give you a practice but also to give you a holistic understanding of the nature of life itself. Whether you then choose to apply these teachings to your own life is up to you; that is personal choice, but we should be aware of what the beliefs were of those who founded the art. If we can understand the art's roots, then we can understand how it grew and developed into what it is; context is everything.

In order to build a foundation in 'health' for our practice, we first have to understand what health is. Health, to the Daoists, included all of the above factors, and so these should be taken into account. Nei Gong training will obviously tackle the issue of physical health, but these other factors should be considered as well. At first, these may seem like elements of our life that we need to directly intervene in, but actually, as we develop in the arts, we often find that they start to take care of themselves as well. In this way, as our inner nature changes, it starts to draw towards us the kinds of experiences and situations we require in order for the nine palaces of health to move into a state of harmony. This is the wider expression of the practice; not only does it build our bodily health, but we should also see it start to spill out into the rest of our life.

That being said, remember that this will not be the case in the beginning. Any change comes from two sources: internally and externally. The practice itself should build the potential for internal change if we are practising correctly, but external change comes from those practical measures we put in place. In the case of the palaces discussed above, we should still seek to make sure we are financially okay, our actions towards others are compassionate in nature, and we express ourselves socially and creatively. A true 'practice' encompasses all aspects of our daily lives, not just the time we are in class or working on our exercises. I often have to remind my younger students of this, as they can have a tendency towards being too obsessive in their approach to the practice. I tell them that it is fine to train hard, but do not become recluses! Go out, socialise, meet people, find your passions in life, or else you will look round and realise you have 'trained away' all of your teen years and twenties. Looking at the palaces above, there is more to good health than just efficient Qi flow. Life is an expression of health.

Innate Potential for Health

Though these arts have great potential for bringing positive changes to our health, we should also understand that we will always have limitations placed upon us by our inherent level of vitality. Chinese medicine states that when we are born, we are given a certain level of Qi and a certain quality of health. As well as this, we have an inherent psychological makeup which is, in part, from our genetic heritage as well as the astrological conditions we were born under. Some of us are born with inherent imbalances and, to be honest, these are always going to be an issue for us. Whilst there is potential for these kinds of congenital problems to change through practice, this is not going to happen until we go incredibly deep into the arts. To put it into context, I have only met a handful of practitioners in my lifetime who have managed to take their art this far. It should not be something we cling to in hope of changing imbalances that we are desperate to seek refuge from. The condition of our health is aptly summed up in the phrase 'We can only play with the cards we have been dealt.'

If we have a congenital defect in the heart or lungs, then it is likely to always be an issue. What we *can* do, though, is support the condition as best as we can by ensuring that we build up as much Qi as possible in the body and open the channels up to serve as a kind of 'buffer' for this condition. For example, I was born with inherently weak Qi in my Lungs. This is clear within my astrological birth chart as well as in my physical body. As a child, I always had asthmatic-type symptoms and would easily run out of breath when I exerted myself. These days, I don't experience any negative symptoms related to my lungs at all unless I am tired. Basically, the level of Qi I have developed and worked with in my practice serves to protect my lungs from even the most unpleasant of environments – conditions that almost certainly would have given me an asthma attack when I was younger. I am free from worry about my lungs. But if I am tired from lack of sleep, too much teaching and travel (jetlag especially), then my Qi level is lowered and, consequently, I re-experience negative health symptoms with my breathing. It is nothing terrible, not like it used to be when I was younger, but it is there nonetheless and serves as a helpful reminder that I am overdoing things and need to rest.

I think of it like a cup with two fluids within it that will not mix. The fluid on the bottom of the cup is the 'reserves' of the body. The fluid on top is the Qi that we can build up. When I 'over-dip' into the Qi/fluid on top, then I touch on the reserves and this is detrimental to my physical health. This idea is summarised in Figure 2.4.

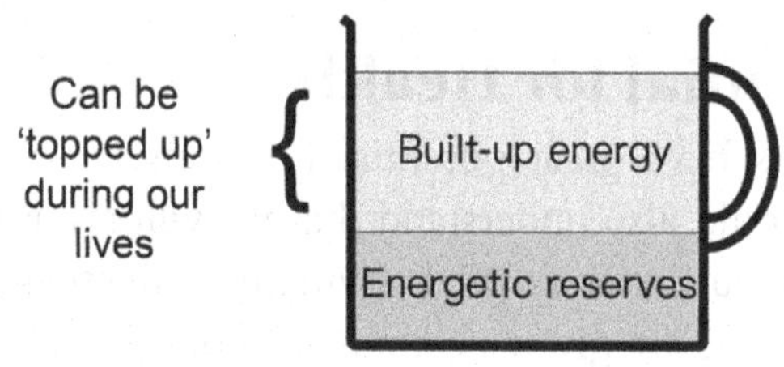

Figure 2.4: Reserves and Built-Up Qi

It is important for me to make this clear to people coming into these arts. There are many unscrupulous teachers out there selling 'cure-alls', generally for large amounts of money. In my experience, there are a lot of people living in discomfort due to the state of their health, and these people are often taken advantage of. We should understand that our congenital makeup is pretty much fixed, apart from in the rarest of cases, and so what we work to do is bolster the body as much as we can and use Qi Gong principles to support and nourish the body. Those conditions that can be changed and effectively 'shed' from the body are those conditions that developed after birth.

Two Types of Disease

According to Chinese medical thought, there are only two main categories of disease: those diseases that originate from outside of our body and those that originate from within us. These are termed 'external' and 'internal' diseases.

External diseases are generally related to climatic effects such as high winds, damp environments or extremes of heat and cold. Included here are contagious diseases as well as injuries that the body sustains through physical trauma and accidents. Internal diseases are primarily related to the mind and how it influences the body. Added to these above causes of disease is an unhealthy lifestyle with regard to food and exercise. The body needs good nutrition and exercise to function well and these two factors should always be taken into account when starting to look at the nature of health.

In essence, externally based disease always leaves a kind of energetic imprint on the body, and these imprints must be shed through the practice. We will discuss this later when we look at the process of purging the body. For now, though, let us focus on what is almost certainly the biggest cause for many people's level of internal disharmony: the mind.

What Is Mind According to Daoism?

It is always difficult to transfer a tradition from one cultural context to another. Linguistic differences mean that directly translating terms from Chinese to English can be tricky, especially as certain terms simply do not exist in English. Added to this confusion is the fact that each teacher is likely to use the terminology slightly differently according to their own understandings and inherent biases. Whilst we can get around this issue easily enough when discussing the body (it is a very tangible and easily label-able thing, after all), it can be confusing when we discuss the mind. For this reason, I wish to make clear exactly how I use certain terms. In the context of Nei Gong, I use 'consciousness' to refer to the shifting, deeper aspects of a human being's cognition. Much closer to the core of 'who we are', consciousness has a close connection to our inherent psychological makeup. The outer mental expression of consciousness, when it has passed through the distortions of acquired layering, is what I refer to as the 'mind'. Our personality and surface emotional layer is expressed through the mind. A third term is 'spirit'; I use this term to refer to a much higher aspect of human life that is closely connected to the divine. 'Spirit' as a term and its application to practice shall be returned to at a later stage when we look at what it actually means to practise a 'spiritual art'. The term 'spiritual practice' is bandied about all over the place these days and, to be frank, very few understand what this actually means. For now, though, let us focus on the mind, its creation and how it influences our health.

The Process of Creation in Daoism

When teaching the Daoist arts, I return to the chart of Chen Tuan (陳摶) time and time again. Commonly known as the 'process of creation', it informs almost all alchemical practices coming out of the Daoist school. Figure 2.5 shows this chart.

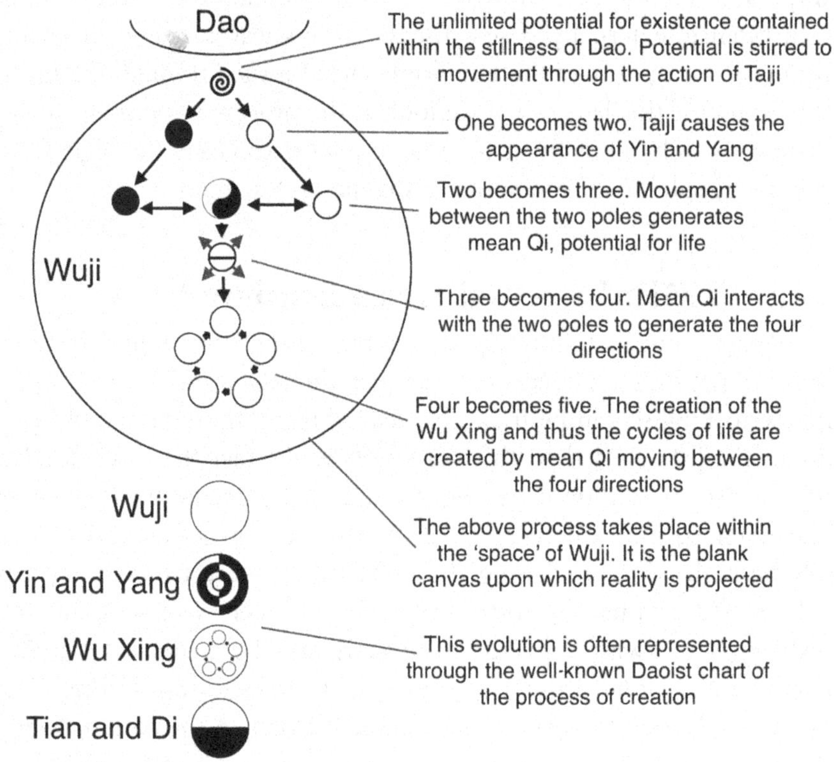

Figure 2.5: The Chen Tuan Chart of Creation

It is a key ethos of Daoism that the external universe is directly reflected within the inner environment of our being. In this way, the macrocosm and microcosm are one and the same. This is summarised succinctly in the popular maxim of 'As above, so below.' What this means is that when Daoist teachers wish to discuss an internal process, they often refer to phenomena taking place within the wider environment instead. This has caused confusion amongst many scholars who have mistakenly believed that Daoists were only concerned with the outer world, when in fact they were a tradition focused almost entirely on inner development. In the case of the Chen Tuan chart of creation, it is the process of the birth of reality that is being used metaphorically to explain how consciousness and mind give birth to our personal journey of development. Since I have previously written about this chart and its application to the birth of Heaven and Earth in my other books (see, for example, *White Moon on the Mountain Peak*), I will focus solely on the 'inner understanding' of the chart here.

Dao and Wuji

Daoism as a tradition has never attempted to define exactly what the nature of divinity is. Though there are many deities in Daoism, there is no one personified creator god. Later, versions of Daoism developed which started to transform it into an organised religion, and the idea of Dao began to change in line with other large religions, but this was never the original idea. Daoism never denied the existence of a creator, nor did it confirm it; instead, it took the very pragmatic approach of simply saying 'we don't know'. Dao is considered to be a state so far removed from our worldly mind that it cannot be understood intellectually; it simply has to be experienced and, ultimately, 'merged with'. I often joke with my students that when people want a definition of Daoism it should really be 'question-mark-ism'.

Dao exists outside of time, and according to classical teachings it is said to 'give birth to the myriad things'. This concept has been taken out of context by scholars who have then said that Dao must be some sort of creative force, but in fact this is only partially true. The creation that is being discussed here is primarily the creation of human consciousness and, from this, mind. This is because Dao can only ever really be experienced in the one place where it manifests into our realm of existence: in the centre of our consciousness.

Dao needs a 'state' in order to manifest within us, and this state is known as Wuji, or literally 'without definitions'. Wuji is generally depicted as a simple circle, as shown in Figure 2.6. The depiction of Wuji in this manner forms the top of the Chen Tuan chart.

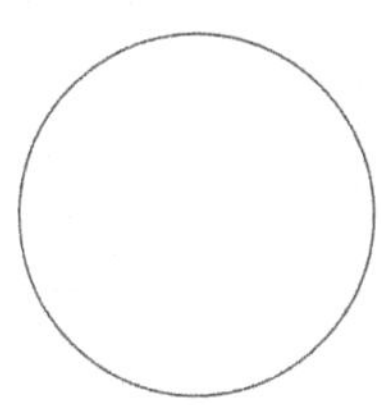

Figure 2.6: Wuji

Wuji can be pictured as a blank canvas upon which nothing has yet been painted. It has no 'projections' and as such is free from definition. When people reach a very still state of being in meditative practice, it is Wuji that they are touching upon. Stillness brings experience of Wuji which, in turn, gives birth to the emptiness that Dao floods into and fills. It is through the development of emptiness that 'mergence' with Dao is achieved.

Wuji is the 'place' within the centre of consciousness where Dao then gives birth to the formation of 'mind'. It does this through the action of Taiji (太極).

Taiji

There is a simple rule in Daoism that nothing can ever reach an extreme without transforming. According to this rule, when extreme stillness is reached, it gives birth to a new movement. A singular point of movement is generated in the centre of the stillness. This is a spontaneous action that arises through the non-action of Wuji.

Taiji is a 'motive force'; it is the bringer of change and the way in which Yin and Yang are first brought into manifestation.

It is a fascinating aspect of nature that almost all life is born in a spiralling motion. From the way in which plants grow, through to the patterning of shells and countless other examples, the spiral is the shape of growth. Daoism recognised this and so represented Taiji as a spiralling line as shown in Figure 2.7. Note that the spiral always travels clockwise as this is the direction for creative energy according to the Daoist tradition.

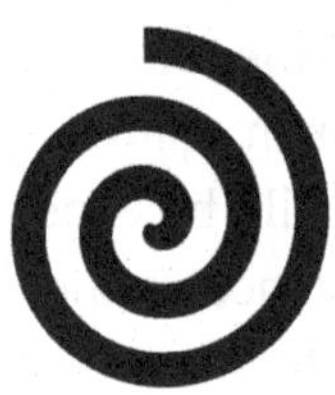

Figure 2.7: Taiji

It is within the microcosm of human consciousness that 'thought' is given birth to. Consciousness can be seen as being like a vast ocean. As the 'wind' of Taiji moves across its surface, it generates waves, and these are the movements of mind. These 'waves' are needed as they give us the capacity for mental activity, but ultimately, it is only through attainment of a state of inner stillness that we can perceive beyond these waves into the vast ocean beneath.

Taiji gives birth to Yin and Yang, and it is here that human mental activity is created.

Yin and Yang

Even those with only a cursory knowledge of Daoism will be familiar with the terms 'Yin' and 'Yang'. Modern popular culture has absorbed these terms and uses them in their most simple form to refer to the feminine and masculine states of being. Chinese medicine uses Yin and Yang as a form of classification as well as a way to understand the process of how disease develops and, in this context, Yin and Yang are ultimately the basis for the way in which the mind works.

Yin and Yang are depicted as the colour black and white as well as broken and solid lines, as shown in Figure 2.8. The linear depiction of Yin and Yang is taken from the Yi Jing (易經) symbolism.

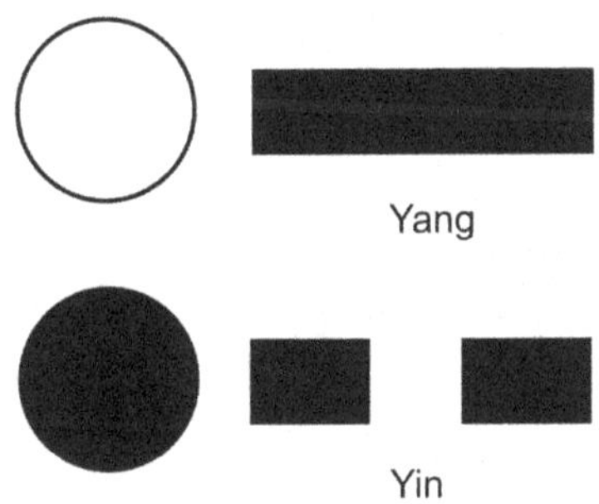

Figure 2.8: Yin and Yang

It is a key tenet within Daoist thought that something can only be identified or understood when placed in the context of its polar opposite. For example, we only know day because of the night. We only understand the direction of up because of down, and so on. Between these two extremes of 'black and white' are then the 'shades of grey' that exist between them. This can be helpful on a practical level, as it enables us to have a cognitive understanding of the world we live in, but it is also the basis for many problems. It is said within the Daoist teachings that we only know beauty because of ugliness. Whilst this is an oversimplification of the issue, it does give us a window of insight into the origin of many inner struggles. If everything is classified according to its opposite, then essentially this brings about ideas of judgement and constant classification. It is these factors that lie at the heart of how our mental condition begins to distort over time. Dualistic thinking in this manner pulls us away from connection with consciousness, and so Daoism talks of 'merging Yin and Yang' within its meditative teachings; an instruction ultimately meaning to take the mind to a place of non-dual perception.

Five Elemental Movements

Beyond the division of Yin and Yang from the source of Wuji comes the birth of the five elemental movements. Note here that the common translation for the Wu Xing (五行) is 'five elements', but this can give the wrong idea. They are not fixed elements but rather a model of how various factors of life cyclically transform into one another as well as control and balance one another.

The five elemental movements are born from the various inter-relations of Yin and Yang when they are combined with the motive force of Taiji. If Yin and Yang produce the potential for thought, then the five elemental movements give those thoughts direction.

The five elemental movements are known as Fire, Earth, Metal, Water and Wood, and they combine into a cycle of generation and control, as shown in Figure 2.9.

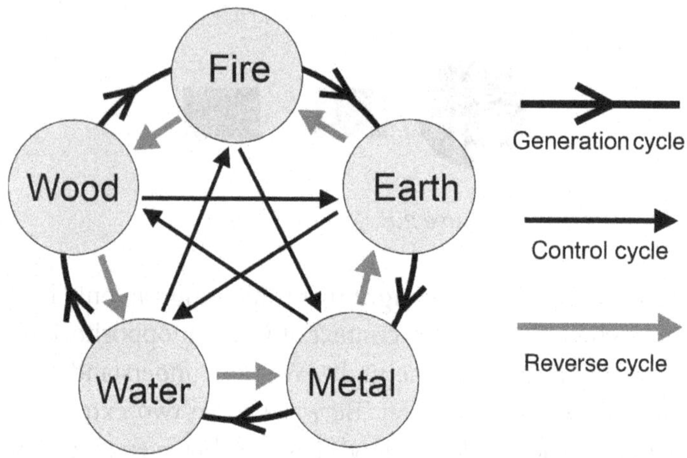

Figure 2.9: The Five Elemental Movements

The generation cycle shows how one energetic movement can produce another, and in this way, they produce a perfect and unbroken cycle. This is reflected within the wider world through the various processes that take place over time, for example the seasons, the ageing process, and so on. These are pure manifestations of the five elemental movements within the physical world. They bring about the concept of constant change and development which are the core principles behind Daoism and the arts that came out of Daoism.

Without the five elemental movements, there would be no change, development or progression. The generation cycle shows the perfect transition from one elemental process to another, whereas the controlling cycle shows how one element can inhibit and manage the growth of another. For example, Water generates Wood, but it is controlled by Earth and at the same time it controls Fire. This keeps the elements in balance and makes sure that one does not become too strong. One slight alteration and this delicate relationship is thrown out of balance.

The elements are best thought of as five movements which can take place within both the physical and the energetic realm. Much of Daoist study (both inner and outer) is aimed at gaining a practical understanding of how all of this takes place within the universe, the mind and the body.

With regard to our thought processes, they essentially give us the distorting layer of emotional attachment. It is here that most issues arise with how our mind influences our personal health.

Heaven and Earth

The final part of the Chen Tuan chart shows the division of Heaven and Earth. Clearly, at this stage in the process, they are referring to the wider creation of the world. The metaphor for how the universe came into being is used to show how from Dao came the potential for duality and this, in turn, generated the realms of Heaven and Earth. With regard to the inner realm of our body, it shows the division of mind and body. In this context, Heaven is representative of the mind, whilst Earth is the physicality of our body. Figure 2.10 shows the realms of Heaven and Earth as they are symbolically drawn.

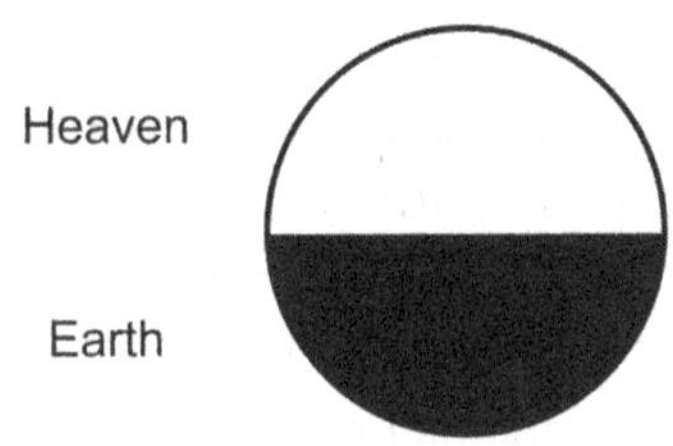

Figure 2.10: Heaven and Earth

If we look at the earliest stages of internal practice, its main/ultimate purpose is to bring the mind into the body. This might sound overly simplistic, but it is a profound detail that many miss. Daoists state that we 'shine our light outside' too much of the time. We look to the outer world and interact with it using our five senses, but we spend too little time allowing our awareness to be interacting with our body; we must 'turn the light around'. By doing this, we initiate a process of bringing Heaven and Earth back together again.

Daoist teachings focus upon a very specific process of 'reversing the course' or 'returning to the source'. Though there are other layers to these instructions, they are primarily referring to the process outlined in the Chen Tuan chart. From Dao and Wuji, the stillness was broken by the emergence of Taiji. The generative force of Taiji created Yin and Yang which are the start of dualistic perception. This, in turn, generated thought and the creation of the human mind. Our mind was then subjected to the five elemental movements which created the emotional distortions of perception – something known as the 'five poisons' in Daoism. As the machinations of the mind continued, we then experienced a 'disconnect' between mind and body, and this began a process of degeneration that we know as ageing. Though we can never fully halt the ageing process (and nor should we want to), we can 'reverse the course' of how our mind works and so be led back through stillness to the source of it all: Dao itself. In doing this, we learn how to adjust our own process of internal development.

Three Divisions of Practice

Within the Daoist tradition there were three recognised paths to Dao that developed out of the various lineages. It was said that the most effective way to progress was through a study of all three but, ultimately, the first path was the most important: Dao could be reached through this path alone. This was the Jin Dan Da Dao (金丹大道) or 'great path of the golden elixir'. The other two paths were the Shuang Xiu (雙修) or 'paired cultivation' path and the Dao Wai Cai Yao (道外採藥) – the 'picking herbs to use as an external way to Dao' path. In modern times, the 'great path of the golden elixir' is the umbrella under which the vast majority of internal practice falls, though we still see remnants of the other two branches of Daoism being practised as well. Nei Gong, Qi Gong and alchemical training most certainly come from the 'great path of the golden elixir', though there are aspects of the other paths present as well. Let us look at these three paths of Daoism individually below.

Great Path of the Golden Elixir

Traditions that focused upon this path adhered to the ethos of working with the three treasures of Jing, Qi and Shen. The 'golden elixir' was the refined spiritual substances that could be developed within the alchemical workshop of the body. Practices developed out of meditation as well as from the shamanic practices of the Wu people. From this root came the practices of Qi Gong and Nei Gong. Essentially, the vast majority of the practices and methods within this book and my other books are derived from the 'great path of the golden elixir'.

Paired Cultivation

'Paired cultivation' comprises various elements, all of which are based on the idea that it is possible to harmonise your own energy system through harmonising it with the energy of another person or aspect of nature. The most well-known aspect of the 'paired cultivation' path are the Fang Zhong Shu (房中術) 'bedroom arts', or 'sexual practices' as they are commonly known. In fact, paired practice with an intimate partner was recognised as only one aspect of this path, along with Cai Qi (采氣) 'gathering Qi'. This method involved using the trees, mountains, rivers and other environmental bodies in order to draw in and realign your own energetic matrix. The practice of Qi Gong with trees is a very important part of the 'gathering Qi' skill and most systems of Qi Gong utilise these methods in some way. Skilled practitioners of this method would also seek out Long Mai (龍脈) 'dragon lines', powerfully conductive regions of the Earth where pure energy could be gathered to aid you in your practice.

Picking Herbs to Use as an External Way to Dao

One classical path of Daoism involved the cultivation and preparation of herbs and medicines that could be consumed in order to regulate the quality of your Qi and Shen. The most well-known surviving branch of this tradition is Chinese herbal medicine, although Wai Dan (外丹) 'external alchemy' is another surviving yet rare branch of this path of Daoism. In the tradition of Wai Dan, practitioners develop herbal formulas and pills that are directly fed by the practitioner's Qi as well as environmental energies radiating from celestial bodies such as the stars and moon. The development of just one of these pills can take many months and only very few have the guarded knowledge of how these pills are made. These pills could be powerful enough to fully consolidate the Jing, open up the body's channels or even, purportedly, help a practitioner develop immortality.

The Formation of Mind

It is said that the human mind lies at the heart of all internal sickness. From what I have seen in my Chinese medical practice as well as in my Nei Going teaching, I would have to agree wholeheartedly with this statement.

In the case of internally generated disease, it is the generation of thought and the quality of this thought that begins to impact upon our health. This follows a simple model which states that movements of the mind generate an adjustment to the Qi, and this, in turn, starts to change the way that the body is evolving. This process is summed up in Figure 2.11. It is a simple model for the nature of the mind/body connection.

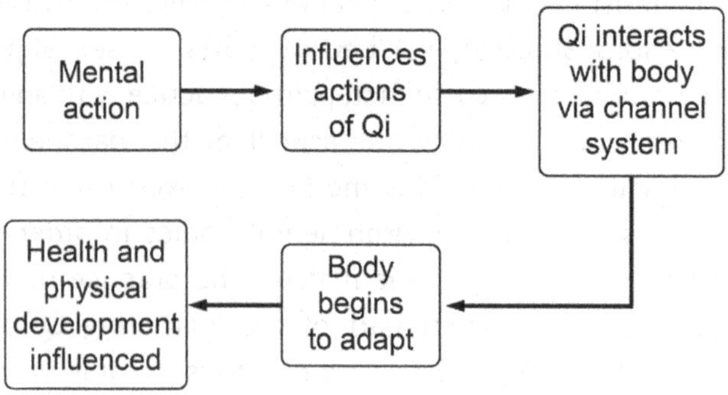

Figure 2.11: Mind Affecting Body

How this takes place is through a series of stages that match the processes shown in the Chen Tuan chart. In this way, with each and every single thought that we have, we are recreating the 'process of creation' on a microcosmic scale. If we just take a second to consider this idea, then it can show us just how important it is to try to cultivate a healthy state of mind.

When we first experience a movement of the mind, it is generated from the centre of the Wuji 'space'. In many Eastern traditions, it is common to ask, 'What is the origin of thought?' Though, of course, each tradition will have its own answer to this enigma, Daoism would say that thoughts come from within Wuji. They are generated from the nothingness of potential as well as a reaction to external stimuli from the sense functions. In this way, perhaps we can say that thoughts come from both inside and outside?

From the potential stillness of Wuji is born a movement, an initiator of mental movement, and this is due to the emergence of Taiji. The 'motive force' of creation exists at the very first point of a 'thought' emerging. In meditative training, when a person begins to move deeper towards stillness, there is often a point whereby the first seed of a thought appearing can be experienced. This 'seed' is quite disturbing, for want of a better word, as once you have become increasingly absorbed into a state that is moving towards awareness of consciousness, every little experience is amplified. It is like turning up the volume on your mental actions. As we grow more still, the appearance of Taiji can feel like a loud echo bouncing around within that mental space. It is here, from this echo, that the first reflections of dualistic thought are born in the form of Yin and Yang.

Yin and Yang are the way in which our mind processes and perceives movements of the mind. As this mental action passes through the lens of Yin and Yang, it starts to be understood according to the biases and conditioned thinking that have inevitably become a part of who we are and how we perceive the world. Dualistic perception is required for the mind to exist, and it is through this particular mechanism that we learn to associate thoughts and experiences with prior learning. By the time we reach a certain age (not very old at all!), we already have a whole plethora of past experiences and conditioned thinking to draw upon, like trawling through a vast database of your life history. We only ever understand anything in comparison to something else. Our mind works on association and, for better or for worse, this then adds a layer of distortion to any thought that we may have. In some cases, this can be helpful; for example, we know that fire is hot and hurts if we touch it, so we don't need to have this experience over and over – we have learnt this lesson previously. In other cases, it can be unhelpful. For example: perhaps you meet a new person and they have a similar look to them as somebody you met in the past who you didn't like very much; it is almost inevitable that you will subconsciously start to judge that person according to your past experience. This is a clear distortion of the acquired mind according to the dualistic thinking of Yin and Yang. These two examples may be slightly oversimplified, but what is important to understand is that each and every thought that you have goes through this same process and it is essentially almost impossible to have a 'pure' thought free from the influence of this particular aspect of mind.

Once a thought has moved through this process, it then starts to pass through the 'lens' of the emotional mind. The Daoists understood the emotional mind according to the theory of the five elemental movements. These five movements are a reflection of five composite parts of your consciousness, but ultimately, how they influence us most is through the actions of the emotions. The ancient view of the emotions is that there were five key emotional responses to life, and these were categorised according to the five elemental movements, as shown in Table 2.1. These are the five broad headings under which all emotions can be listed.

Table 2.1: The Five Emotions

Element	Wood	Fire	Earth	Metal	Water
Emotion	Anger	Joy	Worry	Grief	Fear

When people look at these five emotions, they generally point out, and quite rightly so, that it is a rather sparse model of how the mind works. There is a whole spectrum of emotional experiences which we do not find in this table. Part of the reason for this is that these are simply five key categorisations of the emotions and so other emotional experiences can be placed under these headings. If we expanded the list a little to give you an example of what I mean, then the result would be something like Table 2.2.

Table 2.2: Expanded Emotional List

Element	Wood	Fire	Earth	Metal	Water
Emotion	Anger	Joy	Worry	Grief	Fear
	Frustration	Excitement	Obsession	Sadness	Panic
	Jealousy	Mania	Pensiveness	Loss	Shock
	Envy	Love	Caring	Defensiveness	Addictions
	Control	Lust	Smothering	Attachment	Wanting
	Rage	Embarrassment	Neediness	Possessiveness	Terror
	Annoyance	Sadness	Empathy	Greed	Perversion

This list could obviously be expanded a great deal, and all sorts of character traits could be included as well. Essentially, any character traits or facets to your personality comprise not just the acquired mind and its dualistic perception of the world but also one of the movements of the five elements. This means that each and every thought and aspect of your 'self' is the result of a response to external stimuli that have been passed through the filters of Yin, Yang and the five elemental movements. These are the 'substance' of who you are and what makes you tick.

If we were to take 'consciousness' as existing at the centre of who you are and then depict the various layers of mind, emotional layering and then personality, it would look something like the model shown in Figure 2.12. Though this is perhaps a little over-literal, as a model it should help you understand how the Daoists viewed the formation of 'self'.

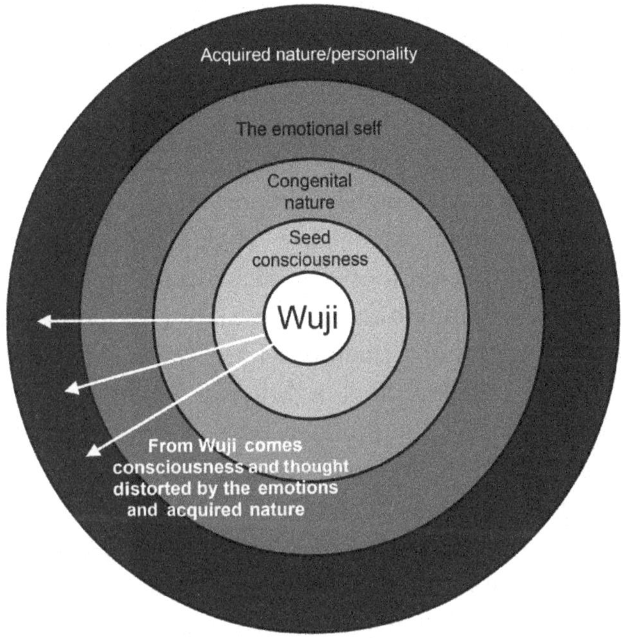

Figure 2.12: The Formation of 'Self'

It should be noted here that this ongoing process of developing the 'self' starts from the second you are born through to the day you die. With every single action of your mind (all of the time!) you are repeating this process over and over again. This does not mean that it is an inherently 'bad' process, though; there is no judgement of this sort in Daoism, it just simply is.

You have seen that the top 'emotion' associated with Fire is listed as 'joy'. This generally raises concerns amongst newcomers to the arts, as they don't see joy as a negative emotion. This is true, joy is fine to experience, we want lots of it in life for life to be fun! Essentially, the elemental movement of Fire is only problematic when there is a 'lack' or an 'excess'. A lack of joy produces another of the emotions listed under Fire, which is sadness. Sadness is often seen as a 'collapse' of the Fire elemental energy. An excess in this area leads to mania or overexcitement; this can be anything from inappropriate levels of laughter to hysteria and even psychosis. In these cases, it is the imbalanced reflection of emotions related to joy that is the issue.

Five Thieves and Five Poisons

If we can understand the process above, then we can begin to see just how we change over the course of our lives. Each of us has a particular emotional makeup; in part, this will be due to inherent differences deep within us, but mostly we change according to the experiences we have. There is no 'fault' in this; generally these experiences are out of our hands, it is just the nature of the rich tapestry of life to provide us with the stimuli which we use to develop the acquired mind.

The Daoists have long been a somewhat overdramatic bunch with a penchant for the extreme, and so this brings us to how they describe this process with regard to our practice. Traditionally, they talk about the 'five thieves' and the 'five poisons'. These are terms that actually appear in other traditions as well; Buddhism and the Sikh tradition have 'five thieves' as well. These are simply the traditions I am aware of; I am sure if I had more knowledge of other spiritual traditions, I would also find such terms appearing. Traditions have long influenced each other, and there probably are some shared roots for these theories, though each tradition will use them in a different manner and name the 'thieves' and 'poisons' slightly differently according to their own understanding of the human psyche.

In Daoism, the five thieves are the senses. We interact with the external world primarily through our sense faculties. We see, hear, touch, taste and feel the world through these five senses and then absorb stimuli in this manner where they are then taken to the mind for processing. Without these senses, it would be pretty much impossible for us to interact with the external world. Of course, there is also the 'internal world' of dreams, imagination and so on, but ultimately, it was the influence of the external world that the Daoists saw as being the biggest influence upon us. Since these five senses draw in information from around us, and it is this information that causes distortions in our mind, they saw the five senses as 'thieves' that would 'steal' from your ability to contact your innate consciousness. The 'theft' of your true consciousness by the senses means that there is layer after layer of acquired mind to trawl through, and this is where the challenge of finding inner stillness lies.

I remember a clear instruction from one of my earliest teachers of meditation: I was told to 'seal the doors and windows of the mind so that the five thieves cannot enter'. As I said before, this may sound a little overdramatic, but it was a straightforward way of making clear to me that I should withdraw my senses and move inwards so that I could temporarily be removed from the outside world whilst I practised.

The five thieves then give birth to the five poisons, which are essentially the emotions and their energetic effect upon the body. As the 'poisons' develop within us, they begin to bring developmental change to our mind, energetic system and body. This then dictates the nature of the 'road of health' we travel along.

The Influence of the Five Poisons

There is an undeniable mind/body link that exists for each of us. Gone are the days when the connection between these two was ignored. When I was a child, here in the West it was seen as kind of mad to think that the mind lies behind most of our physical ailments, but nowadays stress is recognised as the biggest killer of our age, and doctors will openly discuss the emotional root of many sicknesses.

Within Daoism, the mind and the body are connected by one aspect of the inner environment: Qi. Qi is, quite simply, the translator of information between the mind and the body. It is the carrier of 'data' from the mind through into the physical tissues via the channel system and, in return, it draws information back from the body into the mind, meaning that even a physical injury or contagious disease can also influence the nature of mind. This process is summarised in Figure 2.13.

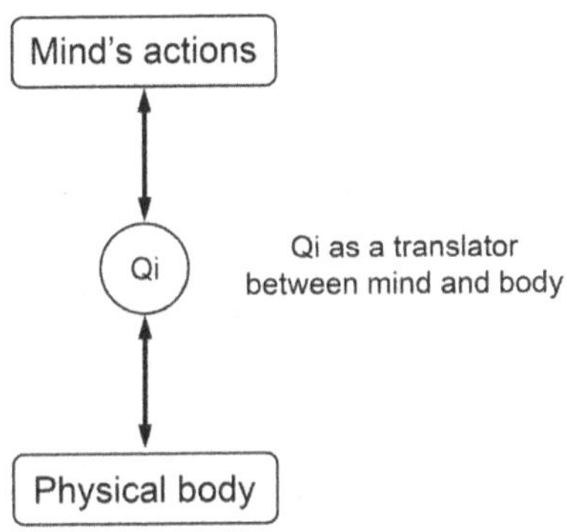

Figure 2.13: Qi as a Translator

We only have to look at Chinese medicine and how it views the body to see just how the mind is said to have an impact upon our physical health. Shared categorisation of emotions, organs, channels and regions of the body shows how our mind will impact upon different regions of our physical form. A full understanding of these kinds of theories can only really come from an in-depth look at Chinese medical theory, but Table 2.3 gives a brief overview of the key correspondences for each of the five elemental movement categories.

The basic mechanism of this process is that as we experience an emotion, it changes the quality of our Qi for the duration of that experience. This Qi is essentially a form of information that is then transferred via the channel system through into the rest of the body. Since the channels run in specific locations, each emotion will resonate with a particular aspect of the body.

For example, people who spend a lot of their lives angry, frustrated and filled with jealousy will, no doubt, start to impact the health of their Liver and Gall Bladder. The channels of the body will deposit this influence into the sides of the torso and around the ribcage where the channels related to this 'poison' have their biggest influence. They are also, with time, likely to experience problems with their tendons which will often become brittle and snap easily, and perhaps start to have pain around their eyes and migraine-type headaches. People with an excess of fear and nervousness will start to injure their Kidneys, and their back will begin to weaken, so spinal issues are common in these types of people. Perhaps this is where the word 'spineless' to refer to cowardly people came from?

Table 2.3: Elemental Bodily Correspondences

Element	Wood	Fire	Earth	Metal	Water
'Poison'	Anger	Joy	Worry	Grief	Fear
Organs	Liver Gall Bladder	Heart Small Intestine	Spleen Stomach	Lungs Large Intestine	Kidneys Bladder
Tissues	Tendons	Blood Vessels	Muscles	Skin	Bones
Sense	Vision	Taste	Feeling	Smell	Hearing
Pathogen	Wind	Heat	Damp	Dryness	Cold
Body area	Flanks	Face	Abdomen	Chest	Back

There are, of course, a multitude of changes that can take a hold on the body over the course of our lives, and none of us is 100 per cent subject to just one emotional type. Over the course of a day, week or year, there are, no doubt, a million different thoughts, each with their own emotional content involved. This means that the body is always being subjected to this kind of transformational information from the mind and, consequently, always adjusting according to this information.

For those of you not familiar with Chinese medical language, the table also includes five pathogenic forms of Qi called Wind, Heat, Damp, Dryness and Cold. These terms can be confusing at first, but essentially they describe the quality of the 'poison' as it is deposited within the body. Chinese medical practitioners will work to clear the body of these pathogens as they can be the root cause of many illnesses.

Recognising Change

Ultimately, none of this process above was seen as something to worry about, because it is completely unavoidable. In fact, worry will damage the Spleen, so that will make it worse! As much as anything, there should be an air of acceptance of what is taking place, and then we work towards changing this process to take us in the most efficient direction. Our body will always go through change, as will our mind. This is something that seems to be missed by many in the alternative community. They talk of initiating 'inner change' as if you would not change without a meditation practice. This is simply not the case; you are changing second to second, all of the time. Your mind and body are adapting, as they have been designed to do, according to the experiences you are subjected to. Change is an inevitability of life. All we are doing is recognising the nature of this change, understanding the mechanism behind it and then adjusting it through our practice so that this 'change' heads in a direction that we wish it to.

Mind/Body Connection

One key strength of Daoism that needs underlining and making clear is that it always recognised the mind/body connection as being the key to training. Each spiritual tradition to come from the East ultimately talked of working with the mind and developing consciousness, but many traditions did this solely through meditative-type work. Through meditation, a practitioner is rarely working with the body but instead engaging with their thoughts and related machinations of the mind in order to attain a certain state of being. In contrast to this, Daoists often work with their body instead to attain similar results. Though there are, of course, meditation techniques contained within Daoism, there are also a multitude of body-based methods which are employed to influence the quality of the mind. Qi Gong and the Nei Gong process are clear examples of this way of working.

The mind/body connection works in a cyclical fashion, as shown in Figure 2.14. In this way, the mind affects the body, and the body affects the mind, through a reciprocal relationship.

As discussed above, the actions of the mind and our emotions govern the quality of information contained within our Qi. This is then sent through the channel system to influence the body's direction of evolution. This means that if we can understand the above theory and work with the body correctly, then we can reverse this process and use bodywork to change the nature of our mind. Anybody who has practised Qi Gong or a similar art such as Yoga for long enough will instinctually understand this process, but it is rarely made clear to beginners how it works. Within our training, we open up the channel system and 'clear' it of pathogenic information. We then fill the body with fresh Qi and circulate it around the system to nourish the organs and tissues of the body. As this happens, it sends a feedback loop of information to the mind which then starts to adjust its emotional makeup to be more in accordance with the body's state. This all, in turn, helps with developing the efficiency of the mind and body's functioning.

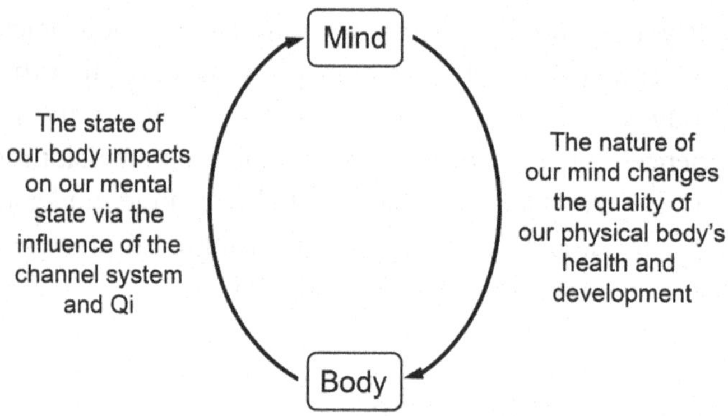

Figure 2.14: Mind/Body Influence

This being said, it is not enough to use Qi Gong or the Nei Gong process to really get to the heart of consciousness itself. It will generally require meditative practice to do this. The use of bodily based systems will help to clear emotional issues and rebalance the mind, but it is rare for it to be enough to get to the heart of who we are and what we are made up of. This is why the deeper aspects of Nei Gong training essentially transfer into meditation and sitting practice. I would like to point out here that in my opinion (and it is just my opinion, so please feel free to disagree), many people dive into meditation to try to work with consciousness at a deep level. The vast majority of these people hit a 'glass ceiling' in their development very early on as they have not managed to work with the layers of the acquired mind to any great degree. The result of this is that many people are stuck simply at the level of deep relaxation without managing to go any deeper. If many of these people added a bodily based system into their training, they would find that it helps to clear a lot of these layers very quickly and efficiently. It is for this reason that I generally tell people that Nei Gong provides an excellent foundation for training in meditation.

Somatic Memory

Another aspect of how the mind and body relate to one another is worth mentioning here: this is the somatic memory of the body. The body is said to be an expression of the nature of mind, and through the discussion above we can start to see what the mechanism involved in this is. The body also 'stores' old experiences within its structure; the majority of people have experienced this quite clearly and it becomes an important part of some of the early stages of Nei Gong training.

It is within the complex matrix of our body's soft tissues that each and every experience is stored. These can be physical trauma, influential events and, most importantly, emotional experiences.

For example, maybe in the past you broke your wrist. Though the wrist may be restored to full function, when you think of the injury and relive the memory of the problem, you are likely to feel an ache in this region of the body. Even many years later, this can still be the case. If you want to test this for yourself, simply place your mind into the body and trawl through some memories of old injuries. Does a tangible feeling of discomfort or aching pop up there when you remember the injury happening? If so, then that is your body's somatic memory. If not, then great! It is hoped that the residues of this old issue have cleared from your body's system. Even in the case of something like this, an old injury, the storing of the information from this problem will cause a change in the quality of Qi in this area of the body. Even though there may no longer be any physical damage, there will still be an energetic 'echo' of the condition and it all adds to the manner in which your Qi behaves in the body.

Another example may be to do with emotional trauma. These types of somatic memory are often the strongest. Perhaps you had your heart 'broken' by an ex-lover. When you think of this person, it brings an ache to your chest. Maybe you have problems with a family member, an old argument that still leaves you feeling upset even though it is in the past? When you think of the event, it may bring a 'knot' to your stomach. People subjected to sexual trauma often still feel an ache in the region of the groin or around the inside of the hips. These are all reflections of the body's somatic memory and an aspect of how just about every event that triggers an emotional reaction contributes to the way in which our body develops.

A great deal of my work as an acupuncturist is based around helping people to clear these somatic memories within the body so that their health can improve and attachment to the root cause of an issue can be alleviated. It is not a classical chart, but Figure 2.15 shows a simple model of where many somatic memories are stored within the body.

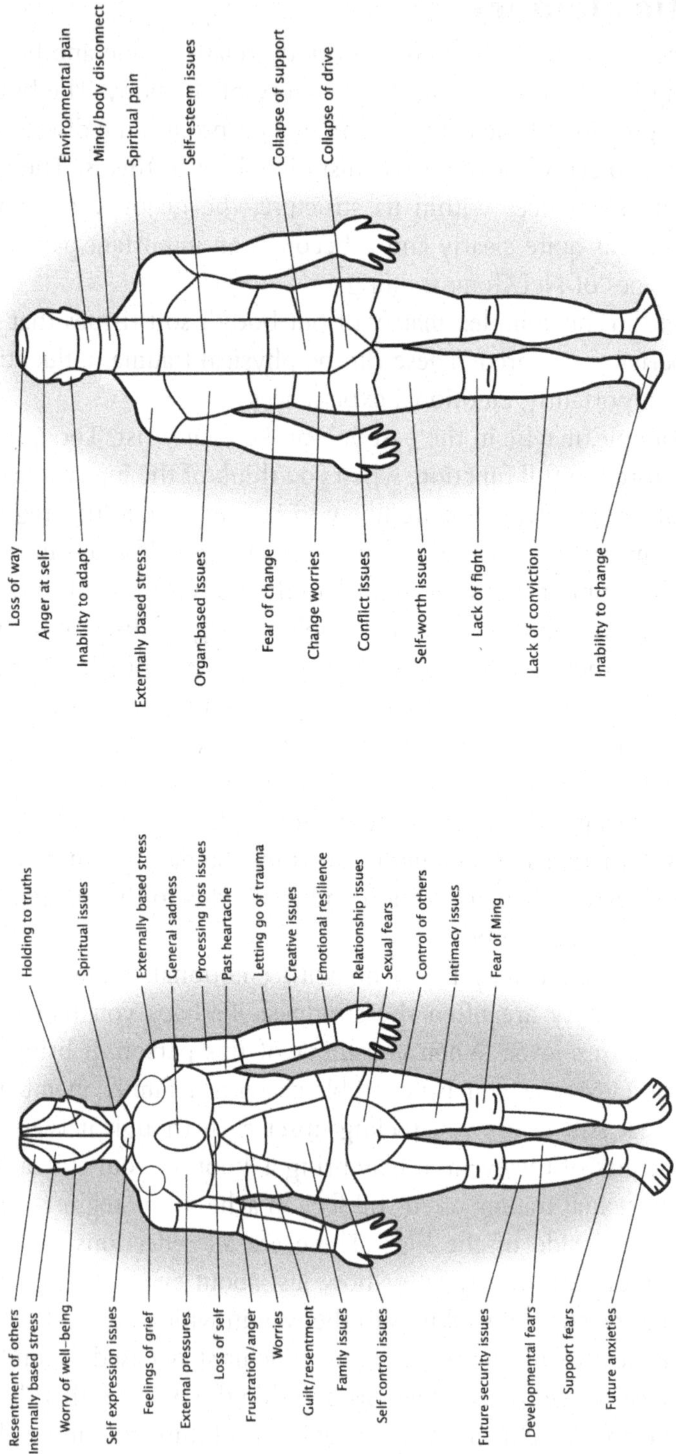

Figure 2.15: Somatic Memory and Body Locations

If you understand the nature of the channel system and the emotions, then you can easily figure out why most of these body regions are connected as they are. On top of this, I have added experience from my own practice as well. Please note, though, any model like this is simply a guide and should not be taken as gospel truth. The mind and body are complex beasts, and to a certain degree each of us will store events in the body in our own unique manner.

A lot of the 'purging' and 'releasing' work in Nei Gong practice is aimed at shedding the energetic root of these somatic memories so that the Qi can flow more easily and the channel system can 'open up'. We will return to this in more detail when we look at the foundation stages of Nei Gong training. For now, it is enough to have an overall understanding of how the mind/body system works and how it contributes to our health.

Letting Go and Attachment

Returning to a statement I made earlier: 'if we overfocus on our health through the training, then we actually hinder our ability to develop'. If we look to the mind as a root cause of many of our health-based issues, we can see why this is the case. A large part of the strength of an art like Nei Gong is that it works to help the body shed many of these somatic memories and thus the energetic root of a problem. Since the 'memory' is stored as a form of Qi in a region of the body, then, when we open up this area of the body in the correct manner, this 'memory' can be let go of and so it ceases to have an impact upon our health and development. It is an aspect of the human mind that it generally does not want to 'let go' of anything. Even if we consciously want to shed our connection to an event or memory, there is a deeper, subconscious part of us that finds this very difficult. Essentially, our experiences have made us who we are, even those experiences we view as being terrible in nature. There is a part of the mind that does not wish to shed its attachment to these events, and the memory of them, since doing so gives it a sense of fear. Though it seems illogical to us, even the most awful of traumas can leave us with a feeling of inner fear once we start to 'let go' of them. I have said this to students before and met a wall of anger from them! It seems to provoke a sense of indignation in many people that you might suggest the mind was wishing to hold on to negatively charged events. I do not say this to insult or inflame in any way; I am simply stating what I have seen. It is, once again, neither good nor bad, it is just how a part of the mind works. Change and 'letting go' can be scary, even if we don't know why.

For this reason, we use the somatic memory as a tool to change the mind. As an example, perhaps I have memories of past conflict with family members anchored into my abdominal region. The Qi running through this area is influenced by these past events and so now I have issues with my digestive system. It leaves me with slight irritable bowel syndrome-type symptoms and difficulty digesting certain foods. If I try to tackle the issues directly by thinking about them and reliving the events that caused them, it is often difficult to let them go. By reliving the event in my mind, I am essentially forming a sort of attachment to the root of the trauma, even though I don't wish to do so. If, on the other hand, I use my bodily based practice to free up the Qi in the region of the abdomen and shed the pathogenic influence from this region through my practice, then my health is more likely to improve. There has been no conscious recollection of the event in the way that psychotherapy may explore the event; instead, I simply focus on my practice and, when the body is ready, it lets go of the somatic connection to the event on its own.

I have watched this take place time and time again in the many hundreds of people around the world I have taken through this process. Though there is no conscious, directed awareness of a particular trauma, it has been able to leave the body through practice. Afterwards, students often realise that the connection to certain past events has left their system and describe it as though these past traumas were 'watched on television' rather than being an event they experienced. Though they can recall the event in their mind, the somatic reaction is gone and there is little in the way of negative emotional reaction to what has taken place.

It is the non-attachment to the process of 'healing' and, instead, a focus upon perfecting the art form for art's sake that has provided the vehicle for 'letting go' to take place. This is the key to gaining the most benefit from Nei Gong training with regard to your health: focus on developing Gong in the art, and let the process unfold for you of its own accord. It is for this reason that, in my own classes, I will rarely discuss medicine or emotional releases with people. I am aware that many Qi Gong teachers are leading the arts in this way but, in my opinion, they are missing the great strength that can come from non-attachment to a process. Let the medicine act upon you in its own way; we simply work to improve the quality of the art form.

The Snowball Effect

Both parts of this process, the accumulation of distortions and the shedding of past information, are taking place all of the time anyway. It is a natural part of life and a normal function for both the human mind and body. Each of us manage it differently and to varying degrees. There is no justice in this; some people seem to shake off even the most traumatic events in their lives, whilst others remain locked in a cycle of stress over even the smallest occurrence. As much as anything, this is to do with our inbuilt resonance with certain energetic qualities.

Every event generates an emotional experience, and we can think of these emotions as a kind of energy. Certain emotional energies are more likely to affect us than others. So, if I am a person who resonates with anger, then when I face an event that generates anger within me, it is more likely to develop a strong influence upon the nature of my Qi. At the same time, if anger is my main 'resonance', then I am more likely to view external events in this way. Whereas the unkind actions of some third party may generate sadness in another person, the person resonating with anger will experience this event through the lens of conflict. In this way, it ends up being like a snowball rolling down a hill; as it rolls down the slope, it picks up more snow and the snowball grows larger. The more anger I experience, the more anger I generate. This then builds more pathogenic Qi related to this organ, and so my anger grows. If this is kept up for a period of time, then eventually I will look out into the world through a thick, distorted lens of anger and frustration.

We will always find it more difficult to 'let go' of the somatic memories and energetic influences pertaining to the emotional quality we most strongly resonate with. This is why in Qi Gong we wish to first deal with the 'surface emotions' stored in the body and then go deeper to find the root of our emotional makeup. Like peeling away the layers of an onion, we continue to go deeper and deeper into our 'self' through the practice. If we become overly attached to any one particular event or stage in the process, then our progress is generally halted. It is for this reason that we focus on the practice rather than its results.

We are 'gifted' a certain emotional makeup at birth. This is, in part, due to astrological influences but also inherited mental qualities from your family line. These will always be the most challenging aspects to change in yourself as they are most ingrained. After this, we have our earliest influences, those that have affected us during our formative childhood years; these are also a challenge to adjust as they are rooted into the earliest stages of our personal development. From here, we then have a whole plethora of distorted layers built up from our life experiences and how the five thieves of the senses processed these events. Figure 2.16 shows this process of mental formation.

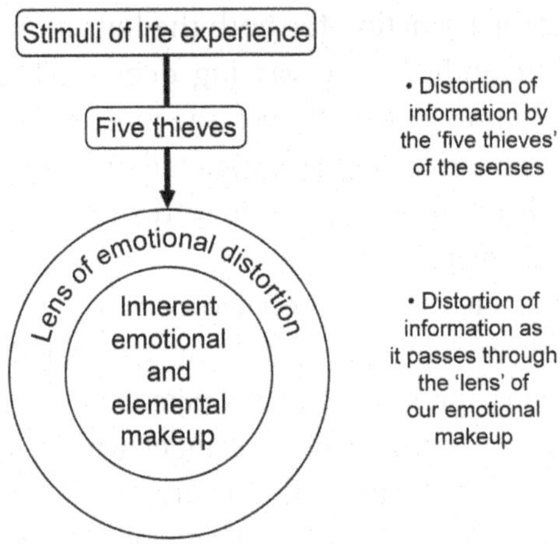

Figure 2.16: Mental Formation Through Our Lives

The view is that these 'lenses' we see the world through prevent us from ever seeing 'truth'. Instead, we have a distorted view of the world according to our own biases. Since all of us on this planet are going through the same process day in and day out, we are all essentially living in a confused state where everything we see and know is distorted to a large degree. At this rate, it is a wonder we ever manage to get anything done at all as a species!

Note here though that none of this is 'wrong' or 'bad'. It is a dangerous mindset to get into if we view this process in a negative light. It is what it is; none of us are any better at it than any other. We are simply a product of this naturally unfolding process, and that is that. The Daoists actually viewed the process with a large degree of humour. They disarmed the process by seeing it as rather ridiculous; how silly that we are all living according to these distortions! Once the ridiculousness of how the human mind develops is recognised for what it is, then any unnecessary gravity or trauma around this process is dissolved. The sooner we can achieve this way of looking at ourselves, the sooner we can get to improving our mind and body's efficiency through our training.

One of the most harmful mental attitudes to these arts is one of 'sin' or 'self-loathing'. This idea of seeing yourself as 'bad' or that something needs correcting in some way is truly detrimental to your training. I have seen this in students sometimes, and they end up using these practices as some kind of self-flagellation. They have often come from a very strict religious background and carried some of the false ideas of sin across into what they are doing. It is always important for these kinds of people to lighten up and learn to enjoy the process for what it is; stop judging yourself, don't focus on the negatives all the time, and simply work on your art! As teachers, we must be wary of these kinds of students as it is inevitably they who run the risk of doing themselves emotional harm with internal practice. I have encountered them over the years in meditation groups, Buddhist schools, Yoga classes and, of course, Qi Gong schools. It is the light-hearted and fun-loving students that generally move through this process with the most ease.

At the same time, there is another attitude on the opposite end of the spectrum which is also incorrect. This is the view of 'There is nothing to change; you are already perfect.' This view is generally propagated by the new-age scene and has now sadly crept its way into the traditional arts of Asia as well. This idea may be good for people with low self-esteem, but it is certainly not the stance that Eastern arts traditionally took. It is a fluffy modernism.

I do recognise that many people come into arts like meditation because they are deeply hurt in some way, their self-esteem is at an all-time low and they are lost in life; I have seen many people of this sort looking for answers through meditation and Qi Gong. The view of 'We are already perfect as we are' is a sensible stance to take in order to help these kinds of students find their footing in life. I agree, build up a person's self-esteem as much as we can so that they can function in life. But I am writing this book for the other kind of students – those who actually wish to penetrate to the core of what these arts are about. If we want to go deep, we must first recognise that there is work to do, but at the same time there is nothing wrong with having work to do; it is a process free from judgement. If we look at the Chinese arts in particular, we can see that Confucianism stated that we needed to 'mould' a person into the right state of being through external cultivation methods. Chinese Buddhism said we must clean the distortions of perception away until we are free from them, and Daoism took the stance that our true self is buried beneath many layers of acquired mind; we must continue to 'shed' these layers until only the 'true and simple' self remains.

Putting It Together

So, if we look at all of this information, we can, I hope, begin to see how the Daoists viewed human health. Figure 2.17 helps to make this clear.

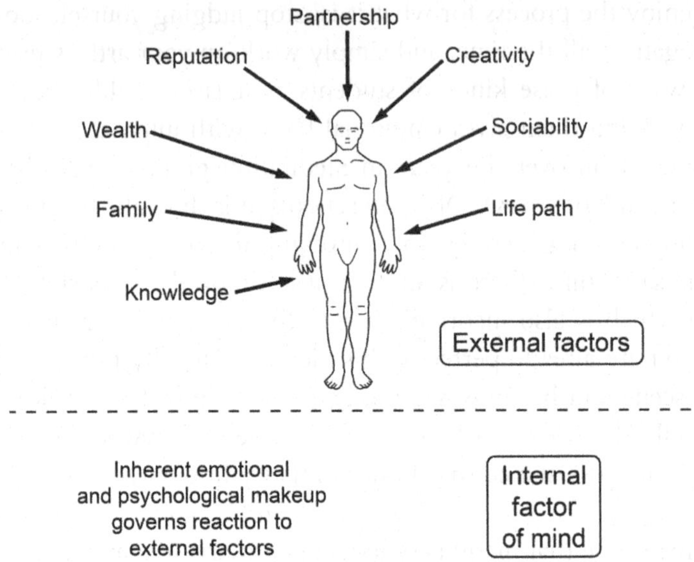

Figure 2.17: The Daoist View of Health

Surrounding the person at the centre of the image are eight of the nine palaces of health. These were essentially said to be the eight aspects of a person's life that should be in a certain degree of harmony in order for the ninth palace of physical health to be positively impacted. This is the basis for health in the external world. The ninth palace then concerns our health, which can be affected by injury or contracted illness but mostly relies on the state of our mind. This is the basis for health within the 'internal world'. If we wish to look at what exactly can give us these developmental experiences – what it is in life that causes these reactions within the five thieves – it is generally something related to the eight other palaces of human health.

Try it yourself, take some problems of your own, some challenges that have had an impact upon your life; you will find that the vast majority of them have their external root in one or more of the eight palaces surrounding the central position of your 'physical health palace'. Between family, people in your life, money stresses and so on, here are the roots for most challenges as well as positive experiences you have had. This is why they factored strongly in how the Daoists viewed human health and how it connects to your daily life.

If we can understand all of this, then we can begin to see what kinds of factors have changed the way our mind and body function. It is these factors that are most likely to adjust through Nei Gong practice. This should start to have a positive effect upon both our psychological and physical health.

Remember, though, that developing one's 'health' was only a foundational stage of practice according to the Daoist way of thinking. It is a platform upon which everything else is built. It is efficiency of the body and mind's functioning that the Daoists sought, and a by-product of this was an improvement to human health. At a later stage in the book, we will begin to look at how these adjustments then affect your wider path in life, but for now we should move on to an understanding of just how the physical body is viewed in Daoism.

Chapter 3

THE QI GONG BODY

All arts, sports or physical endeavours require a certain body type. If somebody tries to carry out a practice with the wrong type of body, then the results will always be of poor quality. We need the 'right' body for the job at hand. Compare the body of a professional ballet dancer to a champion weightlifter or the physique of a swimmer to that of a sumo wrestler. In each case, the practitioner's body has been developed in a very specific way so that it functions as efficiently as possible for the task at hand. This logic is easily seen and applied to more physical practices such as those listed above, but people often find it hard to apply this way of thinking to internal arts such as Qi Gong and Nei Gong. The truth is that just because the changes to the physical body largely take place on the inside, we still need the body to change. An absolute beginner who has never built their body in the correct way for Qi Gong will not get the same results as a practitioner who has spent a number of years putting in the work and transforming the way in which their body is shaped and functions. The Qi Gong body is built in a very specific way, and many of the foundation stages of Nei Gong development involve transforming the physical body in a very particular manner. In the next chapter, we will look more specifically at these changes, how we achieve them and why, but first let us look at the nature of the body and how it is structured according to Daoist thought.

The Sinew-Changing Classic

The basis for almost all Qi Gong teachings regarding the transformation of the body is derived from a set of classical teachings known as the Yi Jin Jing (易筋經). This is a scripture generally translated as the 'Sinew-Changing Classic'. As a text, it has informed almost all authentic Qi Gong systems as well as many aspects of the Chinese martial arts.

As with many aspects of Chinese history, there are disagreements as to when the Yi Jin Jing was first written down. The generally recognised version of the text's history lies with the Shaolin (少林) monastery and a mythical teacher known as Bodhidharma (菩提達摩) who is said to have visited the monastery from India in the sixth century. Whilst staying at the monastery, he recorded the essence of his teachings in two texts, one of which was the Yi Jin Jing. These teachings were then absorbed by the monks at the monastery and formed a part of their martial arts and internal tradition.

Modern scholars disagree with this account and state that it is little more than a fairy tale. They go on to connect the text to various Chinese medicine doctors and Qi Gong practitioners who lived during much later times, whilst some still go on to connect it to several Daoist teachers instead. Indeed, the principles contained within the text are more akin to Daoist teachings than Buddhist, but who knows? Essentially, it does not matter. Personally, I have never been much of a history buff, and I am quite aware that history is often skewed for political reasons anyway, so I tend not to worry about it. For those who want to delve into the discussion around the origins of the Yi Jin Jing, there are plenty of writings online and in printed format.

What we do know, however, is that whoever first outlined the principles, they were certainly absorbed into the methods of the Daoists, and almost all of their Qi Gong systems are based upon the principles of the Yi Jin Jing.

In modern times, there are sets of exercises known as the Yi Jin Jing. They are generally based around flexing and stretching movements. The Chinese Qi Gong Association developed these exercises as an expression of the classical teachings of the Yi Jin Jing, but they are certainly not the original format of the teachings. I have had several teachers who took me through the Yi Jin Jing's principles. Whilst they each had their own, distinct take on what the Yi Jin Jing was all about, they all agreed that it was a set of principles, not exercises.

If we are to summarise the principles of the Yi Jin Jing quite simply, then they are as follows:

- To help the body regain any lost physical vitality
- To enhance blood flow
- To open the channels of the body
- To strengthen the flow of Qi through the body
- To prepare the body for more advanced work involving the marrow and brain

The key aspects of the Yi Jin Jing relevant to practitioners of Qi Gong are opening the channels of the body and strengthening the flow of Qi.

If these two components of the Yi Jin Jing are understood properly, then they can greatly inform your Qi Gong practice and help you along the Nei Gong process.

These functions of the Yi Jin Jing listed above may sound odd considering that the translation of Yi Jin Jing says that the aim is to transform the 'sinews', but this makes more sense when we understand that the channels of Qi travel through the sinews. The 'sinews' are the 'riverbeds' for the channels, whilst the Qi is the river itself. We could even, more accurately, name the scripture the 'Channel Opening Classic'.

If we wish to be able to identify an authentic Qi Gong system based in traditional principles, then we first need to understand the nature of the Yi Jin Jing and how it views the human body. Quite simply, if the Qi Gong system you are looking at does not adhere to the principles of the Yi Jin Jing, then it is not an authentic system, or it may have lost something along the way.

So, before we look in detail at the channel system and what it comprises, let us first look at the various components that make up the physical body according to Yi Jin Jing teachings.

Components of the Physical Body

The Daoists did not view the physical body in exactly the same way as it is viewed in Western biological sciences. Whilst there are certain key understandings that are the same (a bone is still a bone, for example!), there are some fundamental differences in the way that the Daoists viewed the body's structure and functioning. For the purposes of this chapter, I will look at how the Daoists viewed the body, focusing on several key components that must be understood and worked in the correct manner if we are ever to build the Qi Gong body according to the teachings of the Yi Jin Jing.

The components were viewed as being like 'layers' of the body; though they intertwined with one another and, to some extent, shared pathways and regions of the body, they were seen as individual elements that needed to be trained specifically. For the purposes of this section of the book, I will focus upon the following components of the physical body:

- The muscles
- The tendons
- The Jing Jin
- The Huang

- The bones
- The viscera

These are the key components of the body discussed within the teachings of the Yi Jin Jing. Each of these components and how the Daoists viewed them is briefly introduced.

The Muscles

The muscles that are referred to within the Yi Jin Jing are the large muscle groups of the body. They are considered the most 'external' of the layers of the body in comparison to the other elements listed here. They are also viewed as the least important to develop beyond a certain point within the internal arts, though it is also recognised that no muscular strength at all is unhealthy for the body. What is important to understand here is that Qi does not 'conduct' its way through the muscles, and herein lies the reason for the lack of importance placed upon them within the internal arts.

The Tendons

The tendons are cords of strong fibrous collagen tissue that attach muscles to bones. In classical Chinese thought they were also seen as an extension of the energy of the Liver and the most vital part of the body in relation to manifesting strength. Many Chinese martial arts favoured developing and strengthening the tendons over the muscles in order to build power for fighting. Within Nei Gong, the tendons are favoured over the muscles with regard to development, because they have a closer connection to the movement of Qi.

The Jing Jin

The Jing Jin (經筋) or 'sinew channels' are lines of connective tissue that run through and around the muscles of the body. They travel along the same pathways as the meridians of Chinese medicine, and essentially form the most physical aspect of the channel system. Though they follow the same pathways as the meridians of Chinese medicine, they do not follow their directional flow. Instead, they are said to originate on the extremities of the body and travel inwards towards the heart region of the chest. What is important to recognise is that they are elasticated in nature and travel in continuous pathways along the limbs and trunk of the body without being isolated into parts as the muscles of the body are. It is a major part of the body development within Nei Gong to connect the sinew channels together into one elasticated unit. The end result of this is a feeling like you are wearing a kind of biological wetsuit. Whenever you move your body according to the sinew channels, it feels as though you are carrying out a gentle, whole-body stretch.

The sinew channels are less external than the muscles of the body but still only exist on the relative exterior of the body. They are most prevalent around the limbs and torso. They do not run deep into the body.

The sinew channels are said to be like riverbeds for the channel system, and this is mostly because they are very 'conductive' to the movement of Qi. A large part of opening the external channel system relies on locating and working correctly with the sinew channels.

The Huang

The Huang (肓) are often translated within Chinese medical texts as being the 'membranes' of the body, but this is not really an adequate translation of the term, in my own opinion. They are one of, if not *the* most vital components to understand in Nei Gong practice. Despite their importance, they are rarely discussed or taught openly. Many of the deeper components of bodily transformation in these arts rely on working correctly with the Huang. Note that due to a lack of being able to find an adequate translation for Huang into English, I shall stick with the Chinese term for the remainder of this book.

In order to understand the Huang, we should look at how they are described: the Huang are said to exist in all of the spaces of the inside of the body; they uphold the organs and envelop them in a protective layer. They are said to be able to conduct Qi to a very high level and, though only mentioned in brief in Chinese medical texts, are often discussed at length in teachings related to the Yi Jin Jing.

The human body is not actually 'hollow'. If we look at an anatomy book, the organs are usually depicted as floating in space within the torso. Obviously, this is not really the case. If there were indeed a lot of hollow spaces like this in the body, then when we stood up, all of our vital organs would fall down and gather in our lower abdomen! The reason this does not happen is because all the 'spaces' inside of the body are full of the Huang. They extend like a complex web of connective tissues, filling all of the spaces and connecting our body together internally.

The deeper flows of Qi conduct their way through the Huang, and it is here, within this complex web, that many of the deeper aspects of body conversion take place through Nei Gong training. Some may, at this stage, compare the Huang to the internal fascial network of the body. This may be correct; I am not saying that the Huang is not the fascia. The reason I am not drawing this comparison to any conclusive degree, though, is because there are several functions associated with the Huang that I have not yet seen listed associated with fascia in medical textbooks.

The Huang are said to fill the entire body but have their 'origin' within the solar plexus region of the body. This makes the physical 'centre' of our body the middle of this giant organic cobweb of connective tissue.

The Bones

It is interesting to note that many schools of Qi Gong have gone down the route of being all about structural alignments. They have made the methods of the ancient Daoists entirely concerned with deep breathing and postural correction and little more. By doing this, they are essentially focusing almost entirely upon the skeletal system and how the bones are lined up. Whilst it is true that there are many postural alignments that must be adhered to in Qi Gong practice, they are simply something that we work on in the early stages of our training. As soon as the bones have been aligned in the correct way, then it is time to move on. Alignments are the starting point, not the end goal of the arts. We line up the bones in a specific manner, so that all of the above 'layers' of the body can begin to divide from one another; this, in turn, gives us access to the inner workings of the body. This is the main reason for working with the skeleton in Qi Gong practice. In the next chapter of this book we will look at just how aligning the body accomplishes this, but for now I wish to focus on the relationship of the other components of the body according to Daoist teachings.

The Viscera

At the deeper regions of the physical body lie the organs. Chinese medical teachings have a whole library's worth of writings on the organs of the body. How they relate to one another and how they are involved in our mental, energetic and physical functioning has a great impact upon our level of health. The key organs of the body are the Heart, Spleen, Lungs, Kidneys and Liver. These five are said to house various components of our consciousness as well as dictating the quality of Qi within us. Table 3.1 shows the Yin and Yang organs of the body according to Chinese medical theory.

Table 3.1: The Yin and Yang Organs

Yin organs	Yang organs
Heart	Small Intestine
Spleen	Stomach
Lungs	Large Intestine
Kidneys	Bladder
Liver	Gall Bladder
Pericardium	Triple Heater

These organs are paired with one another from left to right in the table. In this way, they function as Yin/Yang couples as well as having complex internal relationships that dictate the level of their functioning.

Since there are many books on the nature of the organs related to Chinese medicine, I will not go into great detail on their functions here. If I included all of this information too, it would become a very long and unwieldy text indeed!

Through Nei Gong practice, we essentially help the organs to purge pathogenic forms of Qi that are negatively impacting their functioning whilst at the same time nourishing them through building and circulating healthier Qi.

I would advise any Qi Gong or Nei Gong practitioner who is not familiar with basic Chinese medicine theory to go and begin some self-study around this topic; it really is vital background information for practitioners. It is also wise for teachers of arts such as this to think seriously about studying Chinese medicine. It really is a useful adjunct to these practices.

External Versus Internal

There has long been a debate running within the internal arts scene as to what actually constitutes an 'internal art'. What is the difference between 'external' and 'internal'? If we wish to reduce it to its most simple definition, it really comes down to which 'mechanism' you are using to move and develop the body.

Externally based movement is generally what we are doing most of the time. Our nervous system sends signals to the muscles, which contract and move the bones of our body like levers. If there is resistance to this force, then muscles grow, as in the case of weight-lifting or working out in the gym.

In this model of movement, you will build the muscles and tendons with little or no development of the sinew channels or Huang. It was not favoured by the ancient Chinese, as the muscles essentially develop in isolation from one another; the body was considered to become disconnected, and thus Qi flow was not developed. Note here, though, that there is nothing inherently wrong with this kind of movement; it is not 'bad' in any way. In fact, it is very good for your health if done correctly; it just does not build the body in the correct way for internal arts practice.

Internally based movement is very different. It is based upon the teachings of the Yi Jin Jing. Some may debate this, but I have yet to see a practitioner of the internal arts (who is doing it correctly) who does not move according to the Yi Jin Jing's teachings, even if they are sometimes unaware of this!

Moving and Developing the Body According to the Yi Jin Jing

As stated above, for a Qi Gong or Nei Gong system to be authentic, it should adhere to the Yi Jin Jing's teachings. Before we start breaking that down, let us look at some of the key components of the Yi Jin Jing. What does it actually tell us?

- The secret to developing one's psychological and physical health is based in the Qi.
- We must cultivate the physical in line with the intangible or there will be imbalance.
- The body must be built in the sequence of Qi, then Huang, then tendon.
- Qi is difficult to understand and build, and so is Huang, but one comes from the other. So, we build the Qi and allow the Huang to form in the right way; this will, in turn, start to develop the tendons.
- The Qi must mobilise; the result of this is the engagement of Huang. This will strengthen the Huang which serves as a platform for the development of health.
- One should keep developing the Qi until the Huang fully stretches and the tendons are strong.
- The result of this is that the channels will open, and the Qi will reach to every part of the body.

These stages above are how we build the body in an 'internal' manner. If we can do this, then the body can operate in a very different manner. The Qi becomes the motive force, the Huang is the mobiliser and stabiliser of the body, and the tendons provide the strength. Once these have been achieved, then we can be said to have successfully built the Qi Gong body, and so we are practising a fully internal art.

The Development of Qi

In order to begin the process outlined above, we must first get our Qi to move. In this case, we are discussing the energetic information that exists within the body. This form of Qi is an extension of the mind that exists in the channel system of the body. It circulates around our body over the course of a day under the direction of several forces, including the direction of the lower Dan Tian.

It is beyond the earliest stages of training to 'build more' Qi. This is a slightly complex procedure that relies on us having developed a solid foundation in our practice first. What is more important is that we learn how to work with the Qi that we already have within our body. This Qi must then be moved in the right way so that it starts to affect the channel system in a very specific manner. This, in turn, begins a purging process which helps the body to clear pathogens from its interior. Only after this work has been completed do we begin looking at building more Qi to any great level.

Our Qi is moved in the foundation stages of Nei Gong training when we learn how to awaken and develop the strength of the lower Dan Tian. This important aspect of the practice serves as an initiator into the Nei Gong process; it can be thought of as 'putting the keys in the ignition' so you can begin your journey.

The movement of Qi goes through three key stages. The first is moving within the channels. The second is purging the body, and the third is starting to influence and engage the Huang. Let us look at each of these three stages in sequence.

Moving the Qi within the Channels

The channels of the body conduct Qi along their length. The movement of Qi in this manner is traditionally likened to the way that the vibration of sound travels along the skin of a drum. When we first start to awaken the lower Dan Tian, this movement of Qi is enhanced so that it can start off a series of reactions within the body. At the beginning of our training, this increased circulation is very important. Without increasing the movement and pressure of the Qi within the channel system, we are held back from ever really passing the first levels of Nei Gong attainment.

Purging the Channels of the Body

Once there has been an increase in the movement of Qi through the channel system, then the channels can begin to clear themselves of stuck energetic debris. This initiates the earliest stages of opening a channel's length. If we think of a channel as being like a river winding its way through the body, then we can think of pathogenic forms of Qi as being like rubbish that builds up in this river. With time, this rubbish builds up, and so a kind of dam is built. This damming of the channels is what we call a 'blockage' in Chinese medical terminology. The natural function of the body's channels is to clear debris on a daily basis, but over time this function is weakened by our emotional state, and so pathogenic information builds up. This is the foundation for disease in the body. By increasing the movement of Qi along the channel's length, we help it to clear some of this 'rubbish' so that the body can function more efficiently.

Influencing and Engaging the Huang

Once the Qi has moved to a high enough level, it will push its way through the channel system. Realistically, for those simply seeking an improvement in their health, this is far enough to go into the Nei Gong process. Once the channels have been freed up of a fair amount of debris, this will ensure that the body functions to a more efficient level. For those wishing to go deeper, however, the Huang must be engaged.

The nature of Qi is that it wants to conduct through the body. It does this by moving along the length of physical structures. Within the body, Qi conducts its way along the length of the Huang and the sinew channels when it is more towards the surface of the body. When the level of Qi has reached a high enough state, it begins to have a very specific effect upon the connective tissues of the Huang. It causes them to engage. As they engage, they start to grow stronger. The strengthening of the Huang then results, cyclically, in more Qi conduction, and so the channel begins to widen. The wider the channel, the more open it is. This is the basis for how the Yi Jin Jing advised opening up the body.

It Is All Internal!

As stated above, Qi conducts its way through certain physical structures of the body. This is a fact of the arts often missed by practitioners. Even though Qi Gong-based arts are primarily concerned with Qi development, they still take the physical body into account as well. The physical body will change in a very specific manner through your training, and this is largely down to the action of the channels.

I remember being a young student and rather naïve in the Qi Gong world. I was probably also a pain in the butt, as I asked too many questions and really felt the need to understand these arts rather than just follow along! I once asked a fairly well-known Western teacher of Qi Gong how far he had gone into his art. He happily told me he was beyond the level of a master now. I asked him how he knew or if he could show me, and he replied that he could not show me his skill because it was 'all internal', and the internal could not be seen.

Now, granted, it was a rather rude question of mine, you will have to excuse me, I was pretty young, but I have since discovered on my path through the arts that what this teacher told me was not true. Though the arts do develop us internally, they also affect the channels of the body, and so there are clear physical changes that take place on the body when we reach certain stages of development. The channels change in shape and feeling and these can clearly be palpated and even seen if somebody is good enough at what they do. When I see my teachers now, one of the first things they do is palpate my arms and torso to see just how well my channels are developing. This is done before they even dream of looking at the quality of my Qi or Shen.

These clear changes – which can be checked – are taking place in the Huang and sinew channels of the body. At the relevant stages of this book, I shall make clear what these tangible changes are so that students can know exactly how far they have come into the process and when enough of a foundation has been built at any one stage.

The Nature of Huang

So, as we have discussed, the Huang fills all of the spaces within the body. It enwraps the organs and various parts of the body and serves to 'uphold' them within the body. This essentially means that we are full up of a malleable substance that connects each and every part of our physical body together. The Huang is where we store the shape of our body. This may sound odd to newcomers to these arts, but anybody who has moved fairly deep into the internal process will know this to be the case. We generally speak of 'muscle memory' being the place where our postural alignments are stored; I would like to make the case that this is not true beyond a very basic level. It is not the memory of the muscles we should concern ourselves with but rather the memory of the Huang. We learn how to lengthen and relax the muscles of the body very early on in our Qi Gong training, but still, in the vast majority of cases, students will retain certain misalignments within their body, especially when they relax and 'sink into their own structure'; as soon as this happens, the memory of Huang distorts your skeletal alignments. These misalignments of the body are generally caused by your daily habits, like long hours on a chair or in front of a computer screen; in these cases, the Huang has changed to suit your habits and built a semi-plastic shape into your structure. We can see how this would happen if we look at the regions of the body where the Huang sits; this is shown in Figure 3.1.

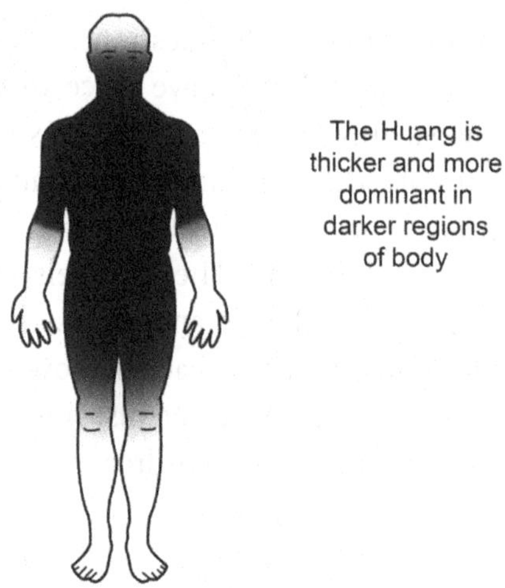

Figure 3.1: Location of the Huang

The Huang fills the entire torso and cavity of the head as well as the majority of the spaces within the arms and legs. It is only near the surface of the body, just beneath the skin, that the Huang converts into the denser elasticated material of the sinew channels.

So, how does the Huang change? The answer is 'stress'. This is vitally important and may seem like an odd word to use with regard to Qi Gong practice. Most teachers are trying to avoid any stress whatsoever in their instructions, but in fact, stress is a precursor to growth when we apply this idea to the body.

The idea of 'stress' being the initiator of change for the body can easily be understood in relation to the muscles and the bones. If bodybuilders wish to increase their muscle mass, they stress the muscles through resistance-type exercises. As the muscles are worked while stress is applied to them, they begin to grow. Bones are the same: as we place weight into our skeletal structure, the downward influence of gravity puts stress into them. The result of the stress is that our bones increase in both strength and density. We can see this in astronauts who have been living in zero gravity for long periods; when they return to Earth, they often need some physiotherapeutic assistance as their bones have become weakened.

This idea of stress is also applied to the Huang. All of the time we are dropping our weight through the body to the floor. Our weight does not just pass through the bones and muscles but through the inside of the body and the Huang as well. As our weight applies stress to the Huang, it changes shape to deal with that stress. The semi-plastic nature of the Huang is such that as we stress it under the force of our weight, it changes shape in order to become more efficient for what we do. If you are the kind of person who spends twelve hours per day sat in a chair with a screen in front of you, then the Huang will change to make your body as efficient as it can be for watching screens! If you are a Qi Gong practitioner, with certain bodily alignment principles being applied to your practice, then the shaping of the Huang under the stress of your standing will build the most efficient shape for this.

Another important aspect of the Huang to be aware of is that it only manifests its inherent shape when stress is applied to it. What this means is that when I wake up in the morning, after several hours asleep, my Huang is actually pretty switched off and loose for the most part. As soon as I stand up and drop my weight through my body, then the 'shapes' and conditions built into my Huang start to show up. This is very important for us to understand.

The art of changing the inside of your body goes in several stages:

1. Align the bones correctly
2. Switch off the external muscles
3. Learn to sink your weight effectively
4. Allow the Huang to change under stress
5. Let the Qi move into the Huang
6. Allow the Huang to transform further
7. The Huang will begin to press outwards into the sinew channels

This will all take place through standing practice of Nei Gong postures if they are carried out correctly and you understand the theory behind the Yi Jin Jing well enough.

A final important aspect of the Huang is that it can 'conduct' your awareness. I liken this to 'water soaking into a sponge' for my students. What this means is that even though you may be able to temporarily and forcibly place your awareness into your body, it will rarely stay there. It will jump around, vary in intensity and generally be unhelpful if you wish to spend prolonged amounts of time becoming 'aware' of the insides of your body. If, on the other hand, the awareness can flow like a liquid through the Huang, it will have a physical anchor within the body and so stabilisation of the mind within your structure is much easier. Figure 3.2 shows this process.

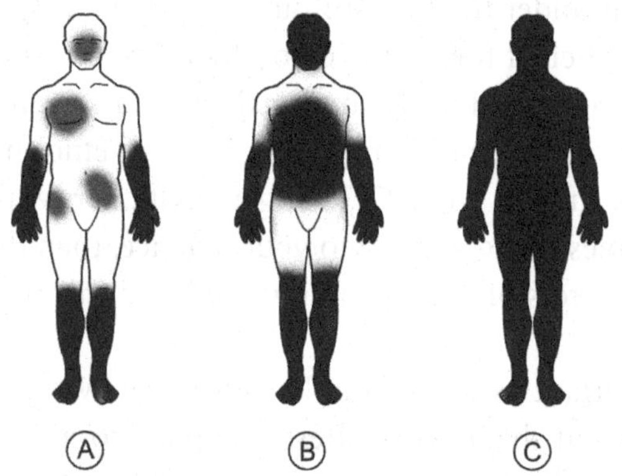

Figure 3.2: Absorption of Awareness into the Huang

As you can see from Figure 3.2, at first, the awareness can only get into certain regions of the body and is essentially disconnected. Over time, the changing of the Huang leads to a greater degree of connection inside. The more 'internally connected' we are, the more 'conductive' to our awareness the body will become. The 'sponge' is being built, and with time the awareness will be able to soak into this sponge like water. As the awareness starts to fill the Huang, it will start to react with it in a series of stages. First, it will cause the Huang to stretch a little under the influence of the mind – we will explore this more in Chapter 6 when we look at the nature of the mind in practice. Second, it will cause the Huang to connect to our intention, and finally, it will actually assist in the production of a very specific type of energy. These later stages are discussed in Chapter 11, as they are quite far into the Nei Gong process with regard to changing the body.

In the beginning, when you reach this stage of absorption, you will find that certain areas are easy to reach and some areas are more difficult. The more difficult areas of the body to 'fill' with the mind are the regions of the Huang that have not yet connected together in the right way. As you progress in your practice, the Huang will connect together more fully, and absorption of the mind into the body becomes easier. As well as this, it is almost always easier for people to absorb the awareness into the outer layers of their body, nearer to the surface and skin. Deep inside the body is very difficult to reach. As the Huang is stressed and built in the right way, it will spread the sponge-like qualities of your inner environment through to the core of your body, and so your awareness will be able to penetrate right through to your centre.

At first, the stretch of the Huang will be subtle, but with time it can become very strong, and the force being pushed from the centre of your body can come with a fair amount of physical power. Many students who I have taken to this stage in their practice have been very surprised at just how strong the internal work of Nei Gong can be on not just an energetic level, but on a physical one as well.

Building the Right Shape

This principle of building the body in the correct manner by shaping the Huang is used throughout our training. Essentially, we are trying to send Qi through the body in very specific directions. The most famous direction of Qi is to send it up the centre of our back and down the front of our body; this circulation of Qi is known as the microcosmic orbit, and we shall return to it in Chapter 8. Most systems of Qi Gong use this direction of Qi movement as a basis for practice; on top of this, there are several other key directions of Qi flow we require in order to progress. The movement of the Qi in these specific directions is developed by shaping the Huang in the right way. As the Huang opens, it causes the Qi to conduct in the right direction, and so we can say that a channel has begun to open.

The flow of Qi through this line causes more of a reaction in the Huang, which also starts to stress and develop more, as shown in Figure 3.3. This cyclical relationship of Qi and Huang is used to exponentially 'grow' the channels in the right way.

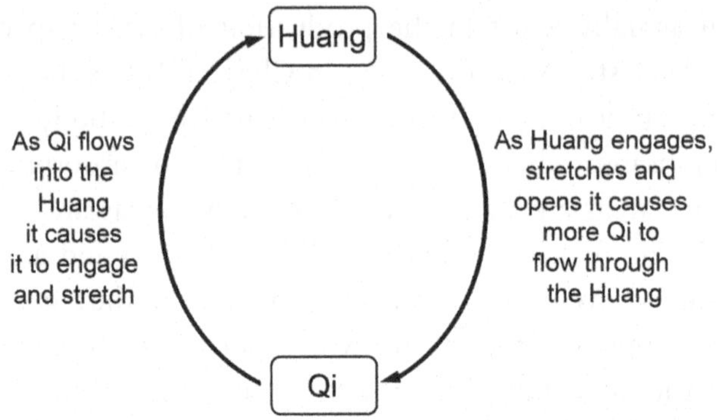

Figure 3.3: The Qi and Huang Cyclical Relationship

The channels have a physiological component to them and this is, essentially, the Huang. The more external channels and their outer expression is then manifest within the sinew channels. The Huang pushes into the sinew channels as it grows; it has to hit a certain degree of 'critical mass', and then its influence upon the sinew channels can be felt. Beyond this, the sinew channels then 'push' into the tendons, and so they grow as a by-product of this process. This means that, according to Yi Jin Jing teachings, the sequence of body development as per an internal model should be Qi first, then Huang; this is followed by the sinew channels (though the sinew channels are not explicitly mentioned in the Yi Jin Jing) and, finally, the tendons. This order of development is summarised in Figure 3.4.

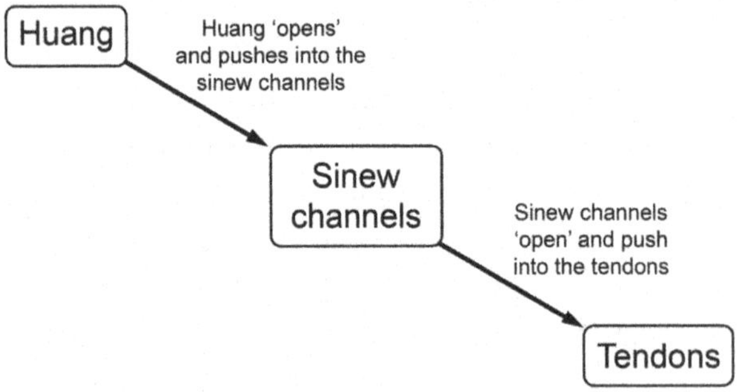

Figure 3.4: Qi, Huang, Sinew Channels and Tendons

If we look back to the original principles of the Yi Jin Jing that were listed earlier, we can see how this fits in with the Yi Jin Jing teachings:

- The secret to developing one's psychological and physical health is based in the Qi.
- We must cultivate the physical in line with the intangible, or there will be imbalance.

- The body must be built in the sequence of Qi, then Huang, then tendons.
- Qi is difficult to understand and build, and so is Huang, but one comes from the other. So, we build the Qi and allow the Huang to form in the right way; this will, in turn, start to develop the tendons.
- The Qi must mobilise; the result of this is the engagement of Huang. This will strengthen the Huang which serves as a platform for the development of health.
- One should keep developing the Qi until the Huang fully stretches and the tendons are strong.

The result of this is that the channels will open and the Qi will reach to every part of the body.

The only aspect that I have added here is the sinew channels. They sit between the Huang and the tendons in the process of development listed within the Yi Jin Jing. They were most likely not alluded to in the Yi Jin Jing because the idea of the sinew channels came later, from Chinese medical teachings. Within the Yi Jin Jing, they would have existed simply as an aspect of the Huang.

If you are confused by some of the theory above, then please do not worry. One of the greatest strengths of Daoism is that it very cleanly connects the theory and practices together as one unit. Theory alone, without practice, is nigh on useless in these arts, but if you go through the training in the correct manner, then you will experientially understand what I have written about. Feeling the teachings in your body is the key to really penetrating the tradition.

Errors in Yi Jin Jing Practice

A final note on the Yi Jin Jing before we move on should be to mention four common errors that it makes a great point of highlighting. These errors are to do with training one aspect of the human body to the exclusion of the others.

Muscle Strengthening

It was understood that the muscles of the body could not conduct Qi through them in a very efficient manner. Rather, it was viewed that muscles trapped Qi instead of letting it flow past. There were some martial Qi Gong schools that attempted to work with muscles to this end and deliberately trapped Qi within the body's muscles in order to make them grow. The problem with this was that when the muscles build, then constriction of Qi flow takes place; it is almost as though the channels are squeezed under the muscles' action.

It was said that building the body in this way, with an emphasis upon muscle growth, would make you strong whilst you were young, but would lead to health problems, including a kind of Qi sickness called San Gong (散功) or 'dispersal of skill', as you grew older. What this means is that, because the channels have not been built properly, your Qi will disperse over time, leading to a breaking down of the body and premature ageing. Muscle was understood to be likely to transform into fat at this stage, and general stagnation would occur.

Tendon Strengthening

It was understood that if the tendons were the focus of the practice, with no awareness of the Huang or Qi, then the inside of the body would become weak. In a similar manner to building solely the muscles, a 'tendon-focused' practitioner would experience health problems in later life. The first and foremost issue that would manifest would be a brittleness of the body, as Qi cannot 'soak' through to all of the right places. This would cause tendons to tear and snap in older age. For a tradition that placed so much importance upon longevity, it is obvious why this would be an issue.

Tendon-focused training of this type is prevalent in many schools of Chinese martial arts. Whilst studying in schools with this kind of practice, I noted that teachers would push the younger students into doing Qi Gong practice alongside these arts in order to help alleviate these kinds of issues.

Huang Strengthening

It was said that in those who only focused upon training the Huang and not the Qi nor the tendons, there would never be any 'stretch' inside. The movement of Qi through the Huang is needed to make them stretch and engage. External stretching will only ever pull the muscles, tendons and sinew channels; the internal body of the Huang will always remain relatively unmoved. The Huang requires the Qi to really stretch as it is engaged under its influence.

In arts that emphasise soft, internal movement, with lots of focus upon the fascia and being as snake-like as possible on the inside, there is likely to be a lack of development of strength. The Huang will not engage under the action of the Qi, and so the sinew channels and tendons will never be affected. This will result in physical weakness and, thus, is detrimental to health.

I have seen this error in some Qi Gong and many Taijiquan (太极拳) schools. They often try to be as soft as they can be, but without an awareness of the Yi Jin Jing process. The result is that they look like wet noodles when they move, and they essentially train themselves to become weaker. I always try to avoid letting my students go down this route. Softness must be built alongside Qi development, otherwise the Huang will slacken.

Qi Development

Probably the most prevalent error across the Qi Gong world is this one: working on circulating and building the Qi without any understanding of the Huang. Essentially, this is Qi Gong without the Yi Jin Jing being involved. Though this kind of practice is relaxing and could be excellent for those suffering with stress, it is going to lead to problems. According to the Yi Jin Jing teachings, this kind of practice will weaken the tendons and lead to only a weak level of Qi being moved through the body. Oftentimes, these kinds of schools end up relying on imagination-based work, as they have not found the key to actually developing the insides of the body in the right way.

I shall leave the Yi Jin Jing here for the time being. I often get questions about the Yi Jin Jing, as there is a great deal of confusion around the subject. Many people feel drawn to it as a practice, but don't know what the practice is. Some think that it is a specific set of movements, and some think it is a whole tradition in its own right. In fact *all* Qi Gong that adheres to authentic principles includes the Yi Jin Jing, as the methods were absorbed into the internal schools way back in history. If you practise Qi Gong in a traditional manner, you already practise the Yi Jin Jing. You should see this become clearer as we progress through the book and into the methods involved in Nei Gong training. For now, though, let us look at some of the components involved in the training: namely, the channel system and the Dan Tian.

What Is a Channel?

The Chinese model of the channel system is divided up into two main parts: the acquired channel system, which comprises the twelve channels related to the organs of the body, and the congenital channel system, which is often known as the 'eight extraordinary channels'. Generally, the twelve organ channels are involved in the health of the body, and medical Qi Gong systems tend to focus on this area of the energetic system. The congenital channels are needed for deeper change and transformative work.

Figure 3.5 shows the pathways of the twelve acquired channels.

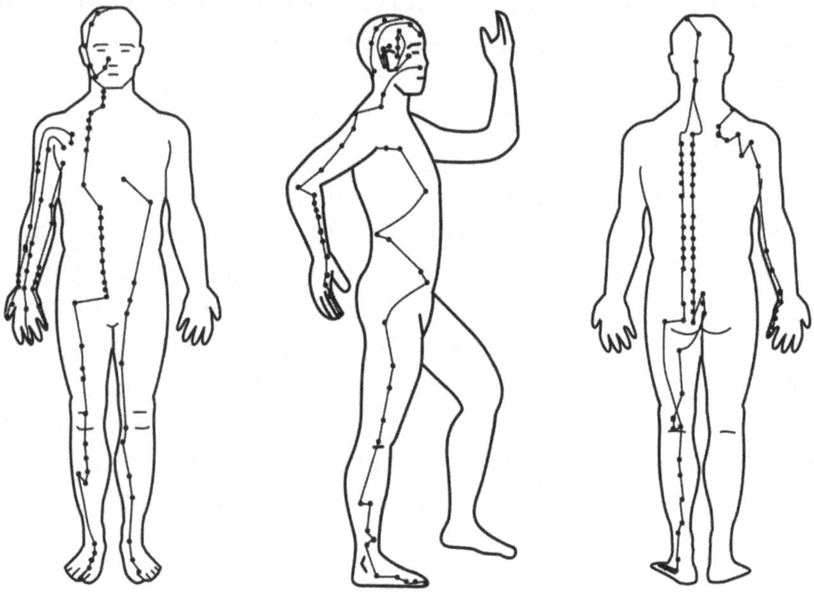

Figure 3.5: The Acquired Channel System

These twelve channels are related to the main organs of the body and they travel relatively close to the surface of the body. It is for this reason that they can easily be accessed through modalities such as acupuncture, where fine needles are inserted for therapeutic benefit along the channels' length. The branches depicted in Figure 3.5 travel primarily through the elasticated sinew channels of the body. As well as this, each of the acquired channels also has a deeper internal branch (not depicted) that travels away from the surface towards the centre of the body. These 'internal branches' run through the Huang of the body instead of the sinew channels, since the sinew channels do not travel inside the body; they run along the body's outer aspect instead.

Figure 3.6 shows the pathway of the eight congenital channels.

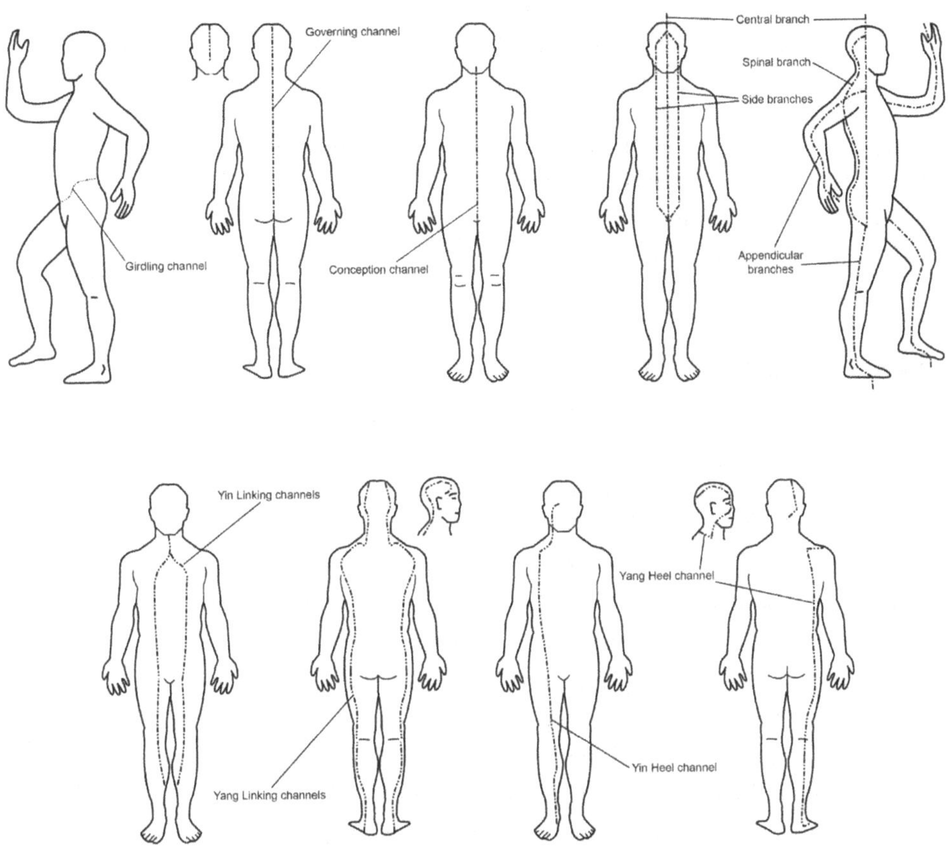

Figure 3.6: The Congenital Channel System

These eight channels run deeper than the twelve acquired channels, with a couple of minor exceptions. They travel primarily through the Huang region of the body and connect deep into the core of our being.

In essence, with Qi Gong exercises we are generally (but not always) attempting to move Qi along the length of the twelve acquired channels, whereas in Nei Gong practice we are aiming to influence the eight congenital channels. In this way, it is seen that the eight congenital channels are like deep oceans within the body. By working with them, we generate movement and a sense of 'overflowing', so that they then spill out into the acquired channels. In this way, the acquired channels are affected as a by-product of the congenital channel work.

The Huang or sinew channels (depending upon which channel or part of channel we are discussing) serve as a physical conductor for the flow of Qi along their length. The less blockages, adhesions and damage to the tissues of a channel, the more it conducts.

These channels each carry Qi, which is an expression of mind, along the channels' length. As discussed in the previous chapter, this is the prime mechanism behind the way in which our mental state starts to affect our physiology. The Qi that travels along the length of the channel is Yang Qi. At a later stage in the book, we will discuss exactly what this means, but for now it is enough to understand that Yang Qi is primarily an extension of the mind through a channel's length. It is a form of information that can often feel quite 'electrical' in nature when we experience it in our practice.

The Lung Channel

To understand what a channel is composed of, let us take one as an example. The Lung channel is generally the first channel you learn in Chinese medical studies, and it is fairly straightforward compared to some of the others, so let us look at it in more detail.

Figure 3.7 shows the pathway of the Lung channel along with the acupuncture points that exist along its length. Not depicted is the internal branch of the channel that travels through the middle of the body, connecting the organs of the large intestine and lungs together, before it emerges at the start of the channel pathway depicted in Figure 3.7. The branch depicted travels through the physical matter of the sinew channel, whilst the internal branch travels through the Huang of the torso.

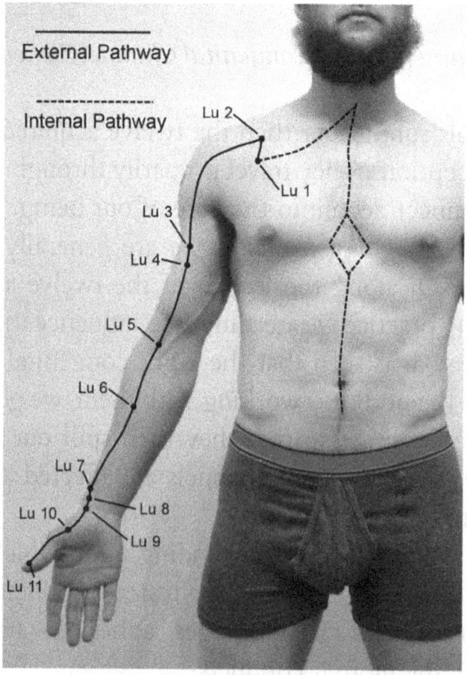

Figure 3.7: The Lung Channel and Its Points

The channel pathway originates on the lateral aspect of the chest in a soft depression just below the clavicle. It then travels along the anterior aspect of the arm and the border of the biceps muscle before continuing down the forearm to the wrist and over the thumb as shown. It concludes on the corner of the thumbnail.

Along its length are eleven 'points' which are regions of the channel that have been identified to have the strongest therapeutic effect when needled or manually stimulated.

Now, this is where there can be a little confusion. This confusion comes with the use of the words 'external' and 'internal'. Because of how we interpret the terms in the West, we understandably jump to the conclusion that it is somehow dependent upon 'depth' or physical location; this is actually not the case. The muscles are considered more 'external' than the sinew channels which, in comparison, are considered to be more 'internal' than the muscles. Confusingly though, the channel shown here actually runs through the sinew channel which travels through and on top of the muscle. The reason for this is that the comparative 'depths' of the tissues relate to their function and the mechanisms involved in their actions. The more 'internal' something is, the closer it is to being driven by the influence of Qi, irrespective of its physical location in the body.

The more we can relax the muscles and open up the length of the sinew channel, the more that Qi will effectively flow. This is summarised in Figure 3.8.

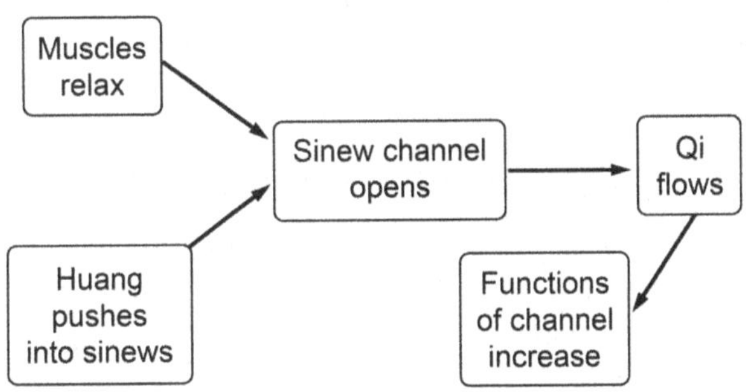

Figure 3.8: The Lung Channel Aspects

Each channel has a distinct role in the delivery of Qi along its length. This Qi then carries with it conscious information from the mind along the channel's length. As this information reaches certain points on the channel, it serves to carry out several important functions. If we look at the Lung channel as an example, we can see in Figure 3.7 that there are eleven points along its length. The Qi at each of the eleven points has the following qualities.

Zhong Fu (中府) (Lu 1) Central Storehouse

Here, the Qi from the Spleen channel converges with the Lung channel. At this point on the body, the health of the Lung channel receives its energetic nourishment. The Qi here is reaching up from deep within the Huang to connect with the Lung channel's origin on the sinew channel pathway.

Yun Men (雲門) (Lu 2) Cloud Gate

The 'cloud' within the name of this point is a reference to the ethereal energy of consciousness. It is here that the Qi of consciousness moves into the channel pathway to begin its descent along the length of the arm. As a point, it can be stimulated to cause a strong reaction within the mind. Because of the Lung's connection to the element of Metal and the emotion of loss, this point will stimulate a person to begin the grieving process if this is something that they need to do.

Tian Fu (天府) (Lu 3) Mansion of Heaven

The use of the term 'Heaven' within this point's name once again likens the Qi here to the ethereal qualities of consciousness. The Qi from the previous point has now travelled down the arm to the anterior aspect of the shoulder. The information from the point can be used as a continuation of the previous point's functioning. If a person cannot begin to grieve or cope with a loss because they are emotionally numb, then this point will help to dissolve the feelings of numbness and bring feeling back to their mind.

Xia Bai (俠白) (Lu 4) Protecting the White

Whereas the previous two points initiated the process of grieving for somebody, this point is a little further down the line. It helps a person to start the emotional recovery process that needs to begin after grieving has ended.

Chi Ze (尺澤) (Lu 5) Large Marsh

A marsh is a boggy place where stagnation is rife. The name of the point indicates that this is the main quality of the Qi here. The Qi has travelled through the previous four points of the channel and now starts to become a little denser. It can stagnate at this point and often becomes stuck. If a person cannot 'let go' of something that is causing them to feel grief, then this point is useful. It also helps to alleviate general stagnation of the Lung channel itself.

Kong Zui (孔最) (Lu 6) Maximum Space

The large depression here is another 'sticking point' for stagnation. The point can be stimulated to nourish and move stuck Qi and Blood in the length of the channel as well as being helpful in moving stuck emotional debris out of the channel's length once more.

Lie Que (列缺) (Lu 7) Imperfect Sequence

If the Lung channel is about processing grief, then the Large Intestine channel is about 'letting go'. It is like a waste disposal chute for the Lung channel. It is here, at this point, that the two channels communicate, and the functions of the Lung channel relating to opening the pores of the body can be accessed, so it is said that this point opens the exterior of the body. Hence, this point can be utilised to let off pressure within the channel and allow the Lungs to relax and the Lung Qi to smoothly descend within the body.

Jing Qu (經渠) (Lu 8) River Ditch

The final sticking point of the channel with regard to emotional debris lies at this point. The name of the point illustrates that it is like a river that has become a ditch. This gives an indication of the level of stagnation that can build up here.

Tai Yuan (太淵) (Lu 9) Great Abyss

This point connects into the deepest reserves of the channel's Qi. The Qi here is dense, very close to the level of our Jing or 'essence' rather than the other end of the scale, the consciousness. It is a strongly nourishing point for the channel.

Yu Ji (魚際) (Lu 10) Fish Border

This point is near the end of the channel. It can help to vent energetic heat and other pathogenic residues from the channel.

Gui Xin (鬼信) (Lu 11) Ghosts Sincerity

The final point causes an opening effect along the length of the sinew channel. The Qi is very faint here, but the connection to the elasticated line of the sinews is strong. Having a needle inserted here, near the bed of your thumbnail, is not always the most pleasant experience, but it is very helpful for moving any stagnation in the channel pathway.

The Channel as a Process

What I am trying to show, from the example of the Lung channel used above, is that each of the channels has a series of processes involved in it. The points of the channel are not isolated entities; they are parts of an ongoing relationship that is dictated by the process that the Qi goes through as it moves along the channel's length. Figure 3.9 sums up the various developing processes inherent within the Lung channel so it is clearer to see.

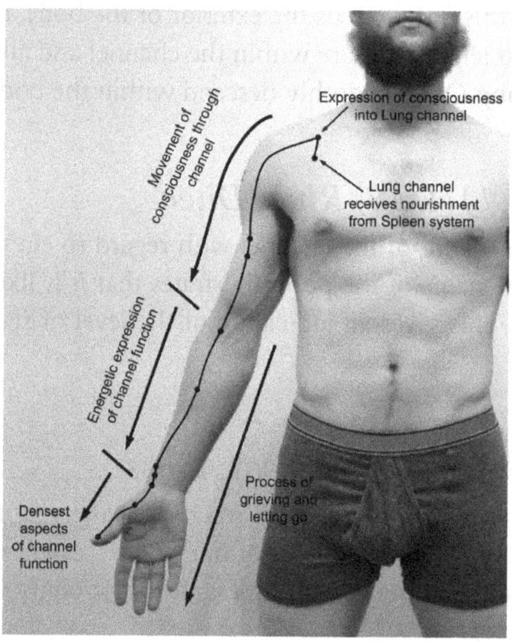

Figure 3.9: The Process of the Lung Channel

There are many other functions of the Lung channel and the points along its length. A skilled Chinese medical practitioner can use these points in a variety of ways to help a patient back to health. I have only focused on some very specific functions for the channel to help you see how the channels work. They extend out of the mind and help the Qi carry out a series of processes and instructions for the body. They are like the circuitry in a machine that carries vital electrical impulses: impulses that ensure each part of the machine is functioning properly.

These channels can become blocked through physical trauma, illness or, most relevant to Nei Gong practice, disharmony within the emotions.

I have used the Lung channel as an example, but Table 3.2 shows the key emotional processes carried out by each of the twelve acquired channels.

Table 3.2: Channels and Emotional Processes

Channel	Psychological process governed by channel pathway
Lung	Processing of grief and any sense of loss
Large Intestine	Letting go and allowing yourself to move on
Stomach	Digesting ideas, problems and life challenges
Spleen	Absorbing new information and life lessons
Heart	Processing heartache and intimate experiences
Small Intestine	Understanding your own sense of 'right and wrong'
Bladder	Having self-esteem in the face of difficulty
Kidneys	Moving effectively along your life path
Pericardium	An extra layer of protection for the Heart
Triple Heater	Effectively and healthily forming social relations
Gall Bladder	Making the right decisions
Liver	Having a dream, plan or life goal and seeing it through

If we have difficulties in these regions of our lives or emotional issues connected to these organ systems, then it can cause the Qi within the channel system to become blocked. At the same time, damage to the channel can cause these aspects of our psychological lives to become adversely affected.

On top of this, there is also the obvious detriment to the area of the body through which the channel pathway runs, as well as to the associated organs and tissues. I have highlighted the psychological qualities of the channel here, though, as it is generally these things which students will notice first when they enter into Nei Gong training and the channels open up. Large changes to their nature and emotional outlook on life can come as the acquired channel system starts to free itself up and Qi moves unrestrictedly along the channel's length. It is for this reason that many students start Nei Gong practice and then, seemingly out of the blue, make large changes to their lives and careers. These changes are often taking place simply because their mind is moving into a more centred place; consequently, they can see that changes need to be made in order for them to be more fulfilled in their lives. This all goes back to the nine palaces we looked at in Chapter 2.

The Congenital Cage

The congenital components of the energetic system include the eight congenital channels and the three Dan Tian. The congenital channels form a kind of 'energetic cage' within the body, as shown in Figure 3.10.

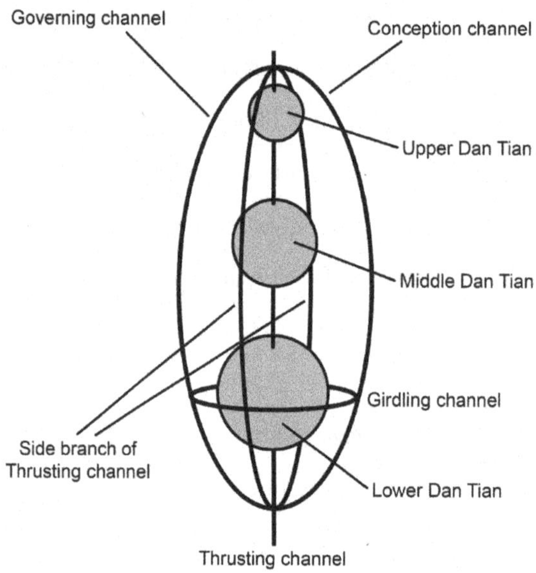

Figure 3.10: The Congenital Cage of Channels

The congenital channels tend to run deep within the body, with the exception of the Governing and Conception channels. They are also not directly related to any of the organs, as is the case with the acquired channels. It is not classically said, but in my own personal opinion, the Governing and Conception channels may, once again, be exceptions to the norm, as I would personally say that the Governing channel is the 'Brain channel' and the Conception channel relates to the Uterus in women.

Within Nei Gong, we are primarily working with energetic flow and circulation within the eight key channels of the congenital meridian system. It is through these channels that we learn to direct information utilising the motivating power of the Dan Tian, and this is, in part, what separates Nei Gong from many systems of Qi Gong.

Daoist theory states that, whilst in the womb, we operate energetically according to the function of the congenital channels. Through these pathways circulate the three key internal substances of Jing, Qi and Shen. The conversion process is twofold, first generating the potential for physical manifestation of a body, and, second, setting in place the physical anchor of human consciousness. All of this is largely motivated by the rotation of the lower Dan Tian which is revolving steadily to generate the necessary power to create human life.

After we are born, we begin to use the congenital channels to a lesser degree. Instead, the acquired channels become active and our health and development is controlled by the relationship of the organs of the body. The lower Dan Tian naturally begins to slow down its rotation, and by the time we are in our early teens, it is hardly moving at all.

As the lower Dan Tian awakens, it begins to start the various microcosmic orbits of Qi circulation which are pretty well known within Daoist esoteric literature. Commonly, you will see writings on only one circulation of Qi, the rotation which moves up the centre of a person's back through the Governing channel and then down the front of the body through the Conception channel. This is the circulation shown in Figure 3.11.

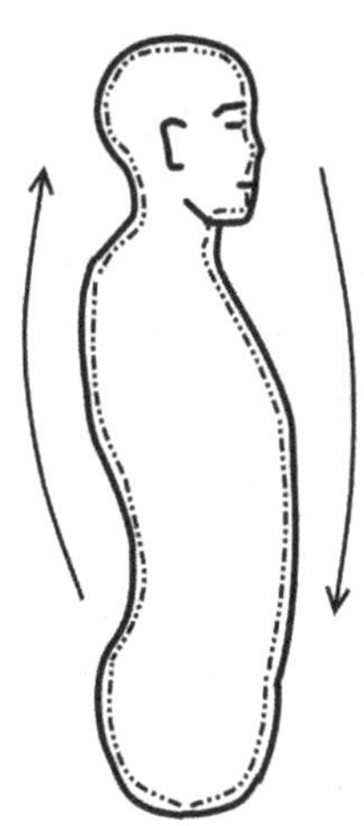

Figure 3.11: The First Microcosmic Orbit of Qi

The first microcosmic orbit of Qi takes place along the length of the Governing channel and then down through the Conception channel. This is the initial rotation which we must achieve if we wish to progress safely and efficiently in our Nei Gong training. It is primarily driven through the initial awakening of the lower Dan Tian.

Whilst it is true that this movement of Qi is very important, there are also other key circulations that need to take place. These are described below.

Women need to understand the nature of the reverse cycle of the initial rotation. This cycle is required in order to extract essence from the menstrual Blood and draw it up towards the chest region where it nourishes the breasts and Heart centre. This rotation is rarely discussed for women who practise the internal arts to any level beyond the basics, but it is essential in their development. This directional flow is not really very important for men and rarely impacts upon their practice.

A second rotation then needs to take place around the length of the Girdling channel which sits around the waist like a belt.

A third rotation needs to take place within the torso between the two side branches of the Thrusting channel. This serves to balance the Qi of the Liver and Stomach. If these two organs are in harmony with one another, then the energy of the body will circulate smoothly.

Further movements generated by these rotations then circulate energy along the length of the arms and legs via extending branches of the Thrusting channel.

Consolidation of this 'cage' is required in order to work effectively with the three Dan Tian and guarantee smooth progression into the deeper stages of Nei Gong training. As a teacher and Chinese medical practitioner, I have met many practitioners from different Nei Gong schools who have developed imbalances through their training. These imbalances have varied between mildly uncomfortable through to completely debilitating. In many cases, these issues developed as the practitioners did not work effectively with the various rotations of Qi listed above. The result of this is that blockages will occur within the body. Blockages occurring deep within the congenital energy body like this will always lead to the development of problems, and in many cases they can be very challenging to correct. For this reason, I always urge practitioners to make sure they fully understand the training and the function of these circulations. Ideally, you should work with an experienced teacher to ensure that these rotations are successfully opened up before moving further into energy work. Please do not underestimate the importance of opening these channels.

We work with these channels in the same way as all other channels within the body, according to the teachings of the Yi Jin Jing. First, we move Qi along their length. This will always be possible as there is always a certain degree of 'openness' in everybody's channels. It might not be enough for going beyond the foundation stages, but it is enough to get things going. We then start to purge these channels to help improve various aspects of our health. Once this is done, then we work the Qi and the body in very specific ways to help the Huang aspect of the channels grow stronger and more defined.

The Congenital Channels

The Governing and Conception Channels

These two energetic pathways form a linked orbit along the centre front and back lines of the body. Essentially, they could be seen to be one channel in charge of regulating the flow of Yin and Yang information throughout the acquired energy body. This happens as, over the course of a day, the circulation of Qi through these channels causes more Qi to be distributed into the twelve acquired meridians. Figure 3.12 shows these two channels.

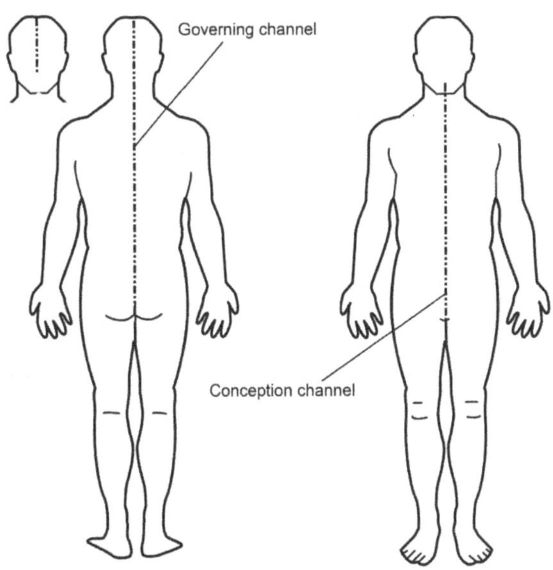

Figure 3.12: The Governing and Conception Channels

Within Nei Gong practice, we use these channels for various reasons. The first goal of our practice is to free them up from any blockages which may exist along their length and increase the efficiency of energy flow. This energy flow should move unimpeded as a circular rotation of information throughout the body. This initially increases the amount of energy and movement within the twelve acquired meridians, which has the advantage of improving our health. On top of this, it is these channels which we will use in our practice to serve as a kind of energetic 'safety net'. Its job is to ensure that any energetic transformation which takes place in an upwards direction has the space to flow downwards again. Without this orbit, any alchemical transformation could be risky. If too much pressure is built up anywhere, then there will be no route for this pressure to escape and sink back downwards again. Many practitioners of the internal arts have fallen foul of energetically based disease through not successfully opening this circulation.

We will revisit these channels in great detail in Chapter 8 when we look at the circulation of Qi that takes place along their length.

The Thrusting Channel

The Thrusting channel is a complex channel that has a number of pathways. As well as the commonly known branch that runs through the centre of the spine, there is also a vertically aligned branch that runs through the core of the body. To either side of this are two side branches which run through the middle of the torso, and then finally there are deep internal branches that travel through the middle of the arms and legs. Figure 3.13 shows the various pathways of the Thrusting channel. Note that the appendicular branches are bilateral.

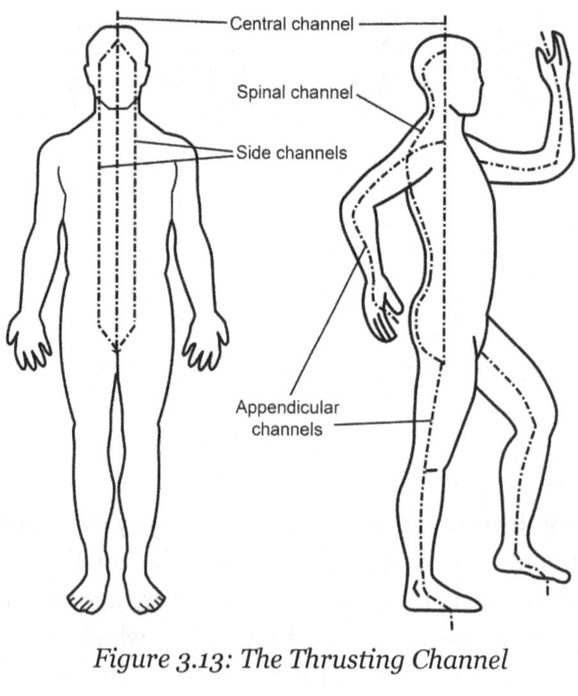

Figure 3.13: The Thrusting Channel

The Thrusting channel is the key channel through which a great deal of energetic transformation takes place. This happens as the conversion of Jing, Qi and Shen is initiated by correct work with the three Dan Tian during Nei Gong practice. It is also the key channel which connects a practitioner into the higher spiritual realms once they have reached advanced stages in their training. It resides deep within the Huang of the body and is known as the most challenging of the channels to fully open. There has to be a very high level of conscious absorption to reach this channel effectively.

The Girdling Channel

The only channel to travel horizontally through the body is the Girdling meridian. It encircles the waist like a belt and dips down slightly on the front of the body as shown in Figure 3.14.

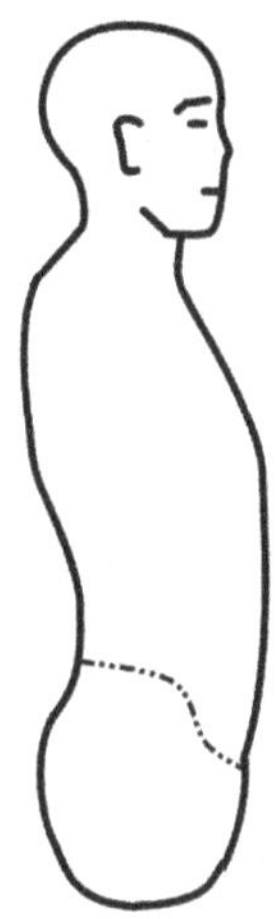

Figure 3.14: The Girdling Channel

This channel is, in part, responsible for the correct direction of rotation for the lower Dan Tian when it is left in a 'neutral' state. The combination of the rising of energy along the Governing channel and the dipping down of the Girdling channel at the front of the body encourages a vertical roll of the Dan Tian which moves Qi into the base of the spine. The horizontal pathway of the Girdling channel then creates a second directional force which stabilises the lower Dan Tian, forming a kind of energetic gyroscope within the lower abdomen.

Every channel also has a function closely related to the psyche; in the case of the Girdling channel, it helps to govern our sense of direction in life.

When it opens up, a sort of psychological 'compass' can be found: a compass that helps us to know what exactly we are supposed to be doing at any given moment.

The Yin and Yang Linking Channels

These meridians run along the length of the body, as shown in Figure 3.15. They serve to connect together all of the Yin and Yang acquired channels of the body.

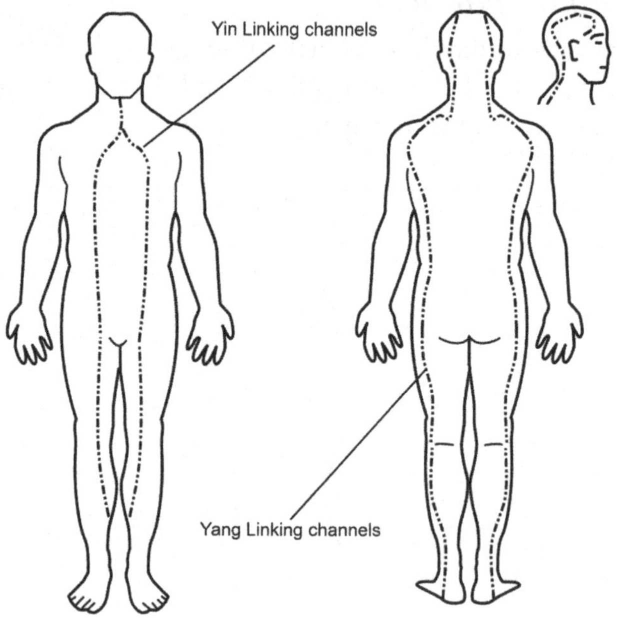

Figure 3.15: Yin and Yang Linking Channels

These channels ensure that any excesses or deficiencies within the acquired meridians are equalised/evened out. If there is any excess energy left after this redistribution, the Yin and Yang Linking channels will help to send this energy back towards the congenital energy body where it is stored. These channels are not used so much within Nei Gong practice but are included here for the sake of completion.

The Yin and Yang Heel Channels

Also included here for reasons of completeness are the Yin and Yang Heel channels; they are shown in Figure 3.16.

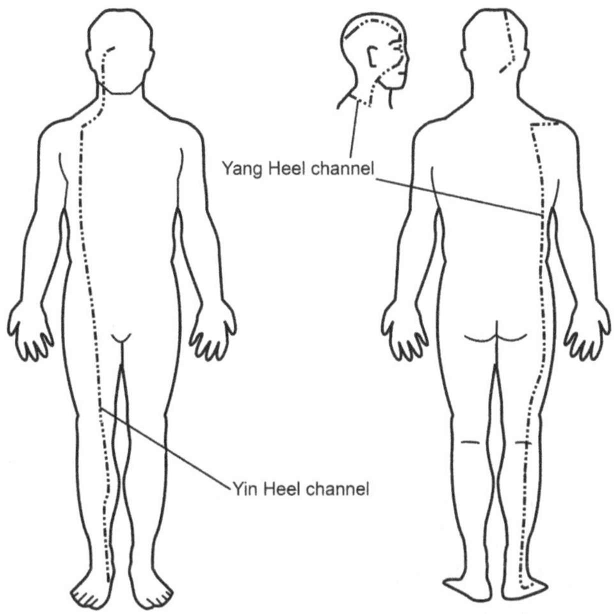

Figure 3.16: The Yin and Yang Heel Channels

These channels can be thought of something akin to an earth wire in an electrical circuit. They ensure that if any sudden excess occurs within the body, it has the ability to drop down towards the planet. These channels will open naturally of their own accord during training and are not focused on to any great degree within this system of Nei Gong training.

The Energetic Cage and the Five Pulses

The channels of the congenital energy body connect together to form a kind of energetic cage as discussed earlier. This cage is where all of the rotations of orbiting energy take place during Nei Gong practice. Within the centre of this cage are five pulses of congenital energy which are rarely discussed but clear to feel by anybody who has moved beyond the foundation stages of their internal practice. These five pulses are different movements of information which correspond to the five elemental movements of Daoism. They work together as a cycle to generate the basis for our emotional and energetic health. As we open up the various circulations of the energetic cage, it becomes much easier to regulate the five pulses. Table 3.3 summarises the nature of the five congenital pulses.

Table 3.3: The Five Congenital Pulses

Element	Movement	Effects
Fire	Expansion	Generates warmth and nourishment
Earth	Division	Generates change and evolution
Metal	Contraction	Generates stability and connection
Water	Cycling	Generates life and growth
Wood	Driving	Generates power and planning

There is little direct work to do with these five pulses, but you can expect to connect with and feel them during your practice. At these times, there will be clear and tangible sensations of these five directional energies moving through your body. As this happens, there are shifts starting to take place within the energy body, shifts which will then have an effect upon the health of your body and organs.

The Dan Tian

The three Dan Tian sit within the core of the body and are connected together via the vertical branch of the Thrusting channel. They are spherical fields of information which vary from person to person in their degree of consolidation. In the vast majority of beginners, you could say that the Dan Tian are there but have the potential be a great deal more powerful. This strengthening process generally takes place as the practitioner's awareness interacts with the energy within the vicinity of the Dan Tian. The mind begins to reinforce the strength of the information field, and so the function of the Dan Tian becomes stronger.

What is often missed by practitioners of Qi Gong is that the Dan Tian also have clear physiological components to them. In the early stages of building and working with the Dan Tian, you are unlikely to encounter the physical side of the process, but at the more advanced stages of practice, this will become clear. The physical side of the Dan Tian exists because, as with the channels, the Qi within that region of the body conducts its way through the Huang. In order to fully build the Dan Tian and turn it into a 'container' and not just a 'driving force', we need to locate and develop the Huang of this region of the body.

The key role of the Dan Tian is to convert each of our energetic substances either up or down. This takes place as the Dan Tian are conversion centres for vibrational states. This conversion happens as the hollow centre of each Dan Tian receives one of the three key energetic substances before transforming it into the next. This conversion process is shown in Figure 3.17.

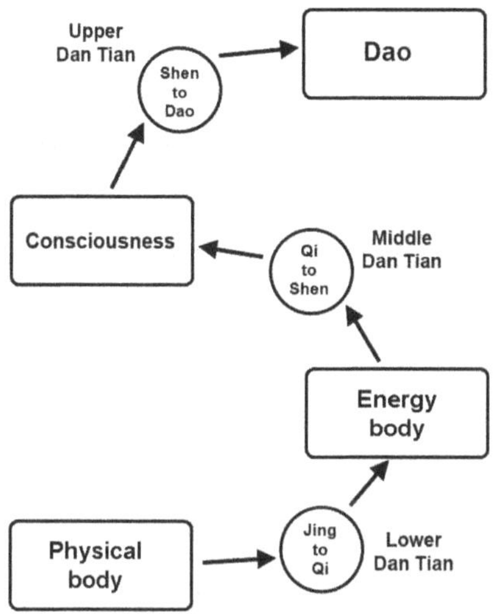

Figure 3.17: Conversion Through the Dan Tian

A lot of work within Nei Gong practice is aimed at cultivating the Dan Tian. They are the key to our practice. There are a number of important principles involved in Dan Tian work, and we shall look at these at each relevant step within this book.

The Lower Dan Tian

The lower Dan Tian serves as our main driving force for Qi throughout the rest of our body. Though it does not build Qi, as many people mistakenly believe, it does drive Qi through the body. It sits within the lower abdomen, below the navel and in line with the vertical branch of the Thrusting channel. Within Nei Gong training, our initial task is to awaken this energy centre, and this is largely accomplished through aiming for a smooth and steady rotation. The lower Dan Tian is in charge of driving energy as well as the conversion of Jing to Qi; as such, it is the energy centre most responsible for dealing with the denser aspects of the energy body. It is generally the simplest to connect with and the focal point for the majority of the foundation stages of Nei Gong.

As with almost all aspects of the Nei Gong process, the lower Dan Tian is developed in a series of stages. These stages are almost always worked through in a clear, linear fashion. There will be a great deal more writing on the lower Dan Tian within the later chapters of this book, but in brief, these are the various stages of development with the lower Dan Tian according to Nei Gong teachings:

1. Locate the lower Dan Tian
2. Combine the three 'initiatory elements' in the lower Dan Tian
3. Consolidate the Jing
4. Rotate the lower Dan Tian
5. Generate the sphere
6. Connect the Dan Tian to the exterior
7. Build the container
8. Develop the centre of the 'gourd shape'
9. Build the Yang Qi
10. Fill the Dan Tian

Some of these stages are foundation stages, whilst others are very advanced and only very few reach these levels in their practice. The trick to managing success at any of these stages is simply making sure that the prior stage has been practised to a high enough stage. Generally, within these arts, if the foundation is solid, then you will find that the body will know when to move on and you will be led naturally into the next stage.

The Middle Dan Tian

The middle Dan Tian sits within the centre of the chest at the height of the Heart. For this reason, it is often known as the Heart centre. The middle Dan Tian is the location for conversion of Qi into Shen, the spiritual energy which governs all aspects of mind from the most mundane thought through to divine comprehension. It is the energy centre most closely connected to our emotions, and this is why the heart has so often been linked to the emotional mind within almost every culture.

It is here, at the height of the middle Dan Tian, that most of our Qi is said within the classics to 'leak'. This happens through the process of excessive emotions. This process is shown in Figure 3.18.

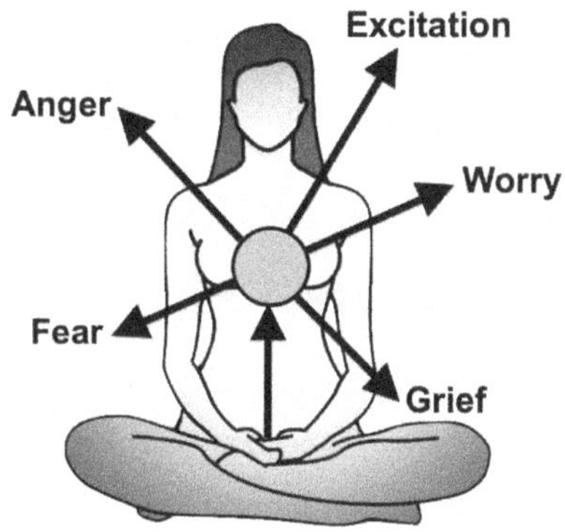

Figure 3.18: The Leakage of Emotional Energy

The emotions cause a great deal of Qi to leak away from the middle Dan Tian. What remains is only enough to empower the strength of the intellect. In order to move towards heightened states of realisation, a practitioner needs to build enough internal energy to strengthen the deeper aspects of human consciousness. This is the way towards connection with Dao and the reason why so much importance is placed upon centring the emotions within the majority of Eastern traditions. The stiller the 'Heart' can be made, the less Qi is lost through it, and thus the more energy is left to feed the process of spiritual elevation. This is all a part of the energetic expression of the five thieves we discussed in Chapter 2.

The Upper Dan Tian

The upper Dan Tian sits within the middle of the skull. It has an exit point which extends outwards to between the eyebrows – a point which corresponds to the concept of the 'third eye'. The upper Dan Tian is the conversion point of Shen into emptiness and the seat of all of the higher-level attainments within the Daoist tradition. There are some direct exercises with the upper Dan Tian, but on the whole, any cultivation here should be as an extension of the lower and middle Dan Tian developmental processes.

Chapter 4

PREPARING THE BODY

The foundations of any art form are, without a doubt, its most important aspect. If we try to build upon poor foundations, then everything we do will eventually collapse. There is often a temptation for newcomers to Nei Gong to try to jump ahead to the more energetic aspects of the practice. The discussion of such elements as Qi, spirit and abilities that can be gained from the practice is often a great draw for people, and this can be counterproductive. Whilst it is true that Nei Gong training becomes very esoteric and fascinating at later stages, we should attempt to put this kind of information out of our head. What is most important is that we focus on the stages of practice relevant to where we are. If we do not build the foundations correctly, then we will hit a glass ceiling in our development. I have seen this mistake time and time again in arts like Qi Gong and Taijiquan. Always know how the foundations of the practice work and revisit them regularly to make sure that your 'base' is solid.

The foundations of the training are built in the physical body. In the previous chapter, we looked at the Yi Jin Jing and several components which we need to work with. Now we need to understand how to initiate this process. The systematic process of Nei Gong development always works in the sequence shown in Figure 4.1. These are the logical stages of progress.

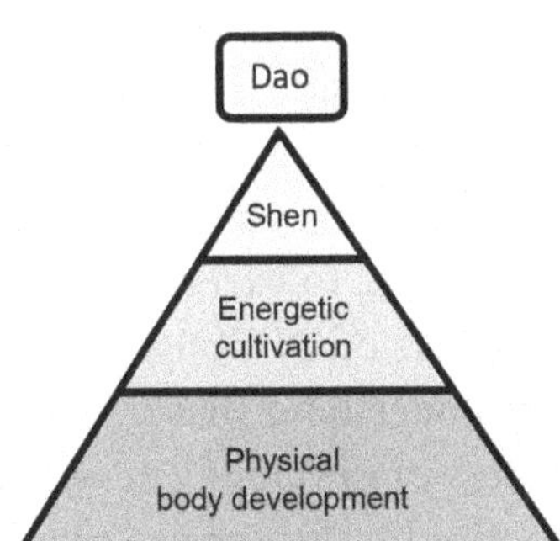

Figure 4.1: Stages of Development in Nei Gong

As you can see, the foundation of the practice is built in the physical body. Our body is our workshop, it is here that we need to carry out our practice. In order for there to be efficient results, we need to ensure that we have built the body in the correct manner. From here, we move onto the energetic system and the circulation of Qi through the channel system. There is obviously a certain degree of crossover between these two stages as they both affect each other during the training, but our emphasis of practice should shift between these two stages as time goes on.

The natural effects of the energetic aspects of the art are that they begin to spill over into the stage of developing the consciousness. These are the alchemical stages of developing the spirit that Nei Gong can lead us towards. What can be done with this level of development is then up to us. There are many roads that Nei Gong can lead down, from medical practice through to martial arts or into the more meditative aspects of the tradition. Nei Gong is the inherent, internal vehicle at the heart of all of these arts; in which direction individual people wish to take their practice is up to them.

Stretching and Strengthening the Body

As was discussed previously, building the physical body for internal training does not follow the same pattern as 'bodybuilding' as we generally understand it in the West. If we create too much chronic tension within our muscles, then it will essentially block the flow of Qi and prevent us from 'finding our insides'. We wish for the muscles to be relaxed and lengthened so that they do not get in the way of developing the channels.

This being said, there does, however, need to be a certain degree of strength. If we are too weak, then we will not be able to support our body in the correct way. In my experience, few people suffer from this lack of strength when they come to class, with the exception of their core muscles and their legs. Many people could do with some extra work building physical power in these areas. For this reason, I often advise new students to take up an additional form of exercise alongside their Nei Gong practice in the early stages if they lack this strength. These should be forms of exercise such as hill-walking, cycling or swimming. Activities like this will build a little strength into the body but not lead to excessive contraction of the muscles.

I am aware that many teachers of Qi Gong will disagree with me on this, but it really is important to understand that health and fitness are not the same thing. Health is a process of development we can accomplish through Qi Gong or Nei Gong practice but fitness most certainly isn't. You can be incredibly healthy, but if you lack a basic level of fitness, then you have another kind of imbalance that needs tackling. For myself, I have a practice of martial arts alongside my Nei Gong training, and this does the job just fine, but if you lack any kind of exercise in your life, then consider one of the activities I have previously mentioned.

Avoid anything that leads to contractive tension in the body, such as weight-lifting or anything with excessive resistance-type work. It is these kinds of activities that will get in the way of your internal development. If you absolutely must do some resistance work (some people seem to need it in their lives), then use your own bodyweight instead of heavy objects as this is less detrimental. The avoidance of contractive-type exercises is especially important at the beginning of your training whilst you are building the foundations. Once the physical body has been built in the right way and you have entered deep into the energetic processes of Nei Gong, then this is not so important any more. It is really at the beginning of your practice, whilst you are building the physical foundations, that you need to avoid developing any extra tension in your body.

Figure 4.2 shows how to understand the right level of 'strengthening' for Nei Gong practice.

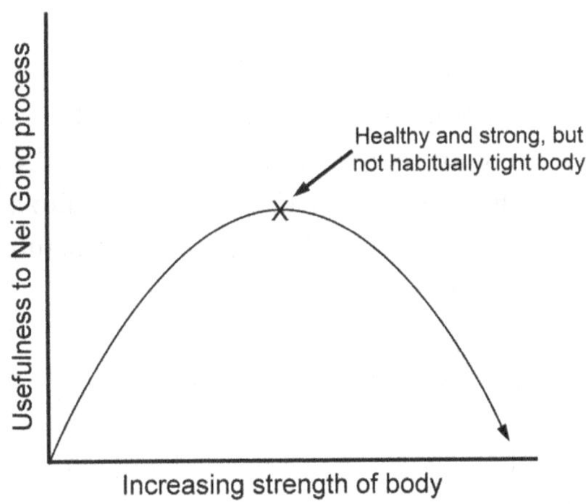

Figure 4.2: How Much Strengthening?

Remember that it is only a healthy level of strength that we require, we don't need to build muscle mass; Chinese arts are more focused on 'tendon strength' as a result of any exercise we carry out. The strength we need is to help us be able to stand comfortably for protracted periods of time and to carry out the various exercises without becoming fatigued.

We also have the question of flexibility. How much physical flexibility do we need for Nei Gong training? The answer is that we do need a fair bit of flexibility, especially in the hips and back. We need to lengthen out all of the muscles around this region of the body so that we can more easily relax them. I was told very early on in my training that 'we can only relax if we stretch, and we can only stretch if we relax'.

In my experience of teaching Nei Gong to many people around the world, it is the stretching that is the 'hard sell'. Many people have a great deal of resistance to this aspect of bodywork within the Qi Gong world. I was shocked to find that many people actually started Qi Gong as they thought it would be an easy alternative to Yoga!

The good news is, though, that we don't need the hyper-flexible acrobatics we so often see in Yoga practitioners today. We simply need to return the body to a level of flexibility that most of us naturally had when we were younger. A regular and simple stretching routine practised daily will help you with this. Some forward bends, some hip mobilisations and a basic floor-work stretching routine will help us open up the body on a physical level in a relatively short space of time.

It is a simple tenet of Daoism that 'We are born soft and pliable, and we die stiff and brittle; therefore, to be soft and pliable is the way of life.'

It is beyond the scope of this book to go into specific stretching routines; stretching the body is quite a big subject. Attending some local Yoga classes for beginners will help you find some basic routines; remember that you don't need to be able to distort your body all over the place; we just need to know how to carry out some simple stretching routines. As with anything in life, it is all about balance. If we overstretch the body into a hyper-flexible state, it actually begins to 'disconnect' our physical structure. If we are on the other end of the scale and we cannot even touch our toes when stood up, then we need to increase our flexibility.

The body will change rather rapidly if you simply adopt a daily stretching routine alongside your Nei Gong training. This is because the stretching practice will lengthen the muscles, and the Nei Gong will help you relax. It is the combination of relaxation and stretching that will open up your body.

Hanging the Muscles

A key phrase that sums up what we are trying to achieve with our muscles is that they should be 'hung' from our bones. Whilst this is obviously not 100 per cent literal – there are small stabilising muscles all over the body – it does give the feel for what we are after. We can basically divide our body up into two main types of muscles: stabiliser muscles and those that generate action. The stabiliser muscles are small, deeply placed groups of muscles that are not used much for developing power – in fact they lack the capability for this; instead, they support the body's structure and help hold our alignments in place. The muscles that generate our movements and actions are the larger muscles that generally (but not always) sit on top of the stabilisers.

The problem is that most people do not have a clear distinction with regards to usage of these two groups of muscles. If you were to think of them as cables and strands through the body, they would essentially be tangled up. This means that some of the stabilising muscles are now being used to generate action and vice versa. The result of this is a lot of tension. As we shall see later, tension prevents you from relaxing your mass to the floor.

One of our earliest missions is to divide up these two types of muscles so that they can each perform their job efficiently. This is generally carried out through standing posture practice within the internal arts. The stabilising muscles will build in the right way, and as we 'hang the muscles from the bones', there will begin a process of 'unbinding' these two muscle groups so that the cables are no longer tangled within the body. When we say 'hang the muscles', we are referring to those muscles involved in carrying out movements and actions.

In Nei Gong training for the body, we align the body in such a way that it can physically relax. Our mass is transferred through to the floor, meaning that it does not 'catch' in the muscles on its way down to the floor. If the body can be relaxed in this way, then the muscles will begin to feel as though they hang from the bones. If they can 'hang' in this way, then they will elongate under the influence of gravity. The more relaxed and elongated the muscles can become, the less they will get in the way of the internal process.

This is absolutely key: the more the muscles contract, the more they stop you from 'finding your insides'. A lot of the alignment principles that you learn at the beginning of your practice are designed to keep your weight off the muscles so that they can relax and lengthen. The more they relax, the more the insides of your body open up.

The Wuji Posture

The first posture to become used to when beginning your journey into Nei Gong is the Wuji posture. This is the standing posture shown in Figure 4.3. It looks simple enough, but it can be surprisingly challenging to get the hang of.

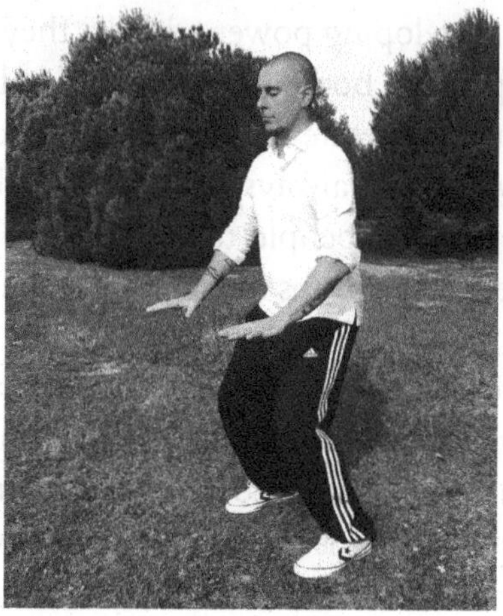

Figure 4.3: The Wuji Posture

As discussed previously, Wuji can be translated as 'without projections'; it is a posture that serves as the foundation of our practice, and indeed all systems of Qi Gong should – and generally do – have their own version of the Wuji posture. The Wuji posture should sit at the core of a Qi Gong system, as shown in Figure 4.4. Understanding the nature of Wuji and how it gives birth to the rest of a system is of key importance for our understanding.

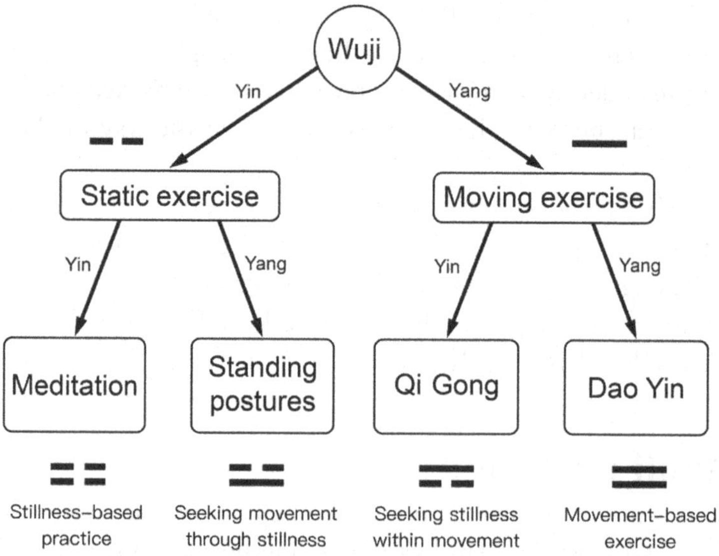

Figure 4.4: Wuji and the Qi Gong System

The reason that Wuji is so important is that it contains the alignment and internal principle 'blueprints' for everything that we do. From the stillness of Wuji are born the movements. The alignments and principles we study in Wuji standing practice should be carried through into all of the other exercises we use; in this way, we could argue that everything we do in a system of Qi Gong practice is nothing more than an extension and abstraction of Wuji's methods. I want to make this clear as it is an error in any practice of Qi Gong to not understand that Wuji is the key. Know your system's Wuji, and you know your system. This is why all systems of practice should really begin with standing practice, not moving Qi Gong exercises.

Learning to Align the Body

The first thing we need to look at is how to align the body correctly for our practice. This kind of alignment work is practised initially through Wuji postural training. The basic alignment principles we need to become familiar with are as follows:

- Correct placement of the feet
- Alignment of the knees
- Usage of the Kua (胯)
- Alignment of the pelvis and lower back
- Lengthening the spine
- Touching the shoulders to the feet
- Sinking the elbows
- Alignment of the head and neck
- Sinking the chest
- Sinking the tailbone
- Opening the sinews

These are the key body alignments that I focus on with beginners. There may be a little variation in this, but in the majority of cases I go through the list in this specific sequence as well. The order of applying these principles into the body has been developed over a decade of teaching large numbers of people. I have seen over time that if the alignments are worked through in this sequence, then they can be developed to an efficient level over a relatively short period of time.

These alignments go through two key stages: the stage of Fa and the stage of Gong. The stage of Fa, or technique, means that you are still actively applying the techniques to your practice. At this stage, you still need to 'make' your body have these alignments in place. This is normal for a very long time in your training. As soon as we drop into our Wuji practice, we go through our checklist and make sure we have these alignments in place.

When we have attained Gong, we have these postural principles inherently built into our body already. At this stage, it is almost impossible to be out of alignment any more since we have built our practice into our body. In this way, our practice has built a Gong, or quality, into it that is at an instinctive level.

Only when we have attained Gong through our practice will we hit the right level in our practice. It is here that the Huang will start to open up, and we will start to engage with the Yi Jin Jing practice that was discussed in the previous chapter.

Let us now look at each of these principles one at a time.

The Nature of the Feet

The feet are our connection to the planet during standing practice. This becomes particularly important for initiating the earliest stages of the Nei Gong process. In understanding the feet, we really need to look at them as having three distinct regions: the front of the feet, the middle and the heel. These three regions are shown in Figure 4.5.

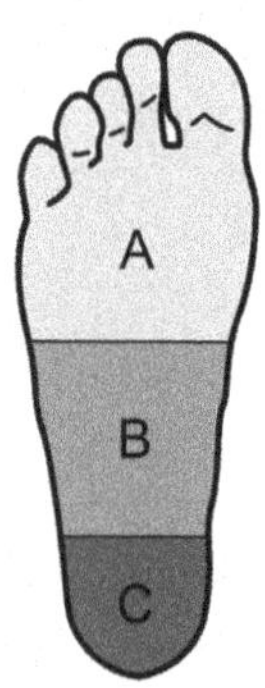

Figure 4.5: The Three Regions of the Feet

Region A is what is classically called the 'surging spring' or Yong Quan (涌泉) region of the foot. Note that in Chinese acupuncture, the names of the points refer to very specific and tiny points on the body. The 'surging spring' point is located on the sole of the foot. It is in a tender depression, one third of the way from the web of the second and third toes to the back of the heel. This is not the case in Qi Gong practice. The point name is used to simply indicate a region of the foot, region A in Figure 4.5. This is the same for many 'points' of the body; the name is used to refer to regions of the body rather than pinhead-sized points as in the case of acupuncture.

Opening the 'surging spring' point essentially means to use your weight to spread the bones of the foot and stretch the Huang that sits between the tarsal bones. It is for this reason that we say region A of the foot opens the 'surging spring' point.

Region B of the foot means to place your weight evenly across the whole foot. Your body mass will then be directed towards the centre of the foot near the highest point of the foot's arch. This region of the foot does not strongly stimulate the 'surging spring' point, as the tarsal bones will not fully open. It does, however, assist us in the intermediate to later stages of standing practice whereby we need to access the Huang of the entire body in general.

Region C of the feet places your weight into the heels. This is a big error in Qi Gong practice. If the weight goes into your heels, then gravity will pull your weight down through the skeletal system. As this happens, your bones will compress downwards and the joints will close. Most importantly, the lower back will become compressed, and this will result in difficulty opening some of the key channels in the back. This is a major error and a very common one throughout the Qi Gong world. It generally happens as people lean backwards into their posture; the structure of the 'back-sway' posture they have created then takes the weight down through the skeleton. This means that the Huang never opens, and these practitioners have, essentially, never really begun the Nei Gong process. They are stuck at the stage of physical body movements.

In the Wuji posture, we place our weight over the front area of the foot so that the 'surging spring' point is stimulated. You will know when you have correctly directed your weight down to the correct part of the foot as the metatarsal bones of your feet will spread open. This will begin to widen the soft tissues of the foot, creating more space for energy to flow into the body. It is normal for the foot to ache when you first start placing your weight here, and some students have even experienced a burning sensation as the Huang around the metatarsal bones begins to open up. This is nothing to worry about and should pass in a short space of time as your body begins to adjust to standing in this way. When the base of the foot fully opens, it will result in a strange sensation of bubbles moving underneath your foot. It is similar to if you were standing on one of the holes through which air is pumped into a Jacuzzi. This is usually a temporary experience and a clear sign of your connection to the Qi of the planet opening.

This process of placing your weight into the front region of the foot works because it stretches open the Huang, as shown in Figure 4.6. This is a very specific line of conduction that we need to 'draw in the Earth's Qi'.

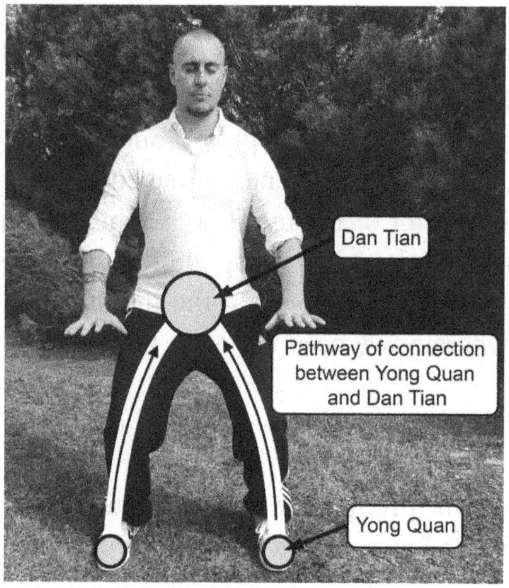

Figure 4.6: Line of the Surging Spring

The Huang stretches under the influence of the tarsal bones opening; the result of this is that it starts to connect a stretch of 'conductive tissue' up through the legs into the lower abdomen as depicted. It is here, through this line, that it was traditionally said we were taking more Qi from the planet.

What Is the Earth Qi?

There are always various phrases and instructions coming from traditional sources that try to describe what we are looking for in our practice. One of the key phrases for Nei Gong is to 'draw in Qi from the planet'; this force is called Di Qi (地氣) or Earth Qi. What is implied is that when we open up the 'surging spring' point, it enables a channel to open that then draws energy up from the planet into the body. This energy is then used as a kind of fuel for initiating the awakening of the lower Dan Tian. This is a more than adequate explanation for what is taking place, as it gives newcomers to the practices a model they can work with. I generally tell most of my new students the same thing, as it is simple, based in tradition and gives them a working understanding of what they are doing; but it's actually not completely accurate.

As human beings, we live in a world full of electrical and magnetic fields. Some of these are man-made in nature, whilst others occur naturally around us. One of the largest magnetic fields that we live in close contact with is the field of the planet. Now, I use the word 'magnetic' loosely here as the field does have some magnetic properties, but it also serves as a vast field of energetic information. The name of this field is the 'Earth's Qi field' and it is essentially Yin in nature. Since the founding of Daoism the tradition itself has always stated that the Earth is Yin and that the purest form of Yin Qi condensed to form the planet during the process of the universe's creation.

We will discuss Yin and Yang forms of Qi in greater detail further into the book, but for now it is enough to understand that we experience Yang Qi as a form of bio-electricity within the body and Yin Qi as a feeling of magnetism. When you feel Yin Qi moving through you, it really is as if there is a vast magnetic field passing through your body. Many of the somatic experiences of pressures and physical displacement that people experience through Qi Gong practice are a result of the Yin Qi reacting with their body. The influence of the Yin Qi is felt primarily within the Huang; it is here, in the Huang, that the magnetic 'pull' of Yin starts to create distortions and stretches on the inside of the body.

We also have another location for Yin within the body, and that is the region of the lower Dan Tian. It is said that the microcosm and the macrocosm directly reflect one another; in this way, the 'field' of the Earth is reflected in the body as the 'field' of the lower Dan Tian. In the majority of people, the 'field' of the lower Dan Tian is somewhat 'dispersed' and consequently it cannot carry out its various functions to a very high level. Since the lower Dan Tian is also considered to be Yin in nature, this means that its 'shape' is ultimately dependent upon Yin Qi. This is because its 'form' is developed as a kind of magnetic field that reacts with the Huang of the abdominal region of the body. More on this later when we take apart the anatomy of the lower Dan Tian in detail.

In order to help consolidate and awaken the lower Dan Tian, we use the theory of resonance. By opening the Huang in the feet, we also open lines of conduction through the legs to the abdomen. This means that we can now conduct through our legs and thus experience the field of the planet. This generally causes a high degree of shaking or vibration in the Huang of the legs at first and then, with time, it reaches the lower abdomen. Here, it causes a reaction in the body, and so the lower Dan Tian begins to develop. One field of Yin Qi builds a second field of Yin Qi; we have used the environment to establish a certain set of qualities inside of the body. This process is summarised in Figure 4.7. All of this process relies upon the feet being opened up in the correct way.

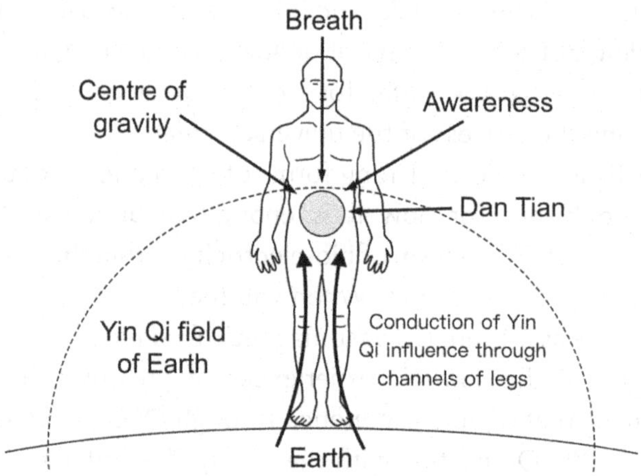

Figure 4.7: Influence of the Yin Qi

To reiterate what I said, though, if the theory above is too complex, don't worry about it. You will understand it as your own body's language of 'feeling' comes into play. Experiential learning must go alongside the intellectual study for it to make sense. For now, if you prefer, you can stick with the first, and more traditional, explanation. After all, these are just theoretical models to guide you in the right direction.

Alignment of the Knees

Once the feet have been put into the correct place, shoulders' width apart, facing forward, with the bodyweight placed so that it causes the tarsal bones to separate, we can look to the knees. The knees are the most common part of the body that people will damage through Qi Gong practice. This is because a few important facts about the knees are missed.

The knees should never support your weight. If you are aligned properly, your weight will transfer *through* your knees to the ground without ever 'catching' in your knees. If your weight does not 'catch' in the knees, then they will never be under any stress.

The alignment of the knees is often dependent upon the alignment of your ankles and your Kua (inguinal crease). In my experience, it is actually the Kua rather than the ankles that is of prime importance, though. In the vast majority of cases, when the Kua opens up sufficiently, any pain in the knees vanishes.

Finally, the knees are under stress for most people as during Qi Gong practice we stand with our knees bent. The bending of the knees is simply to control the height of your centre of gravity, nothing more. Many people are bending their knees too much, and this results in pressure building up.

This all means that, first, we should look to the Kua and understand this region of the body. If the Kua can function properly, then weight will not travel into the knees as it often does for people when they have pain. Second, it means we need to look at why we bend the knees.

The knees are bent so that our centre of gravity can drop down from the upper chest to the lower abdomen; that is all. Over the years, I have heard many odd reasons for bending the knees, some of them based in some kind of logic, whilst others are downright ridiculous! Basically, in order to work with the lower Dan Tian, we need several qualities to be in place. One of the major qualities that we need is our centre of gravity dropped from the chest down to the lower abdominal space. We do this very simply by bending our knees. This means that, in order to find out exactly how high we should be standing in our practice, we need to look to our centre of gravity and make ourselves 'bottom-heavy'. This is summarised in Figure 4.8.

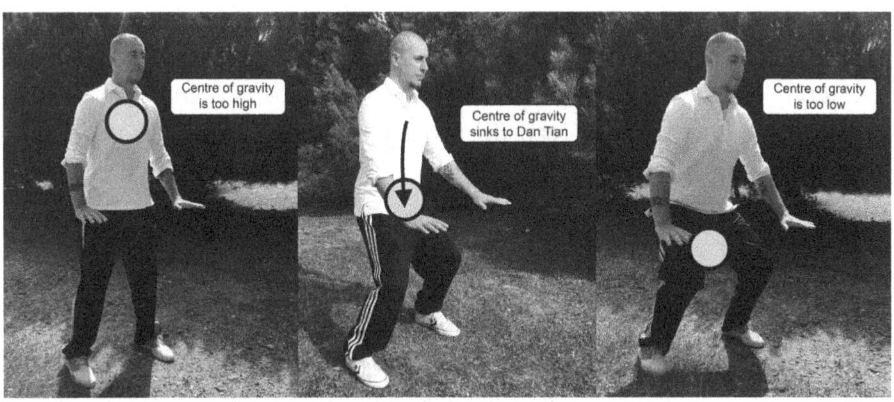
Centre of gravity
is too high
Centre of gravity
sinks to Dan Tian
Centre of gravity
is too low

Figure 4.8: Bending the Knees in Wuji

Shown are:

- standing straight, so that the centre of gravity is in our chest
- bending the knees, so that the centre of gravity drops to the lower abdomen
- standing too low.

In the final posture, where the knees are too bent, the centre of gravity is past the lower abdominal space and therefore not helping us in our practice. On top of this, we have the added complication of the knees now taking pressure from our weight, and we are likely to damage them.

In order to find the correct height, we do need a fair amount of body awareness; people who have danced or practise movement arts of some kind will often be able to find their centre of gravity easily enough, but those with a lack of experience in these kinds of practices will find that it takes a while to actually feel where their centre of gravity lies within the body. For this reason, it is wise to find a teacher who can help you with this; experienced Nei Gong instructors will be able to put you in the correct position until you can feel it for yourself.

So, in summary, to align the knees, we make sure they are not collapsed inwards – that is another common error that generally has its origin in the Kua. We then bend the knees to drop our centre of gravity down to the lower abdomen. For many people this means less bend of the knees than they would expect. Unless you are a particularly odd shape, it should never put your knees into a position where they are protruding over the toes; this would certainly be too much bending of the knees!

Usage of the Kua

The term 'Kua' is usually translated as either 'hips' or 'inguinal crease' depending upon what you read. In my personal experience, it is certainly not the hips. In fact, I tend to try to ban the word 'hips' in my classes as it gives people the wrong idea of how they should be moving. It implies movement from the wrong aspect of the body, the outer aspect rather than the inner soft tissues around the groin region of the body. 'Inguinal crease' may be a more adequate translation for the term, but this implies a certain group of muscles and mechanisms which can be pretty confusing. I keep it much simpler: I would translate the Kua as 'bikini line'! If we picture where the elastic would sit on a bikini, we get an accurate image of the Kua and where it sits in the body. This is shown in Figure 4.9.

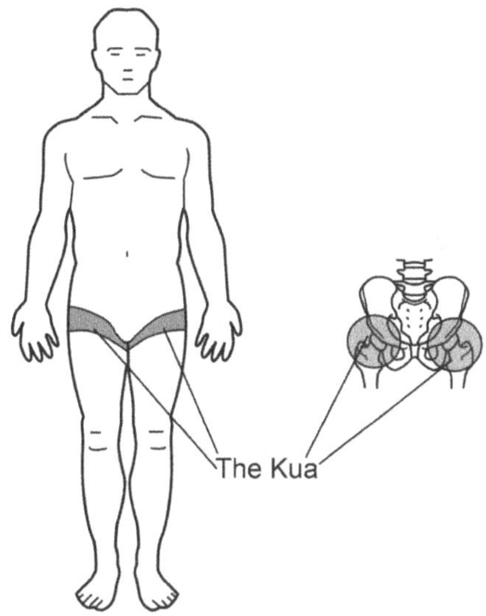

Figure 4.9: The Kua

When most people begin Qi Gong practice, they will incorrectly fold from the hips and lower back when they start to try out standing postures. This builds tension in all the wrong places and essentially messes up your practice. When tension is built around the Kua region in this manner, your alignments are thrown out, you cannot sink your weight, and you will struggle to work with the lower Dan Tian. The prime importance of locating and working correctly with the Kua cannot be overemphasised in my opinion and yet, in many classes, they still do not really discuss this vital region of human anatomy in any great depth.

Figure 4.10 shows how we wish to transfer the origin of power when practising Qi Gong.

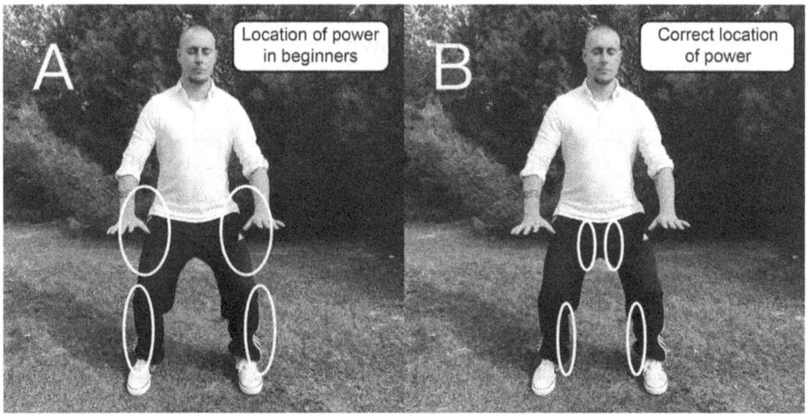

Figure 4.10: Transfer of Power from Hips to Kua

Image A shows the place where people will store their power when they first begin to stand in Qi Gong, and image B is where we wish to transfer it to. If your strength is in location A, then you are using the wrong muscles to hold yourself up and so tension will build up. This will also throw out the pelvis's alignment and make your lower back very stiff. We need to systematically relax the muscles in location A; the result of this will be that you naturally begin to use the Kua instead. When this happens, it will feel strangely familiar, as when you were a toddler first learning to walk, you almost exclusively used your Kua for movement. It was only as you got older and started to change your gait that you changed to using the hips and more lateral muscle groups. Don't worry, though, you won't return to a toddler's clumsy waddle; you can still walk normally, it is an internal shifting of strength that needs to take place.

Sit, Don't Squat

The key to relaxing the muscles of the Kua is remembering one simple rule: 'sit, don't squat'. Funnily enough, I always remember this phrase from a toilet wall in India. I was in a fairly classy restaurant and they had recently installed Western-style toilets, something that was still rare in the region of India I was in. For those who are not familiar with Eastern toilet habits, people there have traditionally used squat toilets rather than sitting down as we tend to in the West. When the posher hotels were installing Western-style toilets, people continued to squat on them and so left dusty footprints on the toilet seats. Consequently, there it was, emblazoned in large red letters on the wall: Please sit, don't squat!

So, how does this apply to standing practice in Qi Gong? Well, it is all to do with which muscle groups are engaging when you sit down versus when you squat. Figure 4.11 shows the difference between these two.

When we squat, we generally know that there is no chair beneath us – we are potentially going all the way down to the floor. The body prepares for this by engaging a number of muscles which serve to support our whole bodyweight. The body does not necessarily know how far we are going to squat down and so simply engages enough muscle to take your whole weight, just in case it needs to. What happens is that, even when we are only squatting down by a few inches, as when we are just bending our knees a little for Qi Gong practice, the body acts as if we were squatting to the floor, and a large amount of unnecessary tension is developed.

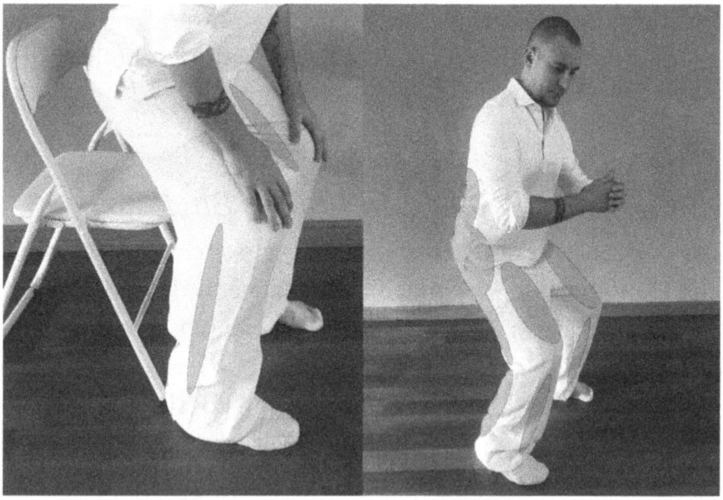

Figure 4.11: Sitting Versus Squatting

When we sit down, it is very different: we are aware that there is a chair behind us, and consequently, a different set of muscles engages. The muscles used are not ready to take your bodyweight all the way down to the floor, as your body knows that it does not need to. It only needs to lower you down so that your butt finds the chair you are aiming to sit in. We have all felt how different this is when we have gone to sit in a chair that has been moved at the last moment, or else we have simply misjudged the distance between butt and seat. The result is that we fall flat onto our backside, generally to the amusement of others.

As a simple experiment, squat down very slowly, as low as is comfortable, and feel which muscles engage. Do it a few times and use your body awareness to become familiar with the mechanism of squatting. Now do the same again, but this time, sit down instead of squatting. Try to feel which parts of your body you are using to sit down (obviously only sit down a little – you have no chair there) – just sit down as low as is comfortable without falling over.

Now, those muscles that you used for sitting down are the muscles you want to use to lower your body in Qi Gong practice. Even though you are only lowering yourself enough to drop the centre of gravity from your chest to the lower abdomen, you should use the muscles involved in sitting down. I generally ask new students to do this a fair number of times until it becomes an ingrained way of settling down into their Kua. If the Kua is used in this way, the muscles of the hips and lower back can relax and the pressure will come off the knees. The mass contained within your torso will also more effectively sink downwards within the body.

At first, this kind of 'sitting' into a standing posture can feel strange, but with practice it will become natural and you will see the benefit of it for yourself.

Alignment of the Pelvis and Lower Back

What many of you will notice from the above exercise is that when we 'sit' into our Qi Gong posture, we immediately reduce the level of tension around our hips and lower back. This is a huge positive, but then the downside to this is that it generally causes us to stick out our rear end somewhat. It is for this reason that after I have got new students to 'sit' into their posture, I ask them to relax the muscles of the lower back and 'let the pelvis fall off'.

By completely letting go of the muscles around our lower back and letting our pelvis drop as if it was going to fall off our lower back, we allow the relaxed weight of the pelvis to do a lot of restructuring for us. This restructuring needs to take place all around the lumbar region of the back.

There is a grave error in Qi Gong which is pretty common: this is to tuck the pelvis underneath yourself in an attempt to straighten the curve in your lower back. For men, it will cause tension and the potential for back problems at some stage in their practice; for women it can be more serious, as it leads to stagnation of Qi in the abdomen and around the uterus. At the very least, as the pelvis is forced under your body, it locks the muscles of the spine and switches off the Kua. To understand this last part, sit into your Kua as per the description above; now tuck the pelvis under, and feel what happens to all that nice relaxation inside the Kua region. That's right: it disappears! It is replaced with tension once more.

The tucking of the pelvis comes from certain martial arts systems where this principle is used for very specific power development reasons. We do not need this kind of power for Qi Gong training, as we are generally not trying to hit anybody whilst we are practising our Qi Gong. We are trying to work with the lower Dan Tian in a different manner from the martial arts, and so we should align our Kua and pelvis accordingly.

There is another error whereby people attempt to deliberately straighten out the lumbar region of the back. This, too, is a grave error for Qi Gong practice. I have even seen methods whereby people actually flatten their backs against a wall in order to completely eradicate the spine's curves. The result of this is a rather stiff and unnatural tension in the torso that goes against any concept of using the body's natural alignments to our benefit.

Whilst it *is* true that the lumbar region of the spine needs to lengthen a fair amount, and it *is* true that the pelvis needs to rearrange itself so that it sits a little more underneath the torso, this cannot be done correctly through the incorrect methods outlined above. It is a simple rule of life that when we try to do things, we tend to do them wrong! Instead, we can simply 'let go' and allow the weight of the pelvis to do the work for us by letting it 'fall off the body'. In this way, we are not really trying to 'do' anything, but the result of the work will be that the spine and pelvis will reshape themselves in the correct manner.

This works by allowing the weight of the pelvis to put a stress into the muscle fibres and soft tissues of the lower back. This stress will start them reshaping over a prolonged period of time. Generally, reshaping the back takes a few months of daily practice; not really that much time in the grand scheme of things. Figure 4.12 shows how the reshaping takes place.

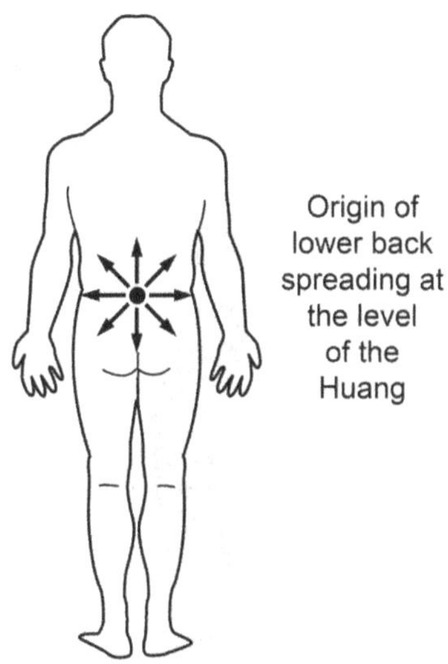

Figure 4.12: Reshaping the Back

If you carry out the pelvis alignment work in this way, over a period of time, then it will happen safely and you will do yourselves no harm with it. Instead, as your body has been given time to change, it will actually enhance the strength and health of your lower back. It is a worthy investment for your future health as well as helpful in your Nei Gong development.

Lengthening the Spine

The above discussion of not deliberately trying to take out the three key curves of the spine brings us to the next point: how then to open and lengthen the spine? The answer to this is that the spine needs to open of its own accord. If we try to lengthen the spine ourselves, that is, essentially trying to increase the spaces between the vertebrae, we will almost certainly do it wrong. Any attempt to purposefully open the back will put unnatural conditions upon the spine's alignments; this will actually serve to close the vertebral spaces and develop muscular tension in the stabilising muscles of the back.

We do need the back to be 'open' in order for there to be a strong flow of Qi and Blood through the spinal region of the body, but this opening must be done in the correct way. We open the back up by relaxing it, over a period of time, in our standing practice. As this happens, the muscles that have previously been contracted will relax, lengthen, and the spine can grow open. It all happens under the direction of our relaxation process. Especially, as the Huang starts to stretch open, it will help the back to expand and the vertebral spaces to widen. If we look at the image of the spine in Figure 4.13, we can see why opening these spaces by lengthening the spine ourselves is so difficult.

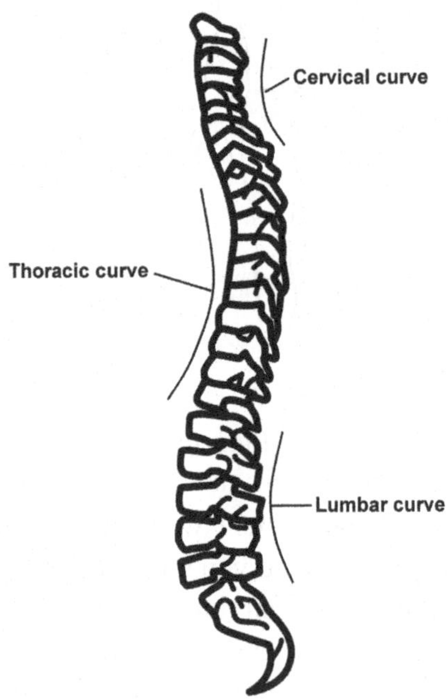

Figure 4.13: Lengthening the Spine

Because of the shape of the spine and its natural 'S' bend, we need to be able to open it in the manner of an arrow drawn running through its centre. If we try to open the spine ourselves, we will almost certainly open it in a 'straight line' on two planes of movement, and this is where the issues develop.

Once again, some schools of Qi Gong transferred the 'straight spine' principle from some martial arts systems, and this should not have been the case. These martial arts were using a straight spine for a very specific reason to do with martial power.

Often, the most difficult alignment for beginners to get right is the positioning of the spine during the Wuji standing posture. This is because the alignment of the spine will actually result in a very slight forward incline of the body. The vertical alignment for Wuji is shown in Figure 4.14. This alignment is based around the spine, rather than the torso.

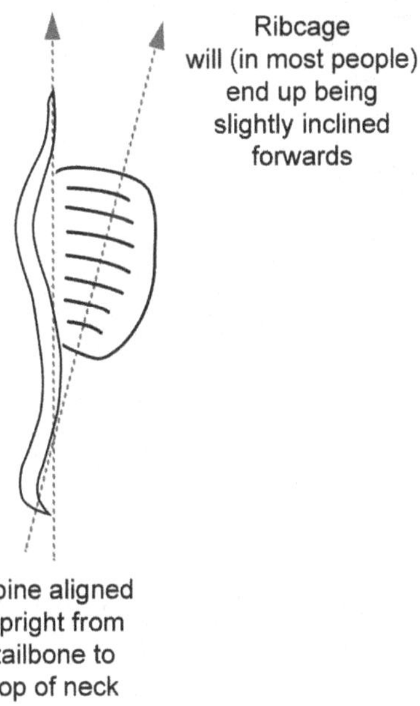

Figure 4.14: Spinal Alignment in Wuji

The reasoning behind aligning the spine, rather than the torso, is that your spinal column actually sits at the back of your body, whilst your ribcage and torso project outwards from the spine. During Nei Gong practice, it is the spine which we wish to have a strong vertical alignment (but still maintaining its natural 'S' curve), not the torso. As you can see in Figure 4.14, the spine actually sits towards the rear of the body, and beginners will almost always wish to align the centre of their torso rather than the centre of their spine.

To align the spine, stretch the top of your head gently upwards, and open up the spine by relaxing the muscles of your back as much as you can. Then ease your body forwards ever so slightly from the Kua region so that the weight comes off your lower back. This will then direct your body mass forwards over the correct area of your feet. If you were to drop a plumb-line down from the region of your chest to the floor, you would see that your body mass is now resting over the frontal region of your feet rather than your heels, which is how many practitioners incorrectly stand. The correct alignment is shown in Figure 4.15.

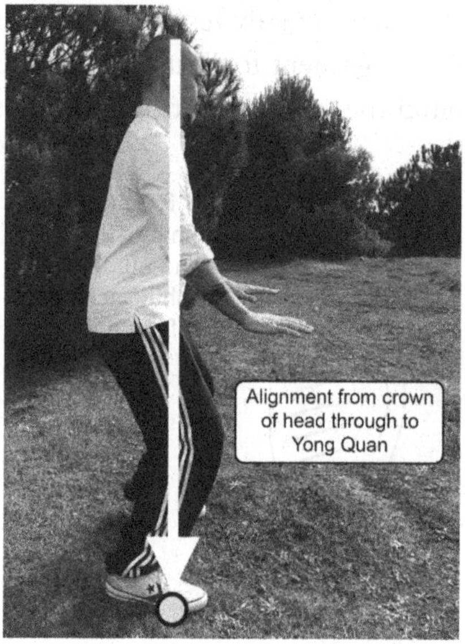

Figure 4.15: Correct Alignment for Wuji

By taking the weight slightly forwards, as shown in Figure 4.15, you will direct your mass downwards to the correct region of your feet. On top of this, you will enable your lower back to relax. The space between each of the vertebrae of the lumbar spine will increase, and with time, this 'opening' will spread its way upwards along your spine. Many practitioners discover that they have actually gained a few centimetres in height as the spine opens; this all happens naturally over time through relaxing into the correct posture.

As you bring the weight forwards, ensure you do so from the Kua and not by bending the spine. If the spine bends forwards, then you will collapse the abdominal region, which will lead to stagnation in this area. This will prevent you from awakening the lower Dan Tian and run the risk of developing other uncomfortable symptoms.

Touching the Shoulders to the Feet

This may sound like a somewhat difficult instruction; it sounds as if it involves some extreme level of flexibility. In fact, it is a very simple and yet very important principle which helps you to sit your shoulders into the correct place. If we do not sit the shoulders in the right way, then we will be disconnecting the upper and lower sections of our body – an issue that will inhibit Qi flow and the opening of the Huang.

Quite simply, when you lower your shoulders down, you wish to 'feel them in your feet'.

When helping beginners to understand this principle, I let them carry out a simple exercise: I get them to lift their shoulders up under their ears and then lower them down again so that they sit in a natural position once again. They do this exercise whilst standing in the Wuji posture. As the shoulders are slowly lowered back down, they should clearly be 'felt' in the feet. This means that there is a pressure increase in the feet. The weight of the shoulders should create this reaction in your feet because, otherwise, it means that the weight of your upper body is not successfully transferring its way to the floor. Instead, it is most likely 'catching' in some of the muscles somewhere in the torso. For the upper body to start aligning itself correctly, the weight of the shoulders has to pass through the body and reach the feet.

This can be difficult at first, but if you practise a few of these slow-motion 'shoulder shrugs' each time you start your standing Qi Gong practice, you should find that you get the hang of it after a few weeks of work.

No Floating Elbows!

After the shoulders have been sat correctly in place so that they 'touch the feet', it is time to sort out your elbow alignments. This was drummed into me by one of my early Chinese teachers who kept yelling (in broken English) 'No floating elbows!' Despite the constant reminders of this sort, it still took me quite some time before I could successfully sink my elbows into the right place during Qi Gong practice.

The elbows have to be 'sunk' after the shoulders are sat; it cannot be done the other way around. This is because the elbows should start to generate a reaction in the shoulders under the action of sinking. If the shoulders are not yet 'touching the feet', then the effect of the elbows will actually generate more tension in the upper body.

'Sinking the elbows' means to relax the weight of the elbows down towards the floor just enough that it starts to pull on the shoulders; if this is done correctly, then, as with the previous stage, there should be an increase of pressure in your feet. You are essentially feeling the weight of your elbows in your feet. To carry out this exercise, stand with your arms in the posture shown in Figure 4.16; this is the Wuji posture.

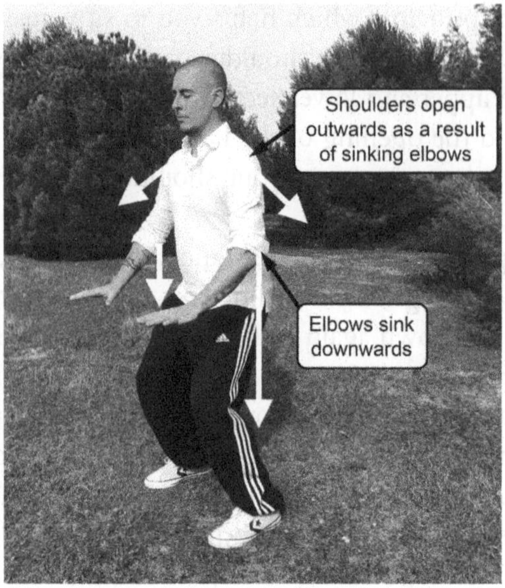
Shoulders open outwards as a result of sinking elbows
Elbows sink downwards

Figure 4.16: The Elbows in Wuji

As you can see in Figure 4.16, the sinking of the elbows causes a very specific pull on the shoulders and, more importantly, on the scapulae. We never force the shoulders down and we never try to align the scapulae under any kind of direction, as this will go wrong and instead create tightness in the shoulders and the back. We simply 'let go' of enough power in the elbows that they start to become heavier. Under the force of gravity, they will pull on the shoulders and start a gradual changing of the alignment of the scapulae. Over a few months (it takes a while with the shoulders!) the soft tissues start to change shape, and the scapulae will change their positioning on the back. Essentially, they will spread out and sit closer onto the posterior aspect of the ribcage. This is important for our practice, as it serves to connect the body together to a higher level as well as opening up the Huang and sinew channels of the upper back; these are vital for opening the upper aspect of the Governing channel.

You will sometimes hear the phrase 'Do Qi Gong like you have a melon under your armpit.' Yes, it is a slightly unusual instruction, but it does sum up the kind of space we wish for under the armpit. As with some of the previous principles, though, we don't 'make' this space for the melon. It will open up on its own as we sink the elbows correctly and thus influence the position of the shoulder and scapulae.

Alignment of the Head and Neck

So, the body should be nicely aligned by now. On to the next major step, the alignment of the head and neck. Anybody who has taught Qi Gong knows that this can feel like 'mission impossible' for a group of beginners. You just get their head sat correctly on their shoulders, and then they relax and their head drops forwards again!

'Suspending the crown and sinking the chest' is an important coupling. It ensures that the correct directional force is set up within the soft tissue structure of the body. This will help with the opening of the Governing and Conception channels which are awakened in the early stages of Nei Gong training. The first aspect, 'suspending the crown', is easy enough, providing it is done correctly. The head must be gently stretched upwards in order to free up the cervical vertebrae. Ensure that you lightly stretch upwards from the correct point on the top of the head, as shown in Figure 4.17. Many people automatically raise their head from a point further forward, which is incorrect. This causes compression in the neck which leads to a blockage of Qi flow along the Governing channel.

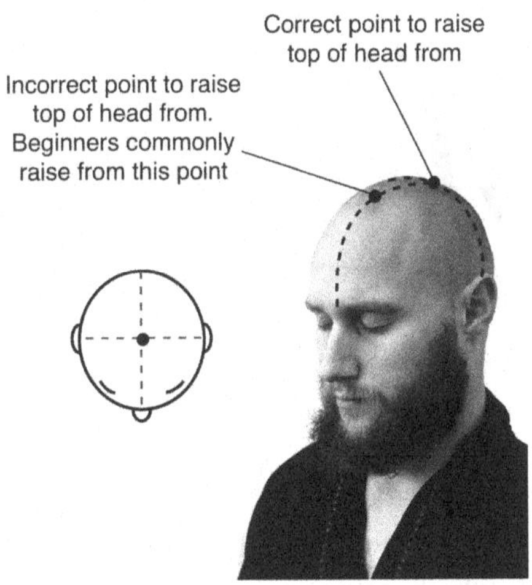

Figure 4.17: Suspending the Crown

The head should be lifted upwards from this point so that the neck stretches ever so slightly. It should not be pulled to the point of being tense but at the same time not relaxed to the point of being slack. This has to be held for long enough that it becomes an automatic postural alignment which does not collapse when you start to relax into your practice. It is a common error for the head to slump forwards when people are new to internal training, and this gets in the way of effective energetic flow.

The balancing principle to the stretching up of the top of the head is the 'sinking of the chest'. This should never be mistaken for 'rounding the chest' which is a common misconception. We never wish for a rounded shape in the shoulders with a collapsed chest as this leads to unnecessary tension and sinking of the Heart's Qi. 'Sinking the chest' involves allowing the Tian Tu (天突) (Ren 22) acupuncture point to be gently released downwards. This release wants to be ever so slight; a drop of a couple of millimetres is enough. This causes the Qi within the abdominal region to begin gently moving down towards the lower abdomen whilst letting go of tension around the Heart centre. The Conception channel also sinks down a little which helps direct the channel to open. This is all shown in Figure 4.18.

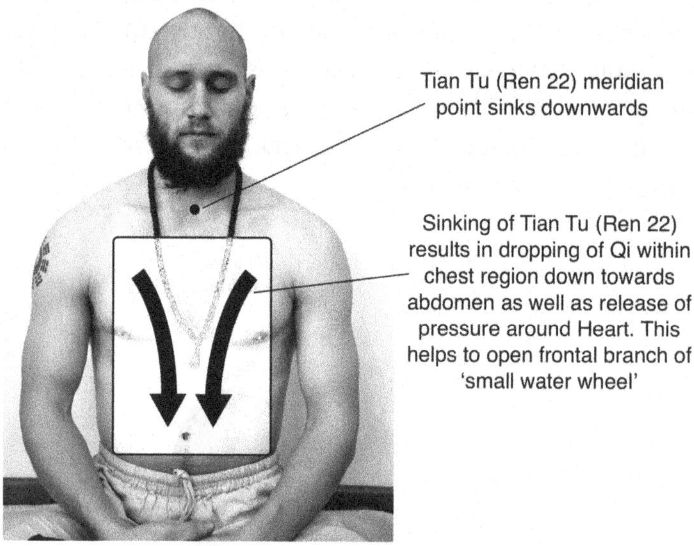

Figure 4.18: Sinking the Chest

When the crown is elevated and then combined with the sinking of the Tian Tu region, it results in a coupled raising of the back channel and releasing of the front channel, which causes a slight muscular link which takes the form of a circuit, as shown in Figure 4.19. This is the muscular basis for the 'microcosmic orbit of Qi'.

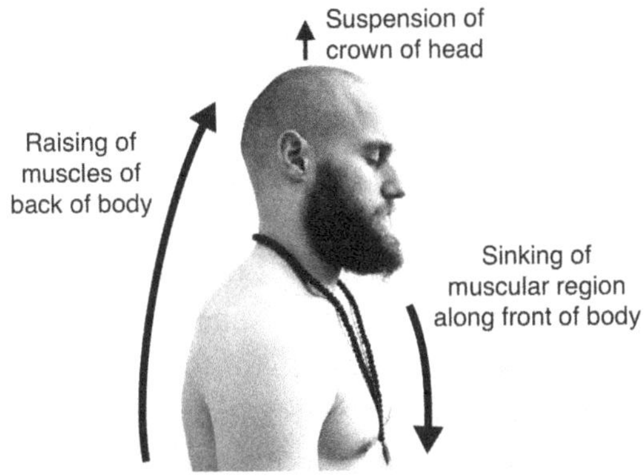

Figure 4.19: The Muscular Link of the Microcosmic Orbit of Qi

At first, this position can feel a little unnatural, but within a short space of time, your tissue memory will change and this will become a natural way to hold your body. Just ensure that the stretching and releasing of these two points is gentle and not forced. The movements should be small, as only a little adjustment is required to get the desired result. Many of the people I have met who have had blockages along these two lines have caused them by making the adjustments too large or with too much force.

Don't Round the Chest

An error that people often make is to 'round the chest' which places the shoulders into a very unnatural position. I used to do this in my early years of practice, and it caused me slight health issues with my lungs as well as making it nigh on impossible for me to sink my Qi through the torso. As soon as I was corrected and shown how to 'empty the chest', I could finally sit my shoulders correctly and understand how to sink through the inside of my body.

Sinking the Tailbone

The final region of the body that needs to 'sink' downwards is the tailbone, right at the very tip of the coccyx. This area is known as Wei Lu (尾閭) or the 'tail palm-leaf' in Qi Gong terminology. The coccyx is very important for a number of reasons, which are given below.

First, it 'locks' the rest of the principles in place within the body. You will feel this for yourself after you have sunk the tailbone down towards the feet. It is as if there is a pulling through the soft tissues of the whole body. As they pull, they serve to encapsulate all of the other body principles you have been applying to your body and holds them in place. If you have been through the above series of alignment practices and have them all in place, once the tailbone has been dropped, you will be able to take your mind off many of them and they will remain in place. It is as if the coccyx is the final key to making your alignment changes, and this is why it needs to be the last part of the body that you drop.

Second, the tailbone sits at the base of the Governing channel. When we sink the tailbone, it causes a 'tug' on the sinew channel and deeper Huang of the channel's base. This is like an initiator for the opening of the channel. The Governing channel almost always opens from bottom to top in the majority of people. As we sink the tailbone, it helps to set up the conductive quality of the channel. When we reach the stage of moving Qi through this region of the body, you will find that it takes little in the way of effort. The coccyx is like a gateway; when we sink it, it opens, and the Qi will start to flow through.

A final important reason for sinking the tailbone is that it helps to support the base of the body. As it drops down, it puts a gentle pull into the Huang around the pelvic floor. This creates a supporting sling which prevents us from 'leaking Jing'; a concept we shall return to in Chapter 7. If we sink the tailbone correctly, then most of the supporting work at the base of the body is completed. It is often said that you should raise the perineum, but there is no need to do so, or anything like this, in our practice. Sinking the tailbone correctly provides all of the support down there that we need.

Sinking the tailbone is carried out in the same way as previous principles. We simply relax those muscles which are preventing it from sinking. This means allowing the muscles around the sacrum to release as if you wanted the tailbone to drop off your sacrum. This will start to pull open the Huang in this region of the body. If you are starting to get good at all of this, you will feel the sinking of the tailbone in your feet, just as you should with your shoulders and elbows.

Opening the Sinews

So, if you have followed all of this, you should have a pretty nice Wuji posture, or, at least, you should be on your way to achieving such a thing. Well done! As you can see, for such a simple-looking posture, there is quite a lot involved in its structure. The final thing we need to do is to stretch it out in the correct way; to do this, we look to our hands. How open or closed our hands are will determine how pulled the soft tissues are throughout the rest of our body. Lengthening the fingers in this way reminds me of tuning a guitar. We have to get the strings tuned just right: too slack, and we will have the wrong note; too tight, and the same will happen.

To find the right level of 'sinew tuning', we start to slowly open our fingers out and spread the palms open until we start to find the absolute beginning of a stretch. We only need that start point of a pull. Once we have this point, we keep the hands in this position and this will be how we hold our hands through all of our practice of Wuji and Qi Gong exercises. You should find that, if you are honestly looking for the absolute start of a stretch, you only need to open the fingers out a little. Over time, you will find that your fingers will open more and more as the body adjusts to these 'fine-tunings'. Once the body is starting to connect together and you can 'find your insides', you will see that the stretch from the fingers will pass through your whole body. It will start to influence the sinew channels not just in your hands but also your legs, torso, neck and face.

This 'start of a stretch' throughout the body is very important as it serves as a strong impetus for change. It is as if we are slowly teasing out the length of the soft tissues so that they can begin to restructure in a very specific way. If we put too much force into the stretch, it will cause stagnation; if we do not have any stretch, and instead hold our body in a state of 'slackness', then the sinews will not be inclined to transform as we wish them to.

The Location of the Lower Dan Tian

Almost every system of internal work from within the Daoist tradition will, at some point, discuss the importance of the lower Dan Tian. It is generally the start point for all other energy practices and considered to be the first aspect of the energy body that a person should learn to work with. This sounds easy enough in theory – placing the awareness on the lower Dan Tian – but it is generally more challenging than that. A great number of practitioners fall down in the earliest stages of their development, either because they don't know how to locate the lower Dan Tian, or they work with it in the wrong manner. If you miss the lower Dan Tian with either your body mass or, later, the mind, then this will obviously slow down the practice, and if you focus on it incorrectly, it can lead to the development of internal stagnation.

The exact location of the lower Dan Tian will vary a slight amount from person to person. This is partly due to body shape and also due to people's energetic nature. Within textbooks it is usually said to be a few centimetres below the navel, when in fact it is a little more complex than this. In order to locate the lower Dan Tian, we need to follow a few steps.

We first use two key acupuncture points as references to locate the lower Dan Tian. These points are Qi Hai (氣海) (Ren 6) and Hui Yin (會陰) (CV 1). Qi Hai sits in the front midline of the body, two fingers' width below the lower border of the umbilicus. Hui Yin sits on the base of the body between the opening of the anus and the edge of the genitalia. Figure 4.20 shows how these two points can be used as a cross-reference for locating the lower Dan Tian's location.

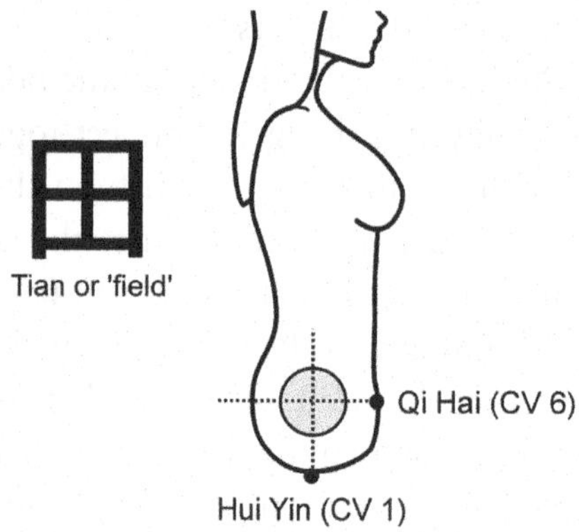

Figure 4.20: Location of the Lower Dan Tian

Alongside the diagram is the Chinese character for Tian, as in Dan Tian. Looking at the character, we can see a nod to cross-referencing these two points in order to locate the lower Dan Tian. The point at which these two lines cross each other gives the rough location for the centre point of the lower Dan Tian. From here, we then need to move our awareness around a little until we find the exact location.

When attempting to understand how far back in the body the lower Dan Tian is located, remember that it sits directly upon the line of the vertical branch of the Thrusting channel. This channel travels like an upright bar through the core of the body. This is why the lower Dan Tian sits directly above the Hui Yin (CV 1) acupuncture point. The majority of Qi Gong practitioners I have met actually place their mind too far forward within the body and so miss the Dan Tian by quite some distance. The awareness is a curious thing, as it likes to have certain locations to 'grab onto'. If you ever try to put your awareness into a single point within a large space, you will see what I mean. Those of you with enough internal sensitivity to know where your awareness actually is will find that it quickly seeks to attach itself to a physical point of reference within that space if there is one. If you want an easy experiment, just extend your index finger and then try to focus on the air an inch or two from its tip. What you will find is that, in the majority of cases, your awareness is very keen to shift across onto the tip of the finger, and only a focused level of concentration will keep it where it is. If your mind wanders for just a second, your awareness will be on the fingertip. Locating the lower Dan Tian can be similar, as within the space of the lower abdomen you basically have two points which the mind will be able to attach itself to. The first is the true lower Dan Tian and the second is the false Dan Tian. These two points are shown in Figure 4.21. The false Dan Tian corresponds with the Qi Hai (Ren 6) meridian point.

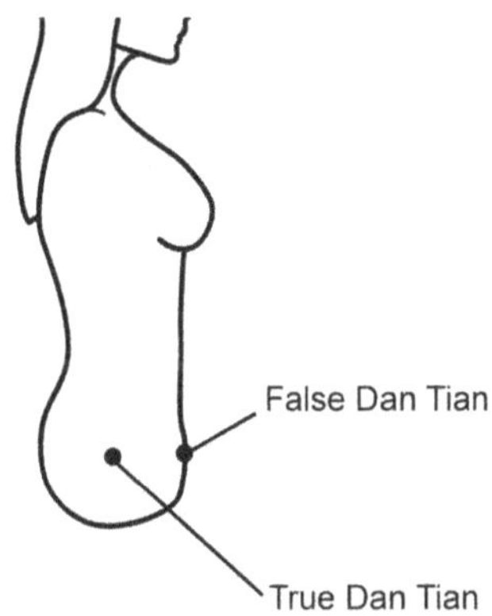

Figure 4.21: The True and False Lower Dan Tian

The true location of the lower Dan Tian is what we seek. If we are able to find it, then our awareness will have a 'tangible' spot to attach itself to. If we cannot find this exact point, then it will almost always have a tendency to attach itself instead to the false Dan Tian point which sits on the front of the lower abdomen.

When new students come into our school, we generally ask them to place their mind where they think their lower Dan Tian is located. We then ask them to contract the muscles around the region of the perineum a few times. From this muscular contraction, they can find the Hui Yin (CV 1) acupuncture point. If they then trace a line up within the core of the body from this point, it gives them the line of depth which the lower Dan Tian resides upon. In nearly every case students are surprised to find that they have had their focus too far forward – their mind has instead been resting on the surface of the lower abdomen in the location of the false Dan Tian. The Daoists long recognised the mind's tendency to travel to this point and so it was known as an early hurdle in a person's practice.

If a practitioner focuses upon the false Dan Tian for any length of time, they will find that they start to develop energetic stagnation within the region of the lower abdomen. This will generally lead to physical swelling and weight gain in this region of the body, because your awareness is leading Qi to a point in the body that it cannot be circulated away from. Though the acupuncture point will initially stimulate and increase in vitality (the point is used for this in acupuncture) it will, over time, slow down your development.

Once you have used the height of Qi Hai (Ren 6) and Hui Yin (CV 1) to find the approximate location of the centre of the lower Dan Tian, you need to then move your awareness lightly up and down along the pathway of the vertical branch of the Thrusting channel. Move your awareness gently up and down along the length of the line shown in Figure 4.22. Move slowly in order to give your mind a chance to translate any sensations which take place during this practice.

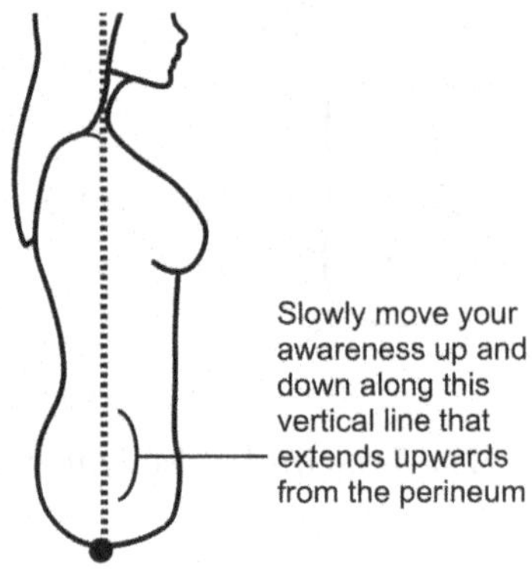

Figure 4.22: The Line of the Lower Dan Tian

You should only have to trace your awareness up and down along the portion of this vertical branch indicated in Figure 4.22. The most that your lower Dan Tian location should deviate from the height of Qi Hai (Ren 6) is an inch or so.

Stick with this practice until you experience one of two different sensations. There does not seem to be any pattern as to why certain people experience one of these over the other, but it does not matter as both are positive signs of success. The first sensation is one of heat, and the second is a pulling feeling, as though a deep muscle is gently contracting. As your mind runs over this spot, you will find that there is a point which is hot and, sometimes, if you are very healthy, slightly bubbling like boiling water. The second experience is that when your awareness touches the correct point, there is a gentle tightening of something inside the abdomen. It is an unusual feeling as there is no actual muscle there which is tightening, but the feeling is nonetheless quite distinct; this tightening is taking place within the Huang of the abdominal cavity. Either of these will only come when your mind passes over the exact right point. Do not worry if this takes some time, though – learning to feel for the Dan Tian's location can take a while.

At first, this practice can be a little tricky, but persevere and take some time to explore the region of your lower abdomen in this manner. Keep trying regularly until you successfully find the point of the centre of the lower Dan Tian. Once you have found it a few times, it starts to become easier to do. Your mind learns that this is a point it can 'grab onto', and before long you will be able to simply drop your awareness down onto this point straight away with no risk of it moving forwards onto the false Dan Tian. As a rough guide to progress times, most students seem to manage this within a few weeks to a few months if they practise the exercise every day.

Settling into the Lower Dan Tian

By this stage, you should have an understanding of the physical structure of the Wuji posture; this is the basis for our entire Qi Gong practice system. As stated before, all of our exercises, whatever they may be, are born from our method's Wuji practice. You also now have a method for locating the lower Dan Tian. We just need to put these two together to complete the exercise. This is done by lowering yourself down, sitting into the Wuji posture so that your centre of gravity moves to the place where you have located the lower Dan Tian's centre. This is shown in Figure 4.23.

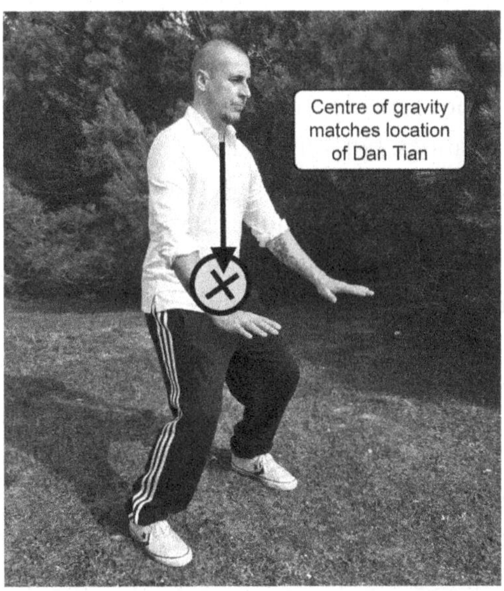

Figure 4.23: Connecting Wuji and the Lower Dan Tian

The more exactly you can place the centre of gravity upon the place you have identified as the lower Dan Tian, the better. There are likely to be some small adjustments you need to make in order to find the right place. It is quite common for people to lower their centre down and then find that it is too far forward, closer to the 'false Dan Tian' than the actual point we are looking for. In this case, don't worry, it is quite normal – just start to explore the nature of the Kua alignments once more; it is almost certainly guaranteed that the issue lies here somewhere.

It is worth spending some time making Wuji practice an 'active' process rather than simply a static exercise. What I mean by this is that you should keep hunting out the correct alignments; make increasingly subtle adjustments with your body to help yourself find the correct spot.

Throughout all of this, ensure that your weight is still directed to the right place on your feet: far enough forward that the bones spread open but not so far forward that you are off balance or that your heels are lifted.

Opening and Closing the Posture

'Opening' and 'closing' are two terms that you will hear a lot if you ever study the internal arts. Each art has its own use of the terms and, to some degree, their own definitions of what the terms are referring to. You should be careful not to cross over a definition of the terms from one method to another; I made this mistake for a long time, and when I discovered that each system was completely distinct in its use of terminology, it made my practices more effective. An example of this that you will often hear is that 'Taijiquan is Qi Gong'. This is not actually true in my experience. Yes, there are quite a number of shared qualities, but Taijiquan and Qi Gong have enough distinct differences that it makes them very different subjects. Understanding one does not necessarily mean that you understand the other.

In the case of Nei Gong, when we refer to 'opening and closing', we are referring to the position of the body's centre of gravity in relation to the lower Dan Tian. The 'open' version of a posture is when the centre of gravity and the lower Dan Tian location do not match – they are apart from one another; essentially, they are like two parts of a hinge that are away from each other. The 'closed' version of a posture is when the lower Dan Tian and the centre of gravity are on top of one another. Their location is shared. In this case, the centre of gravity and the location of the lower Dan Tian are like two ends of a hinge that have been brought together. This concept is shown in Figure 4.24.

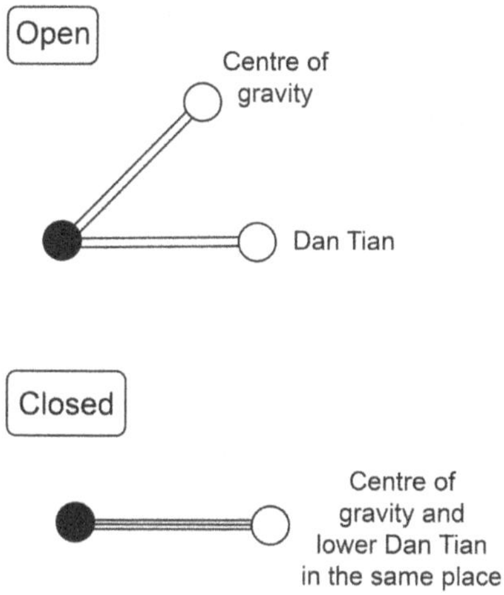

Figure 4.24: Opening and Closing

Many have mistakenly thought that the terms 'opening' and 'closing' within Qi Gong practice means to open and close the body's joints. This is most certainly not the case. Whilst it is true that our joints must function under the action of our exercises, this is not what the classical teachings were indicating; they were discussing internal dynamics, not external movements.

A simple exercise to practise is to move between the two positions shown in Figure 4.25. This is a very simple exercise to get the hang of 'opening and closing'.

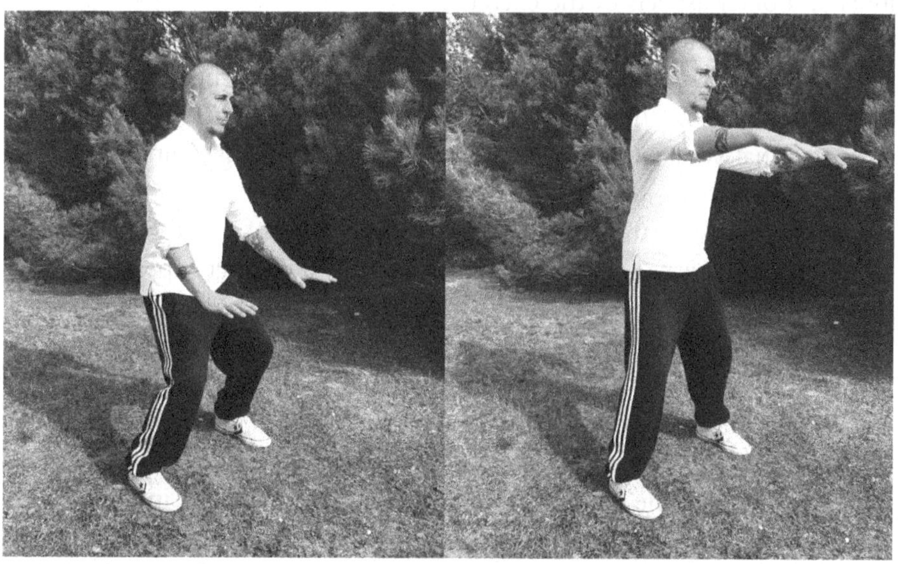

Figure 4.25: Opening and Closing Exercise

First, we begin the Wuji posture with our lower Dan Tian and centre of gravity in the same place; this 'bottom-heavy' posture is the 'closed' aspect of the exercise. We then inhale and slowly move into the second position shown in Figure 4.25. Our hands rise up to the height of the chest, and our centre of gravity should move upwards towards the chest as well. When our centre of gravity is in the centre of the chest cavity, we stop and allow our hands to remain at this same height. We then exhale and lower our hands and centre down together, as one unit, returning to the Wuji posture. We then repeat this exercise, over and over, until we are comfortable with the principles of opening and closing.

It may seem like this is an easy enough exercise but, almost without fail, when I teach newcomers this exercise, they need some assistance with it. In order to help you, below are some pointers for you to consider whilst you are practising.

First, you should retain all of the alignment principles discussed within this chapter whilst you are moving up and down. It is almost certain that you will lose some of the alignment rules when you first start to move; it will take time for you to maintain them in your body whilst moving in and out of Wuji.

The height of the hands must match the location of your centre of gravity. As your centre rises to the chest, it passes through the torso; the location of the hands must match this completely. If you do not match the hands and the centre of gravity as they move, then you are essentially disconnecting the inner and outer aspects of the exercise.

You must retain your weight on the correct part of your feet as you move up and down. Most beginners will find that their weight shifts from the front to the back of the foot as they move; it can take a little bodily control to ensure that your weight is helping the 'surging spring' point stay active during the exercise.

You should start to try to develop an awareness of exactly where your centre of gravity is as you move. There is actually a distinct experience to be had at the place where your centre resides within the body. As you 'open' and 'close' with the exercise, you should find that this point moves through you. With practice and effective absorption of your awareness into the body, you will find it.

If you have practised this exercise for a while, you should see that you have two heights: the upper height whereby your centre is in your chest, and the lower height where your centre of gravity is in the lower abdomen. These are the two heights you will use for almost all standing and moving Qi Gong practices. In exercises where you move up and down, you are supposed to be moving between these two postures. There really is no need to go any lower or to stand up higher as in the case of many modern systems that are very stretched out. The changing of the height of your body is simply to help the Di Qi have an influence upon the two key centres of your body, the lower Dan Tian and the middle Dan Tian. Keep this in mind when you practise any moving forms of Qi Gong that are intended to take you through the Nei Gong process.

In Conclusion

When you first start out in Qi Gong practice, it is said that there are three regulations you should look at. These are the regulation of the body, the regulation of the breath, and the regulation of the mind. What this means is that we have a series of foundational qualities we need to instil into these regions of our practice in order for healthy progress to take place. This chapter has looked at the basics of regulating the body; in the next two chapters we shall look at the other two regulations.

Chapter 5

REGULATION OF BREATH

Once we have looked at how to structure our body for Qi Gong training, we next need to look at the way in which we breathe. Effective breathwork is an essential part of all internal practices; it carries out a number of vital functions, and without regulating the quality of our breathing, we will struggle to access many aspects of the Nei Gong process.

The basic process of regulating the breath is based upon a simple procedure: we first look at how we are currently breathing, then we make some adjustments, and finally, we return the mechanism of breathing back to our body.

The reason for this is that, within Qi Gong teachings, we are generally taught to 'breathe naturally', which would be okay if most people's natural breathing was of a healthy standard. In the majority of people, this is just not the case. For this reason, we need to get involved and start to try to improve our breathing habits. Herein lies one of the biggest issues, though: how to change our breathing without forcing it? This is very important, as our breath and our mind are inextricably linked. If we begin to make forceful, heavy changes to our breathing over a short period of time, then we can stress the mind, and this will adversely affect our practice. This means that we follow two simple guidelines when working with the breath:

- We work very gently with our breathing to make changes to it over a long period of time. Short sessions of practice are better than longer sessions at first. Practising the methods within this chapter for short periods of time but frequently is better than hammering away at it. This will give the body time to change. Between these practice sessions, if we wish to continue our breathing practice, then we use gentle awareness of the breathing. Simply observing it without getting involved between practice sessions will actually help it to change of its own accord.

- All changes to the breathing should be based in 'relaxation and release'. If we keep this in mind, it will stop us from 'forcing' the breath, a common error.

Throughout all of your breathing practice, keep these two rules in mind. If you stick to this ethos, your breathing patterns will improve greatly, and this will bring you along, both in your practice and your overall well-being.

The Basic Functions of Breathing

Our breathing is an intricate system that affects the entire body and many aspects of our mind. It would be difficult to identify either a physical or an energetic system of the body that did not, in some way, rely on the quality of our breathing to function properly. That being said, these are the key functions of our breathing that are important for our practice:

- To bring oxygen and Qi into the body
- To expel excessive amounts of carbon dioxide from the body
- To assist with circulation of blood
- To regulate the emotional mind
- To regulate the internal pressures of the body
- To assist with absorption of awareness into the body
- To release the bindings of the Huang and sinew channels
- To guide the Qi passively

It is these key functions of the breath whose efficiency we wish to increase.

Bringing Oxygen into the Body

Oxygen is taken in through the airways and lungs, passes into our blood stream and there, via the red blood cells, reaches every muscle, tissue and cell of the body. We require this oxygen to survive, and maximising the level of oxygen within our practice will obviously increase the efficiency of the body's functioning.

Many chronic sicknesses that build up within the body are due to a lack of oxygenation of the cells. If they cannot receive the oxygen they require, they begin to decrease in health; this means that they no longer carry out their individual functions adequately. If we look at cells, the energy they produce is vital for the continuation of life; only around 25 per cent of the energy produced in our cells is used up through physical activity, the remaining 75 per cent going into all of the automatic processes going on within our body, from hair growth to organ function. To maintain life, we need this oxygen; the more effectively we can manage our breathing, the more efficient these processes will be. In short, poor breathing leads to poor health.

Within Chinese medicine theory, if we look at the Chinese character for Qi, we can see that 'air' makes up one of two parts of the character. This character is shown in Figure 5.1.

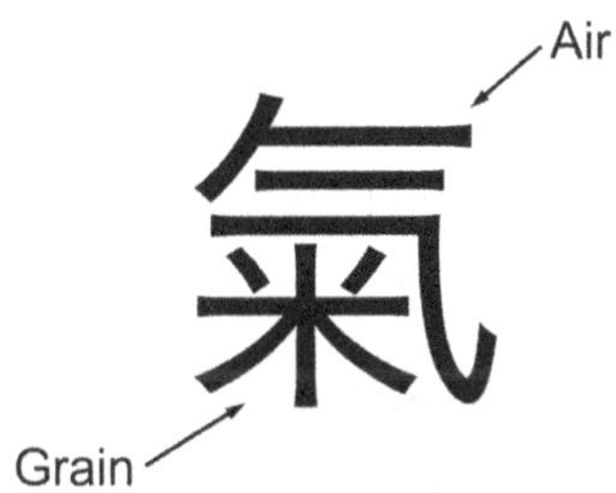

Figure 5.1: Chinese Character for Qi

The other aspect of the character is the symbol for 'grain' or 'food'. One way of looking at the character is that in order to produce a healthy amount of Qi within the body, we need a good quality of food and intake of air. This is the key breakdown of the character from a simple, medical standpoint; as with everything in the Daoist arts, we can go deeper. In Chapter 9 we will look at a deeper definition of this character.

Expelling Excessive Amounts of Carbon Dioxide from the Body

If there is an excess of carbon dioxide within the body, our breathing will speed up in order to expel this gas from our blood stream. If this continues for too long, then our breathing naturally becomes much shallower and higher up within the chest. This is counterproductive as it essentially means that we never fully expel all of the carbon dioxide that we should. An excess of carbon dioxide means that brain function diminishes, along with our physical stamina and overall health.

That being said, we also have the added factor of too little carbon dioxide within the blood stream being an issue. Carbon dioxide is also involved in the function of cells as it is the presence of carbon dioxide within the body that causes the blood cells to distribute their oxygen effectively. This means that our cells require carbon dioxide as well as oxygen. Too much of this gas and our body will become stagnant and toxic, too little and we cannot internally produce the energy that we require. This means that both oxygen and carbon dioxide must be balanced in the right way in order for efficient functioning of the body – for it to produce energy as it should.

This is important, and it was understood by the ancient Daoists who had a very clear rule for their exercise: when training any form of physical exercise, we should 'sweat but not pant'. Light sweating indicated that the Qi was moving as it should, right to the surface of the skin. 'Panting' or being out of breath from the exercise meant that we were essentially hyperventilating and thus changing the balance of oxygen and carbon dioxide within the blood for the worse. It was too Yang a state, meaning that we received no Yin or nourishment internally.

Assisting with Circulation of Blood

The action of deep, regular breathing assists in the circulation of blood through the body. As much as anything, this benefit to the body's functioning comes from the way in which we relax when we learn how to breathe efficiently. It is traditionally said that Qi and blood flow together; they are the Yin and Yang of our body's vital substances. Qi provides the life, whilst blood provides the nourishment. If we look at cellular habits, as blood flow increases and carries oxygen more effectively to the cells, they produce more energy, a function that will assist in the production of Qi internally.

Regulating the Emotional Mind

Our breathing can take us pretty deep into the internal processes of Daoism due to its connection to many aspects of both our mind and consciousness. In the early stages of practice, though, what we are primarily concerned with is regulation of the emotional mind. Figure 5.2 shows the cyclical relationship of our emotions and our breathing.

It is easy to see how people experience shifts in their breathing patterns when they are in a heightened emotional state. Extreme anger produces short, rasping breaths that are high in the chest; sadness makes people draw in long, sighing breaths as though the body is struggling for air. We can see these switches to the breathing habits of the body when a person is in an extreme of an emotional swing; they are very clear, but of course these changes to our breathing are happening all of the time. Any emotional response to stimuli generates a change in the breathing somewhere along a sliding scale of 'slight' to 'extreme', as in the examples above. All of these changes affect the internal environment of the body, from circulation to energy production, and so start to transform our health.

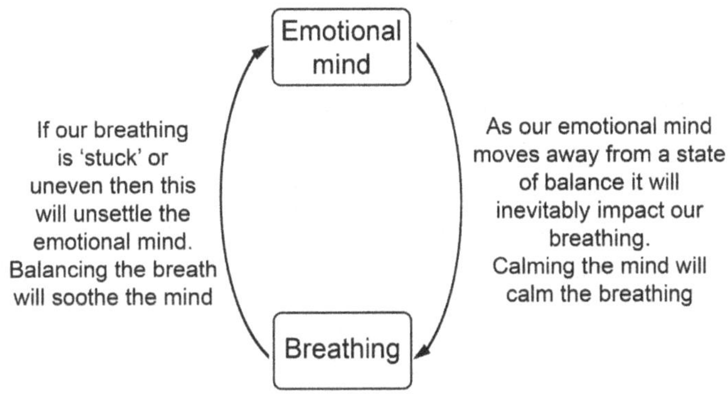

Figure 5.2: Breathing and the Emotional Mind

The connection between our breathing and our emotional mind is so strong that we can use our breathing 'in reverse' to the process described above and so use it to calm the emotional mind. The transient emotions move like waves over the vast ocean of our mind. Through regulation of the breath we can help to calm this ocean and return it to stillness.

In the case of chronic stress, an affliction which affects countless people every day, our body remains in the 'fight or flight' state, a condition that makes the body far too Yang in quality. Qi flow is impeded and we are essentially burning up the fuel of our Kidneys at an increased rate. Regulating the breath can help calm a person and take them out of this 'fight or flight' state. For some people, even if they never progress past this stage in their practice, it can be a literal lifesaver to learn how to calm down in this way.

Regulating the Internal Pressures of the Body

Our torso is physically divided into two main regions known as the thoracic and abdominal cavities. These two regions are shown, along with the diaphragm, in Figure 5.3.

As we breathe, the large muscular sheet of the diaphragm is raised and lowered. This is the primary mechanism behind the action of breathing. The movement of the diaphragm generates an alternating pressure within the body that rhythmically squeezes and nourishes the regions of the abdomen and chest one after the other. This serves to help shift Qi through the body as well as working as a kind of internal massage for the body's insides.

This is one of the reasons why overly forceful breathing, an issue common to many internal systems, will damage the body. Aside from any problems around excessive forcing of Qi through the body, the aggressive nature of the changes in internal pressure can damage the physical organs. This can be especially problematic for the Heart and the Kidneys, organs I have seen people damage considerably through forceful breathing exercises.

In many people, the diaphragm is quite 'stuck'. Stress has led to tension building in this region of the body, and so it does not move as it should. The result of this is that general stagnation will build in the body's two main cavities and our breathing is impaired. Regulation of the breath and increased relaxation levels will assist in the 'unsticking' of the diaphragm so that it can move properly once more.

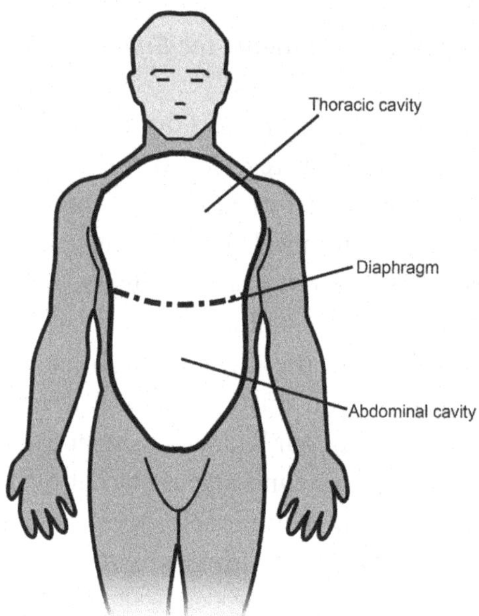

Figure 5.3: The Cavities of the Torso

Assisting with Absorption of Awareness into the Body

One of the most challenging aspects of internal training for newcomers is to actually get their awareness into their body. Whilst this may not sound like a very difficult thing to do, it can be a real challenge. This is because when most people place their awareness into the body, they cannot find anything to 'lock onto' with their awareness. The result of this is that the mind will jump around inside the body; then, starved of stimuli, it will start to produce a whole host of thoughts. These thoughts prevent you from finding the level of stillness needed to connect with your internal environment and feel what is taking place in there.

As you start to regulate your breathing, it can help with absorption of awareness into the body. This is because the action of your breath helps to stir Qi, and this Qi then moves through the Huang. On top of this, the Huang will also react to the rhythmic quality of the internal pressure changes coming from the movement of the diaphragm.

As the fibres of the Huang start to react to the movement of your breath, they will begin to generate subtle internal movement. This movement generally begins as small waves and undulations inside whose origin is difficult to pinpoint. It is as if the whole of the inside of the body is starting to come to life and move in waves with your breath. As this process unfolds within you, there is the start of the release of tension between the layers of the Huang. This, in turn, gives a 'space' for the awareness to move through. This is the beginning of the absorption of awareness into the body.

There is nothing to 'do' to assist in this process. It will naturally unfold of its own accord as you practise your breathwork. It is a pleasant part of the process, the usefulness of which in connecting the mind and body cannot be overstated.

Releasing the Bindings of the Huang and Sinew Channels

Carrying on from the previous function of our breathing, as the Huang start to move, they will start to unbind. Regular, smooth, even breathing serves as a kind of 'divider' of the layers of the Huang; this will then begin to spread to the sinew channels as well.

The binding of the Huang comes from tension, both physical and psychological; this then traps Qi that would otherwise travel through this region of the body. The trapped Qi leads to stagnation and sickness, and so we wish for these bound-up layers of Huang to let go and be got rid of. There are several factors involved in the process of unbinding, but one of the earliest ones we encounter is through the internal relaxation generated as a result of effective breathing.

Guiding the Qi Passively

This final key function of breathing is very simple: it helps to move Qi! Qi circulates both through the channel system and, in the form of waves and fields, through the Huang. There are many factors involved in its movement, and one of these is the action of our breathing.

It seems to be something that is missed in many Qi Gong methods that we want our Qi to move all of the time. Too many people seem to be focused upon setting aside some time each day to 'move their Qi' or 'circulate it'. This is okay, but what about the rest of the day? We really want to set up our body and its mechanisms in such a way that when we relax and get on with our lives, our Qi continues to move. As we learn to regulate the breathing, we will establish one of the key catalysts for continued movement of Qi that pulses through the body on a subconscious level.

The Keywords of Qi Gong Breathing

The Chinese arts are generally described through the use of 'keywords'. These are lists or chains of descriptive words contained within traditional teachings. The function of the words is to show you what qualities you should look for within your practice. Every system, from martial arts through to meditation, within the Chinese schools has these groups of keywords.

With regard to Qi Gong breathing methods, different systems have their own words; some schools use more or fewer words, depending upon how they were taught. I was taught five keywords by my own teacher that apply to how we should regulate our breathing; these are:

- Jing (靜) or 'quiet'
- Shen (深) or 'deep'
- You (悠) or 'at ease'
- Huan (緩) or 'slow and gradual'
- Mian (綿) or 'cotton soft'

As with many chains of keywords in the Chinese arts, they form a kind of causation chain. This means that only the first in the line of words needs focusing upon; the result of this quality being achieved is that the next term in the chain will start to manifest of its own accord. This is something worth remembering if you are going to explore the classical teachings of any of the Chinese arts. I, like many others, missed this key aspect of classical Chinese linguistic structure for a long time. Consequently, I was working towards each quality as if I was trying to complete a checklist. This kind of practice led to a 'stuckness' in what I was doing. As soon as I understood the 'causation chain' nature of the lists, the efficiency of my practice increased greatly.

These qualities should be understood, though; if you understand them, you will know what you are looking for and have a clearer idea of how your breathing practice is developing.

Quiet

The first quality we wish to seek is quietude. Shortly, there will be an introduction to the two main categories of breathing methods within the Daoist arts; whichever method you use, the principle is the same: it should be quiet.

The word 'quiet' applies to the outer expression of breath as well as the inner. The outer expression of 'quiet' means that nobody should hear your breathing unless they are incredibly close to you. We breathe gently in and out through the nose during our practice and aim for a gentle, calm practice. If your breathing pattern is loud and forceful, to the extent that people around you can clearly hear it, then you have not attained the quality of 'quiet' yet. To develop this quality, look to the inner.

Since our breathing and our psychology are so intimately connected, we can use this to our advantage. If we quieten our mind, then we will quieten our breath. This is the prerequisite to attaining the first keyword for Daoist breathing methods. Simply allow your awareness to absorb into the process of breathing and from here be gently led into the body. To help the mind grow quieter, do not try to 'do' anything; simply allow your awareness to become absorbed into what you are doing and, over time, it will start to become quiet. At this stage, we are not looking for a profound state of emptiness or anything so advanced. We are simply looking for a shift towards the mind and breath becoming increasingly quiet. You will know when you are coming close to achieving this as the by-product of 'quiet' will be the next word – 'deep'.

Deep

As you begin to grow quieter, you will find that your breathing begins to deepen. First, the length of your breath will naturally begin to extend, and then it will start to change its point of origin. This point will be within the lower abdomen.

Babies and young children naturally breathe from low down in the abdomen. As we grow older and our emotional mind begins to get involved, we change this natural habit and start to breathe from higher up within the body. When a child breathes from their belly, they are doing so as a natural continuation of how they absorbed Qi within the womb; this took place via the action of the lower Dan Tian. As we age, we draw most of our energy from our food and our breathing. As discussed above, we do not use the lower Dan Tian to the same degree and consequently it is no longer the focal point for our breath.

For our Qi Gong practice, we wish to return to using the abdomen and the lower Dan Tian for our breathing. When we can do this, we can successfully start to study the two main categories of breathing: passive and active breathing.

As you quieten the mind through absorption of awareness into the body, you will be led to a deepening of the breath. You will naturally find with time that you are breathing from much lower down. The deep muscles of the lower abdominal cavity will have become involved and you are now 'belly breathing'.

At Ease

When the breathing has become deep enough and you have reached the lower Dan Tian, there is a very specific reaction that takes place. You will find that your breathing has now reached the stage of being 'at ease'. This means that it now feels anchored into the lower Dan Tian. This is now your natural place of breathing. The result of this is that your mind and body will begin to enter into a state of relaxation that many people are unable to feel in their daily lives. The tissues will begin to unwind, the Huang will begin to 'unbind', and the mind will grow increasingly calm.

The level of calm you achieve in your mind tends to bring with it a sense of joy or fulfilment. As you breathe in towards the lower Dan Tian, it can generate a feeling I have previously called 'tranquillity' for lack of a better word. As you breathe out, there is a feeling of deep 'release'. The result of this stage, feeling 'at ease', is deep abdominal breathing that is your natural method of breathing; you will feel as if you 'breathe in tranquillity' and 'breathe out tension'.

Slow and Gradual

In order to try to translate the experience of the word 'Huan', I have used two English words. 'Huan' is a mix of being 'slow' and 'gradual'.

This is referring to a resultant feeling of Qi movement through the body that will come when you have attained the quality of being 'at ease'. The movement of Qi out of your lower abdominal space will be like gentle waves that move slowly and gradually through the Huang of the body. As these waves pass through you, they will release interior tension and so the unbinding of the Huang will reach a new level. This is all increasing your level of interior relaxation as well as helping to passively move the Qi through your body.

It is at this stage that a bridge has been made between your breath, your Qi and your physical body. The previous stages have been leading you towards a certain level of relaxation, but now the effects of your breathing are distinctly starting to unfold various processes in your physical tissues.

Many practitioners of Qi Gong do not realise that their practice has the potential to do this; they don't know that we need to keep absorbing the awareness into the breath until not only our Qi moves, but also our physical tissues. This is a shame as this is where much of the deepest change takes place. We should keep working regularly with our breathing in this manner until we reach the stage of 'Huan' – 'slow and gradual' movement of Qi and release of tension.

Cotton Soft

The final result of this unfolding process is that you will find that your body feels like it is made of 'cotton soft' layers that slide across each other with ease when you listen to the insides of your body. All binding will have left the body, and the Huang are free to move around. Interestingly enough, when we look at the more advanced stages of training in Chapter 11, you will see that this 'softness' has been replaced by something quite different. At the far extreme of softness comes a special type of 'hardness'. We will discuss this in great detail later, though. For now, at this stage in your development, it is the 'cotton soft' quality you are looking for throughout your body.

If you can increasingly move through these keywords and understand the qualitative changes that come from simply allowing your awareness and breath to become quieter, then you will have built a solid foundation in your practice of regulating your breath.

The next step, beyond here, is to look at the two main types of breathing used in Qi Gong practice, passive and active breathing.

Passive and Active Breathing

There are many types of breathing practice within the Daoist tradition. Some are very simple and based in improving your health, others are more complex and aimed at developing powerful alchemical change within the body. There are breathing methods such as 'Song breathing', 'turtle breathing', 'pore breathing', 'embryonic breathing', 'the firing breath' and so on. If I were to explain each breathing method in detail, it would take up an entire volume, and these are only the breathing methods I am personally familiar with; there are, no doubt, countless others.

In order to simplify it down to the absolute basics, though, all of these breathing methods can be divided up into two main categories: passive breathing and active breathing methods.

Passive breathing methods are all variations on the practice of 'abdominal breathing', whilst all active breathing methods are a variation on the 'reverse abdominal breathing' method. Let us look at the differences between the two.

Passive Breathing Methods

Passive breathing methods are based upon deep abdominal breathing, or 'belly breathing' as it is sometimes called. This is the standard breathing method of all forms of Qi Gong. Before anybody attempts to work with the other breathing methods of Daoism, they should be well versed in abdominal breathing; it should have reached a stage in your development whereby this is your normal, everyday way of breathing. If you have not yet reached the stage of automatically breathing in this way throughout your daily life, then you should never think of moving onto more 'active' or advanced forms of breathing. Even if you have practised for a few years and are still not able to breathe abdominally as a subconscious function of the body, do not move on. I cannot emphasise this point enough; many people underestimate the connection between mind and breath. If you start to hit the more complex or assertive forms of breathing too early, you run the risk of frying your nervous system and sending too much Qi to the wrong place in your body – generally upwards! I have seen this issue with many practitioners of forceful Qi Gong methods as well as in some Yogic traditions; the result is a build-up of tension, emotional swings and the possibility of psychological health problems.

Passive breathing methods such as abdominal breathing serve to circulate the Qi that we have within our body in a healthy and relaxed fashion. It is the primary breathing method we need to calm the body and place it into a state of 'rest'. It stimulates the parasympathetic aspect of the nervous system which helps the body to move out of a state of stress and into a state of recuperation.

Active Breathing Methods

More active breathing methods are all variations of the 'reverse abdominal breathing' method which some people will know as 'Daoist breathing'. This kind of breathwork is designed to move Qi to a far higher degree through the body, stimulate the Dan Tian and ultimately create more 'action' inside of our system. It is the breathing method used as the catalyst for change in many Daoist arts including alchemical meditation.

The downside of this type of breathing is that it can put stress onto the sympathetic aspect of the nervous system, which is stressing for both the body and the mind. If we use it too much, it can lead to 'burnout', both mentally and energetically. It is a highly stimulating form of breathing and should only be used at specific times and for specific purposes. It should also only ever be used once regular abdominal breathing is your subconscious breathing method.

You can think of active breathing methods, based in reverse abdominal breathing, as being like putting your foot on the gas in a car. Sometimes it is needed and useful, it gets you going to places, but it uses up gas.

Table 5.1 shows the comparative differences between abdominal and reverse abdominal breathing.

Table 5.1: Passive and Active Breathing Comparison

	Abdominal	**Reverse abdominal**
Categorisation	Passive	Active
Action	Calming	Stimulating
Effect on Qi	Circulating	Driving
Dan Tian effect	Regulating	Compressing
Nervous system	Parasympathetic	Sympathetic
Polarity	Yin	Yang

The five keywords that we have previously looked at should be applied to both breathing methods, but essentially, if you carry out some regular practice of absorbing the mind into the breath and looking for the unfolding of these qualities, it should lead you naturally into the abdominal breathing method. This is because you used to breathe like this when you were very young, and it is linked to feelings of calm and relaxation. As you relax the mind and sink the breath, the body should remember this way of breathing and re-establish it for you within the body.

Abdominal Breathing Technique

Abdominal breath is based upon inhaling down into the lower abdomen so that the lower Dan Tian is the focal point for your breathing. When you inhale, the lower abdominal cavity should naturally expand a little, and when you exhale, the abdominal cavity will contract slightly. This is shown in Figure 5.4.

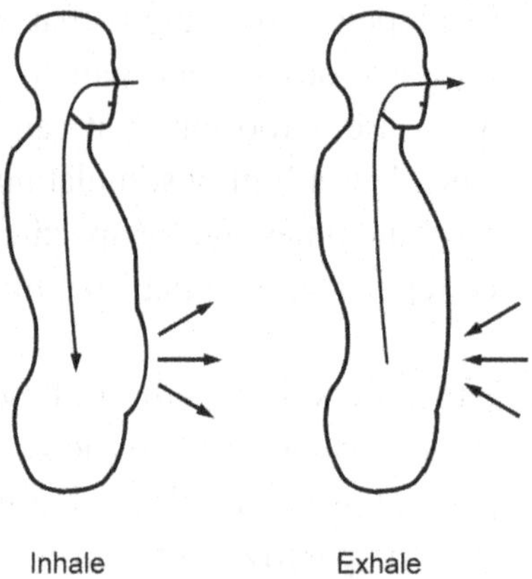

Figure 5.4: Abdominal or 'Belly' Breathing

Though the diaphragm is obviously still involved in the respiratory process, it is as if the abdominal muscles are leading and controlling the process of breathing. There is an important thing to note here, though: you should not aim to achieve this; it should happen of its own accord. Please make note of this, it is very important. The transformation of your previous breathing method to the deep abdominal breathing of Daoist Qi Gong should be an automatic process; you are simply an observer. There are schools that aim to train you to breathe abdominally in various stages; they inevitably end up with students having a very stagnant quality to their Qi. To attain deep abdominal breathing in the correct way, we just need to sit quietly, absorb the awareness into our process of breathing and relax as much as we can. The result of this will be that we start to be led through the five qualities of quiet, deep, at ease, slow and gradual, and cotton soft. By the time we hit the second stage of this process, the stage of 'deep', we are starting to return to abdominal breathing.

There is just one minor adjustment that may need to be made once you have managed to attain abdominal breathing as a skill. This is to do with the highest point of your inhalation. Many students have a slight error here and it is mostly to do with tensions within the body.

Breathing to the Correct Point

When we inhale using the abdominal breathing method, our diaphragm moves downwards and the lungs expand to a high degree. The front part of our abdominal wall then expands (and to a lesser extent our lower back) and so we then need to identify which of three regions of the lower abdomen is the highest point of our breath.

There are different opinions on which point of the lower abdomen we expand and breathe into; they generally vary between the navel itself, the acupuncture point known as Qi Hai (Ren 6) and the acupuncture point known as Guan Yuan (Ren 4). These points are shown in Figure 5.5.

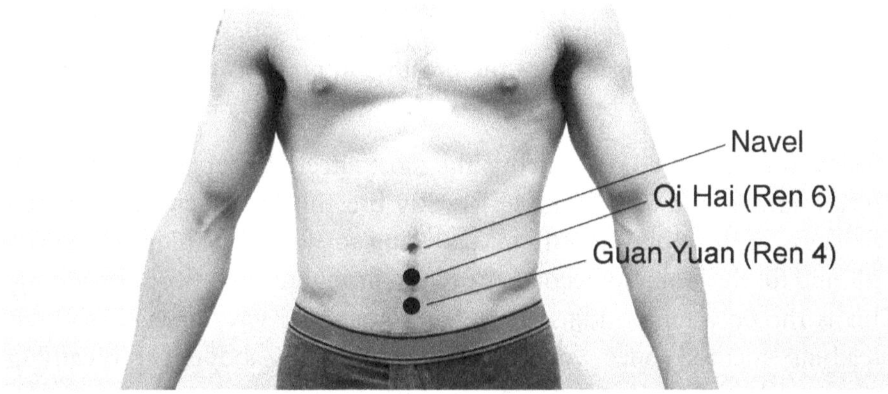

Figure 5.5: Lower Abdominal Acupuncture Points

In my personal experience, it is most efficient for our practice to breathe into the Qi Hai (Ren 6) point. If you wish to feel why, then take your index finger and place it onto each of the three points shown in Figure 5.5. Now take a few deep breaths and make an adjustment so that your lower abdomen expands into each of the points one at a time. Examine your body and feel what is taking place as you breathe into the points.

- **The navel:** Breathing into the navel means that the lower abdominal muscles are expanded unevenly with an emphasis on the upper abdominal muscles. The diaphragm tightens on the front of the ribs and the Qi does not sink fully down towards the lower Dan Tian region of the body. As a result, the breathing should feel as if it sticks higher than in the other two points discussed here. Those with a high level of internal sensitivity will also find that the temperature of the lower Dan Tian gradually drops as you breathe into the navel, as it causes Qi to move away from it. This is not good for our practice.

- **The Qi Hai (氣海) point:** Breathing into this point means that the emphasis on the expansion of the lower abdominal muscles is evenly spread. The space created in the abdomen should enable the diaphragm to fully expand downwards, which will, in turn, lead the breath and Qi down towards the lower Dan Tian. This should feel like the smoothest point to breathe into and create the most comfortable feeling on inhalation. The name of the Qi Hai point means the 'Sea of Qi', which refers to its close connection to the flow of Qi emanating from the lower Dan Tian itself.
- **The Guan Yuan (關元) point:** Breathing low into the abdomen, into Guan Yuan, unevenly emphasises the lower abdominal muscles, meaning that tightness is created in the sides and rear of the diaphragm. This restricts the breath and prevents the breath and Qi from effectively being led into the lower Dan Tian.

Once you have settled on which is the most effective acupuncture point to breathe into, spend some time just gently breathing and having a relaxed awareness of this point. It will not take long for your breathing to adjust a little and for this point to become the focus throughout all of your breathing. This is the only minor adjustment that you should have to make to your breathing method once you have developed the abdominal breathing technique through relaxed absorption of the awareness.

Breathing and Release

As you move through the five keywords of the mind, you will find that the body naturally begins to 'let go' of various layers of energetic stagnation. This is a natural progression of abdominal breathing, a further form of breathing that falls under the 'passive breathing' category. At this stage, you will begin to understand the energetic process of Song (松) or 'letting go'.

This removal of stagnation through Song then helps us to physically relax and ensure a healthy flow of Qi through the channel system as well as the Huang of the body; this serves to free up emotional tension from the mind. If we can reach a high enough level in our practice of this method, then we actually train our breathing to become a form of letting go.

Understanding the nature of tension is important for any practitioner of the internal arts. Tension is essentially stagnation; they are one and the same. Nothing can exist purely within the physical realm; it also has to have an energetic pattern and a 'consciousness' component, especially in the case of facets of human existence. If there is tension somewhere within the physical body, then there will also be a related blockage within the flow of Qi as well as an aspect of the acquired mind which is 'stuck'. More often than not, this 'acquired mind tension' is actually the root of the issue. These 'tensions' then transfer around our mind/body system in a circular fashion: physical tension will transfer into the mind, and mental tension will transfer into the body; this takes place via the channels of our energetic system which serve as a bridge between the two. This is demonstrated within the 'tension cycle' shown in Figure 5.6.

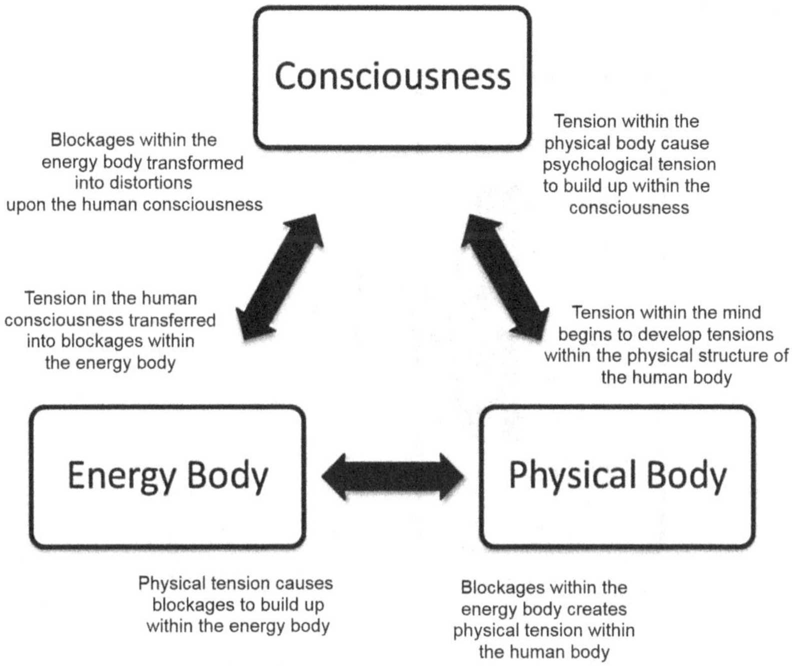

Figure 5.6: The Tension Cycle

By letting go of the tension (stagnation) on any of these three levels, we break the cycle which leads to the development of imbalance. When the body begins to let go of these blockages, we begin to find that our body is more relaxed, our health improves and the acquired mind begins to become more peaceful. This is particularly important because your biggest difficulty in the early stages of Nei Gong training is going to be dealing with an overactive mind that wants to wander from its allotted task.

In the earliest stages of this 'letting go' process, you will notice tensions within the physical body beginning to ease away. These tensions disappear first from within the large muscle groups. From here, we begin to relieve tension from within the Huang and sinew channels. The deepest stages of physical relaxation involve releasing stuck tensions from deep layers of the Huang surrounding our organs. During this process of letting go of tension, stuck energetic pathogens are released as well as old emotional patterns, which can be released through the experience of sudden mood shifts during your practice. This is because of the multi-layered nature of existence and the direct connection between the three bodies involved in the 'letting go' process.

As you grow used to the process, you will find that the tensions in the body as well as emotional baggage within the acquired aspect of the mind are leaving as a vibratory wave through your tissues. This is the passing of tension from the three bodies via the energetic realm as shown in Figure 5.7.

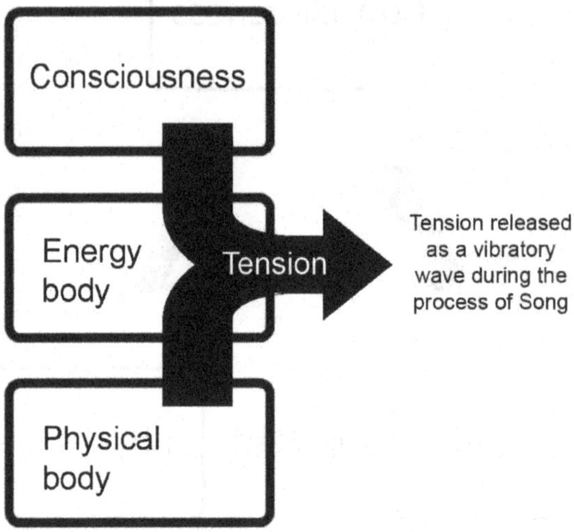

Figure 5.7: 'Letting Go' as a Vibratory Wave

This vibratory wave is a form of Qi, an expression of the movement of 'mind' out through the channel system. This vibratory wave serves to store 'information' from a variety of sources. All you need to do to find this wave is to go through the process of attaining abdominal breathing as discussed previously and maintain the process of absorption into your body. As you go deeper into the practice, the quality of letting go will begin to manifest for you. As this happens, the vibrations are very clear and tangible; it is as if a small shaking within the tissues begins to move through you and out of the body. In many cases, there will be small shudders and tremors in your soft tissues; don't worry about these, they will pass, don't focus on them, just let them come and go of their own accord.

As you move deeper into the process of letting go, you will become aware of a variety of somatic experiences. These can fall into the types of experience described below.

Some areas of the body will have feelings of pain or discomfort. These pains can vary from very sharp through to very subtle and slightly deeper. This feeling is often as if somebody is gently pressing on a bruise. In the case of bruise-like pain in the depth of the muscles, you are feeling an area of stagnation which needs releasing from the physical body.

The second group of sensations can exist within the energetic layer of the body. This means that as your mind passes over the area, there are sensations of unexplained cold, warmth, pressure, tightness or tingling. It is normal for your awareness to also become slightly stuck on these areas as though it is catching on something as it tries to pass by. These are areas of energetic stagnation which your awareness has tuned in to. If you gently become aware of the area of the physical body, you are likely to find feelings of being bruised in the same location. It is just that your mental frequency has shifted from the physical to the energetic.

The third sensation is an area of stagnation within the body which corresponds to an aspect of acquired mind which needs releasing. The 'glue' which bonds this stagnation into the body is always emotional in nature, so connecting with this stagnation will result in the experience of an emotional shift. You may suddenly become slightly sad or angry, or start to smile. It is normal for students to reach this stage and begin to unexpectedly weep or laugh. This is nothing to worry about, your awareness is just touching upon an area of stagnation whilst being tuned into the frequency of the emotional mind.

The body actually stores these tensions in the form of a complicated web, meaning that one tension will often hide another. Through maintenance of 'absorption of awareness' into the breathing process you will clear these areas, only to find that yet more areas of tension pop up! This is a result of moving deeper into the various layers of which your body is made up. Do not become frustrated at this, as the 'letting go' process is something that is never fully completed!

A Change of Perception

Upon hearing the term 'absorb the awareness into the breathing process', many people assume that it is referring to simply watching as your breath moves in and out of the body. Whilst this is true, it is simply the first stage; there are also countless other layers to this process. In order to fully explore some of these processes, it is necessary for the mind to be able to change its level of perception so that it can follow some of the processes which are taking place within the energetic matrix of your body. This will begin to happen naturally and takes no real focus or method. Your breathing can serve as a form of intermediary between the physical and the energetic realms as your awareness begins to tune into ever-deepening layers of your being. As you 'observe the breath' for longer, you will naturally start to become aware of the nature of Qi moving within your system. At first, this takes the form of various tingling sensations along the surface of the skin, waves of warmth flowing through the limbs, and then small movements inside the Huang of the body. At higher levels, it enables you to become aware of the movement of the auric field; this is a useful stage of energetic sensitivity to reach. You will begin to feel that the field of energy surrounding you contracts inwards upon your inhalation and expands outwards upon exhalation, as shown in Figure 5.8.

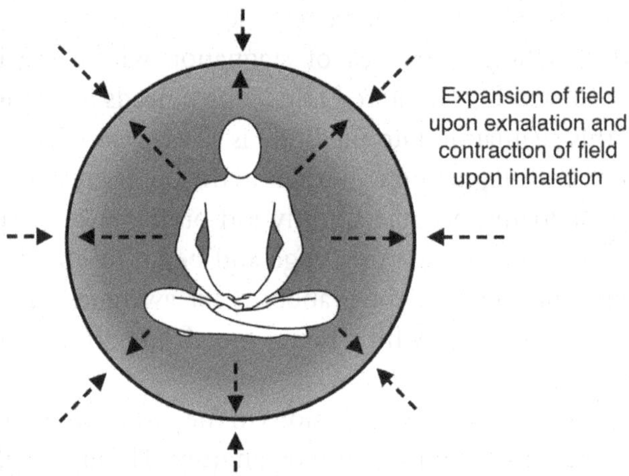

Figure 5.8: Breathing with the Auric Field

As your awareness is naturally led to this stage, you will find that you can clearly experience the place at which the auric field and your body interact. This is within the pores of the body all over your skin. It is an experience much like an energetic tide washing over your body as you breathe in and out. This is called pore breathing in Daoism, and it is a natural development of abdominal breathing once it has hit a certain level of efficiency.

Concluding Abdominal Breathing

So, if we look at all of this information, we can begin to see how different breathing methods and results can develop naturally out of one another. In the examples shown above, we can see that abdominal breathing gradually develops into Song breathing, and then from here we develop into pore breathing; both of these further developments of the breathing process are evolutions of the passive breathing type.

Of course, it is possible to manually train these types of breathing by specifically focusing upon their method and 'doing' this type of breathing practice. There is nothing inherently wrong with this; however, anything we 'do' will not be built into the deepest layers of our being. Only when we can start with the simplest exercise of absorbing the awareness into the body and increasingly relaxing our mind will we enable the evolution of our breathing processes to lead towards a true state of Gong.

Breathwork is deep. It takes a long time and there are always further layers of refinement involved. No matter how long I have studied these arts and no matter what other processes I am working on in my daily practice, I always save a little time for observing the breathing process; here, in the fundamental skills of passive breathing, lies enough material to keep you busy for your entire lifetime.

Reverse Abdominal Breathing Technique

The final breathing technique I wish to look at in this chapter is the more 'active' method of reverse abdominal breathing. In reverse abdominal breathing practice, we do the opposite of abdominal breathing methods. When we inhale, we draw in the lower abdomen, and when we exhale, we relax and allow it to expand once more. This process is shown in Figure 5.9.

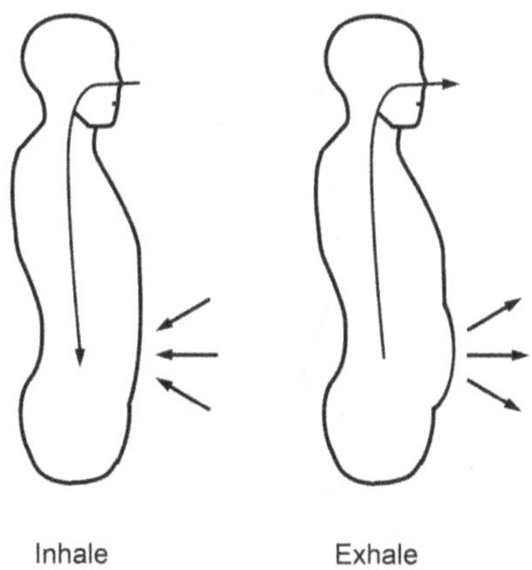

Figure 5.9: Reverse Abdominal Breathing

This means that we need to intervene a little in what the body is doing to ensure that we get the method right. Note that by this point you should have managed to develop your natural breathing to the stage of deep abdominal breathing as already discussed. You should not move on to any form of reverse breathing until you are sure you are at the right stage. This is for one simple reason: if you have not yet attained the right level of abdominal breathing, when you use reverse abdominal breathing, your diaphragm will go the wrong way. This is something that is missed by many practitioners; naturally, when you breathe in, your diaphragm should move downwards to create space in the chest cavity and to pressurise the abdominal cavity. This is exactly the same for both abdominal and reverse abdominal breathing. Many mistakenly believe that 'reverse abdominal breathing' allows the diaphragm to move upwards on the inhalation; this is simply not true. If this happens and you use reverse abdominal breathing in the wrong way, the raising of the diaphragm on the inhalation will raise Qi to the head and damage your lungs. This is the main reason why many have had problems with this method in the past.

There is very little you can actually do to control the direction your diaphragm takes when you inhale, it is too deep within the body to easily govern; instead, we simply wait until we have moved through the above stages of abdominal breathing before we 'reverse' the breath. This will ensure that our diaphragm moves in the right direction.

The same point of Qi Hai should move in on the lower abdomen; it is still the 'peak' of the abdominal movement. Essentially, this point moves back towards the rear of your body and passes through a line of connection that travels through your lower Dan Tian; this is shown in Figure 5.10.

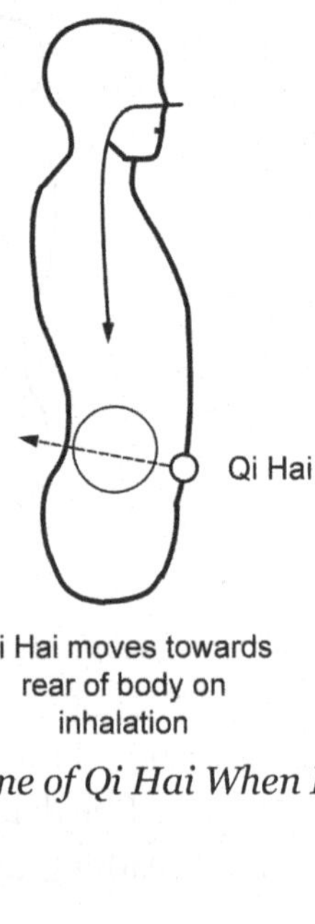

Figure 5.10: The Line of Qi Hai When Reverse Breathing

As this happens, the Qi of the lower Dan Tian is squeezed and so this serves to stimulate the Qi to a higher degree of movement throughout the body. It is a breathing method that helps to move things along in your practice and should be used for short periods of time.

Energetic Mechanism of Reverse Abdominal Breathing

When the breathing is reversed and the lower abdomen is drawn in, the lower Dan Tian is stimulated to a higher degree than in passive forms of breathing. Essentially, the whole of the abdominal cavity is squeezed from all directions when we breathe in this manner. The abdomen is drawn in, the diaphragm descends, and the rear is supported by the natural shape of your lower back. Within alchemical meditative practices we also draw the perineum up a little to support the base of the abdomen, but this is really not required for basic-level reverse abdominal breathing in standing or moving Nei Gong practice. In fact, it can cause stagnation, as the perineum can 'lock' the cavity in an unhealthy manner unless you are very open around the region of your Kua. This is a part of the reason it is primarily used in sitting practices; if a person can sit correctly in a meditation pose, the lower aspect of the body and the hips are naturally held open; this makes it more appropriate for the perineum to become involved. When we are standing, the perineum being raised can lead to a lot of tightness that is really not helpful for what we are trying to achieve.

As the lower Dan Tian is squeezed, it is like pressurising a liquid within the lower abdomen. Obviously, this is not literally what is happening, it is just easier to think of it in this manner. When the liquid in the lower abdominal cavity is pressurised, it will want to move, to lessen the pressure. The result of this is that it will begin to move towards the nearest 'escape point'. If the diaphragm is being lowered in the correct way, then the escape point for this liquid is going to be the lower back, specifically the sacrum and the lumbar region of the spine. This is the origin of the Governing channel which we will use later for establishing the first of the key rotations of Nei Gong practice. Figure 5.11 shows the different movements of these paths, both correct and incorrect.

Here lies some of the danger from incorrect reverse breathing practice. If the diaphragm is not yet moving downwards on your inhalation, then the easiest 'escape point' will be upwards through your body. Instead of moving into the Governing channel, the energy that raises will increase the level of activity through your body. You will start to go into a more Yang or 'hyper' state. This will overstimulate the nervous system and the emotions and, with consistent practice, start to negatively impact the health of the Liver and the Heart. Since this usually happens over a lengthy period of time, practitioners will not necessarily be aware of this increase in the quality of Yang, as they learn to normalise it. The mind and body will compensate for the change of internal state and so you can slowly burn up your health without necessarily being aware of it. Eventually, though, your error will catch up with you. To make sure that this does not happen, we check that we have built a solid enough foundation in the five keywords of breathing and developed the skill of abdominal breathing to a high enough degree.

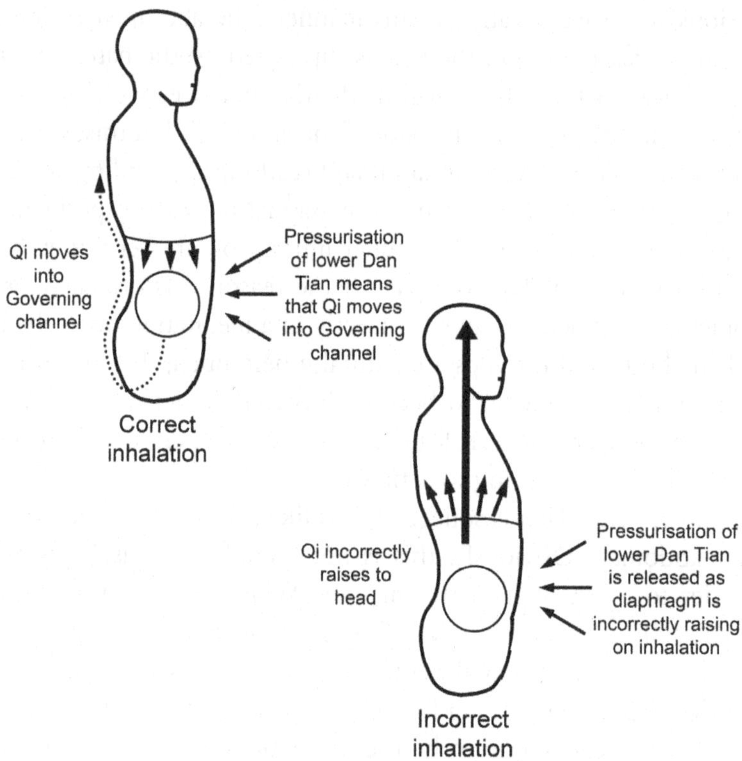

Figure 5.11: Different Results of Reverse Abdominal Breathing

Deflate the Abdomen, Don't Squeeze the Muscles

I will not discuss reverse abdominal breathing too much here, as we shall return to it further into the Nei Gong process. I will make clear at which stage of the process reverse abdominal breathing can be helpful. I just want to give an overview of what it is and how it works. Most importantly, I wish to bring to your attention a major error that many people make when they start this breathing: they use their abdominal muscles. In fact, you should 'deflate' the abdomen instead. This might sound like a minor detail, but it is a really big deal. There have been many people who burnt themselves out and did themselves harm with overuse of this breathing method; if they had made sure that they deflated the abdomen to begin the method and combined this with a diaphragm that travelled downwards, they would have been fine and no problems would have occurred.

What I mean by this is that there are two ways to initiate the contraction of the abdominal cavity. The first and most instinctive method is to contract your abdominal muscles; if not instructed otherwise, almost everybody will do this. The second is to slowly 'deflate' the abdominal cavity as you inhale. This might sound strange, but it is as if you are sucking the air out of your abdomen as you inhale through your nose! If you overthink it, it sounds odd. If you simply give it a go, it is not that difficult. Basically, I inhale through my nose and allow the inside of my abdominal cavity to decrease in size. The result of this is that the abdominal wall is brought in and I have not had to use any great amount of muscular contraction in the abdominal muscles to achieve this.

If you breathe in this way, there is no major build-up of pressure – a pressure that can be overstimulating – and the abdominal wall only moves in by a couple of centimetres. This is all we need for the method. We are not trying to suck our guts inwards as in some Yogic cleansing methods; the movement of the lower abdomen is very slight.

Concluding Reverse Abdominal Breathing

As stated above, we shall return to reverse abdominal breathing when it is more relevant to the process; this has just been a short introduction to the method.

If you are working through the material in this book, then do not hurry onto the reverse breathing technique. Take your time and develop a strong practice of deep abdominal breathing first; do not rush. The more time you spend on the foundations, the better.

As a final note, after you have been practising reverse abdominal breathing, always take some time to check that you have returned to regular abdominal breathing afterwards. You don't want to get stuck in the reverse pattern as it is too stimulating to become your normal breathing method; you will end up feeling like you have just drunk several coffees and your Kidneys will suffer.

A Note on Sweating but Not Panting

The phrase 'sweat but not pant' was mentioned above, but it would be wise to return your attention to it once again as it is a very important guideline for practice. Within Nei Gong theory, the opening of your pores and the generation of light sweating is a result of the circulation of Yang Qi. Within Chinese medicine, this is a little different: there are other factors involved in sweating, but for Nei Gong we use a much simpler model. We want the Yang Qi to circulate within the body, so it is considered healthy for your practice if there is a light sweat during your training. Note here, though, that I said a 'light' sweat. A heavy sweat usually indicates something else; if it is all of the time, then it can indicate a chronic imbalance, but if it is in short, acute bursts, then it can be down to a pathogenic release.

It is for this reason that the Daoists never liked to practise Qi Gong in draughts or outdoors in windy weather. If the pores are open, then the energy body is more receptive to the outside environment. This means that when you train, you have the possibility of absorbing the quality of the wind into your body; this can disturb both the Qi and the Blood.

If you are out of breath or gasping for air, then there are several factors to be aware of:

- First, you are upsetting the energetic pattering of the Heart. This will make it much harder to regulate your mind.
- You are also messing with the balance of oxygen and carbon dioxide within your body; this will impact your body's ability to process and produce Qi.
- The strenuous work that your lungs are carrying out during your 'panting' means that the Qi within your body is rising; this will mean that the lower Dan Tian is not the focus of your practice.
- When you are breathing in this way, you are changing to an 'external' model of movement; the 'internal' has become lost. Whilst this may not be an issue to a person who is pushing the boundaries of their fitness for physical gain, it is no good for people wanting to build up their internal state.

If sweating and panting are balanced correctly, this will enable you to draw the most benefit from your training.

The Daoists' only exception to this guideline was very elderly or weak people. The Yang Qi was better for these groups of people; it was maintained within the body so that it could nourish them and help them recuperate some lost vitality. For this reason, there was a slightly different rule for them: 'no sweating and no panting'!

Practising the Breath Regulation Exercises

Practising the exercises in this chapter can be done during moving Qi Gong exercises or during static practice, but they can also be isolated out into sessions where you are just lying on your back or sitting, either in a chair or on the floor. Make sure that you maintain a good posture if you are sitting down, just as you would when standing in Wuji.

If you are new to this kind of work, I would suggest working on the passive forms of breathing; sink your awareness into the body and try working with your breath until you feel that the five keywords are starting to manifest through your practice. Practise short sessions at first, and only let them stretch out into longer practice sessions once it feels natural to do so. Don't force anything, don't try to impose your will on your breath; stay relaxed, be kind to yourself and, through gentle application of your awareness, allow your breathing to evolve of its own accord.

Chapter 6

REGULATING AND SHAPING THE MIND

In the previous chapters, we have looked at the basic regulation of the body and regulation of our breathing. The third regulation is that of the mind. When these three aspects have been sufficiently regulated, then we shall have all of the ingredients we need to successfully delve into the world of Daoist Nei Gong practice.

There is obviously a vast wealth of teachings coming out of Asia that are focused on developing the mind and spirit. We only need to look at the sheer amount of writings that have been produced upon this very subject to see just how much exploration of the human psyche has taken place over the centuries. Within the practice of Nei Gong it is no different; there is a great deal of work to do that is 'mind-focused'. Much of this takes on a very alchemical quality to it and we shall return to this in the later sections of the book when we look at the differences between cultivating the mind and elevating the spirit. For now, though, we are still at a foundation level in our practice; we simply need to look at two factors – regulating the mind so that it can effectively move into Nei Gong training, and 'shaping' the mind so that it can connect with the tradition of Daoism.

Regulating the Mind

Essentially, at these early stages of training, regulation of the mind is closely connected to regulation of our breathing. In the previous chapter, we looked at the five keywords of breathing. These words describe a series of developmental stages that your breathing goes through as you develop effective abdominal breathing. Essentially, these words can be applied to the mind as well. If you have started to work on the previous breathing exercise already, then you will have noticed a change starting to take place in your mind. Let us return to these five keywords.

Quiet

As we allow our awareness to absorb into the body along with the process of our breathing, it should naturally start to grow more still. There is a calming effect that the breathing has upon the mind. As discussed previously, our emotional state and our breathing are inextricably linked. As the breathing starts to become quiet, so does the mind; in the same way, as our mind grows quieter, the breathing follows. It is this linking of mind and breath that has formed the foundations of many meditative systems.

There is another aspect of quietening of the mind to be aware of here: this is the strength of 'absorption'. To be absorbed in something means to be fully mentally engaged with it, lost in the practice or experience that is unfolding for you. To be fully absorbed in any activity means that the mind is content; it loves absorption!

Remember that what your mind craves all day, every day, is stimulation. It needs stimulation to develop and grow in the way it is desiring to go. The more stimuli it can feed on, the more it can carry out its natural function, which is keep developing your acquired self. This is how it learns.

We can see this is the case if we have ever tried to meditate. Perhaps you are experienced with this practice already and have developed some Gong in meditation, but I am sure you can remember your earliest attempts at any kind of quiet sitting practice. You sit down, close your eyes, and 'boom', there goes your mind. It races through a whole stream of pointless thoughts, one after another. It is as if somebody has amplified your mental activity and ramped it right up to its maximum level! Of course, with practice, this situation changes, but this is what happens in the early days of meditation practice.

As much as anything, what the mind is doing is providing itself with a form of stimulation. You have shut off your senses, the five thieves have been taken away. Starved of its stimuli from the outside world, the mind instead starts to produce a random stream of thoughts. If we ignore those thoughts, then they disappear, generally to be replaced by other thoughts. There is a lengthy process of one thought fading and another taking its place. Here the mind is giving itself a series of options, like presenting dish after dish for a fussy customer until one of them looks appetising enough to start eating. As soon as one of the thoughts looks interesting, then you become involved; the sheer action of getting involved with the emerging thought feeds it energy, and hey presto – you have a thought stream! The thought expands into a stream of thoughts and so the mind has what it wants, it has engaged you. By engaging you, it can start to carry out its role of helping build your acquired self.

The ancient Chinese talk of the mind as being like a monkey in its behaviour. The monkey is hyperactive and attention-seeking. It is jumping up and down right there in front of you all the time. One way of training the monkey is to give it a banana. The 'banana' we give it is our breath. Absorption into our breathing is the distraction that the mind is given in our practice. Yes, it is still a stimulus of sorts, so it is not perfect, but it is enough to satisfy the mind enough that it does not need to tempt us over and over with a stream of random mental activity. It is a stop-gap for sure; later we must use more refined methods, but it will serve our purposes at this stage.

As we become adept at this, we should find that the mind grows more still; the monkey-mind is satisfied for now, and so we can allow the quietness of the mind to grow. This serves to assist in the quietening of the breath as well as setting us on the path of regulating the mind.

Deep

As with when they are applied to breathing practice, the keywords follow a sequential order based upon a naturally unfolding causation chain. This means that in order to develop this second quality of 'deep', we simply continue to quieten the mind.

When the breath starts to become 'deeper', it means that it slows down. The length of our breathing generally extends and more of our lungs are being used. It also, most crucially, sinks downwards so that we breathe from the lower abdominal region. This also helps to 'deepen' the place from which our mind operates. The mind is slowed and functions according to the qualitative properties of the lower Dan Tian. Within Daoism the ancient Chinese talk of three 'types of thought' and where they come from. These are shown in Figure 6.1. As you can see, they correlate with the approximate locations of the three Dan Tian.

When our thoughts are based in our upper Dan Tian region, they are cerebral, intellectual and very cognitive. This is useful for problem solving and practical skills such as study and learning. It is not helpful for our Nei Gong practice, though. The location of your thoughts for reading this book, for example, is in this region. Very cerebral people, scholars and such like, spend most of their lives operating from this place. This is why one of the first instructions given to me when I began meditation was to 'get out of my head'! This meant to start to sink away from this place so that the quality of my mind could change.

The second region of thought is the Heart. Here we have emotionally based thoughts. Memories of loved ones and influential experiences, both positive and negative, are based in this location. Often, when we start to practise sitting meditation, you will experience the same process: phase one is a whole process of random mental activity. Here we are still 'in our head'. Phase two involves sinking the mind's location a little, and then we shift into emotional experiences and more 'memory-based' movements of the mind. The final phase is the sinking to the lower Dan Tian.

The third region of thought, the lower Dan Tian, is a more stable place. The thoughts here are more steady and quieter. It is as if your mind is more 'grounded' from this place. This is where we wish the mind to go to, this is the deepening of the mind that comes with deepening the breath.

When you have practised for a while, you will find that the mind is able to stabilise in this location. Every now and then, your mind will rise, though, and you will feel the change of conscious location as well as the change of the nature of your thoughts. It is interesting to note that you can tangibly feel the change of location and often your breathing changes accordingly. This is a good thing, though – the more awareness you have of the process, the more it will unfold in the right direction.

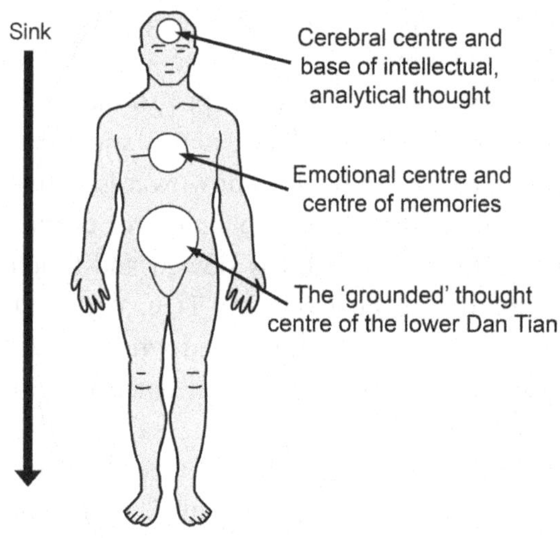

Figure 6.1: The Three Regions of Thought

At Ease

As the breath and mind deepen in their quality, they will start to reach the stage of being 'at ease'. The result is a feeling I can only describe as 'stable tranquillity'. The mind will like to stay rooted into the lower abdomen at this stage and the whole practice will feel very pleasant indeed. It is here, at this level of mental regulation, that you are able to let go of many things you are holding on to. It is here, at stage three in the process of moving through the keywords, that true calm will start to change the quality of your mental state.

This feeling of being at ease cannot go hand in hand with racing thoughts and emotions. Whilst we do not require profound levels of stillness at this stage, we do require the mind to have reached a deep level of inner calm; it needs to be at ease with itself.

Slow and Gradual

Once your mind is at ease, it will begin to spread out through the body. It will move like gentle waves, following the ebbs and pulses of your Qi until it can suffuse into the Huang, from the surface of your body through to the deepest levels. This 'slow and gradual' movement of the mind will unfold naturally and bring about a high level of mind/body connection.

Cotton Soft

The final development of the mind that will unfold through the regulation process is that it will develop a soft quality to it. It is like a fine mist that spreads over the body, it is all-encompassing and is now fully absorbed into the body. This is a high level of Gong if you can reach this stage.

The Intellectual Versus the Absorption Method

As we can see from the process discussed above, the key to regulation of the mind within Nei Gong comes from absorption into the breath and thus the body. The interconnectedness of body, breath and mind becomes our tool for helping develop our mind in the right direction. It is a simple, and yet surprisingly intricate, method for helping us build a solid foundation in this area of our practice. It is a method we should return to many times, over a long period; the attainment of true Gong relies on having absorbed the mind into the breath and practice for a long time.

I should point out a clear trap that many fall into when looking to regulate the mind. Do not confuse actual regulation of the mind with 'intellectual trickery'. What I mean by this is that there are a countless number of books that talk endlessly of the philosophy and nature of 'stilling the mind', what this means and how you do it. Whilst this is not inherently negative (this very book is, in part, also a discussion of stilling the mind!), you should not mistake actual practice with simply reading about and cognitively tricking yourself into thinking that you have achieved it. 'Understanding' and 'doing' are two very different things. Intellectually understanding the regulation process means that you are 'still in your head'. This is a place we need to start at, for obvious reasons, but then we need to transfer this theory into practice and 'get out of our head'. If we wish to look at the difference between 'doing' and 'understanding', we can say that the 'doing' is the regulation of the mind aspect of our practice, whilst the 'understanding' is the shaping of the mind. They are quite distinct from each other and we shall now look at what it means to shape the mind.

Shaping the Mind

Shaping the mind for Nei Gong practice takes place in two ways: through externally trained methods, and through internally cultivated qualities. If we look back to Chapter 2, we discussed there the three aspects of spirit, consciousness and mind. Generally, it is very difficult to contact human spirit for a very long time in our practice, apart from in very fleeting moments. Consciousness is also difficult to work with; we will return to this in Chapter 12 when we look at what it means to study a spiritual practice. What we will engage with first in our practice is the mind, the outer expressions of our conscious makeup. Figure 6.2 shows a summary of the various layers of spirit, consciousness and mind.

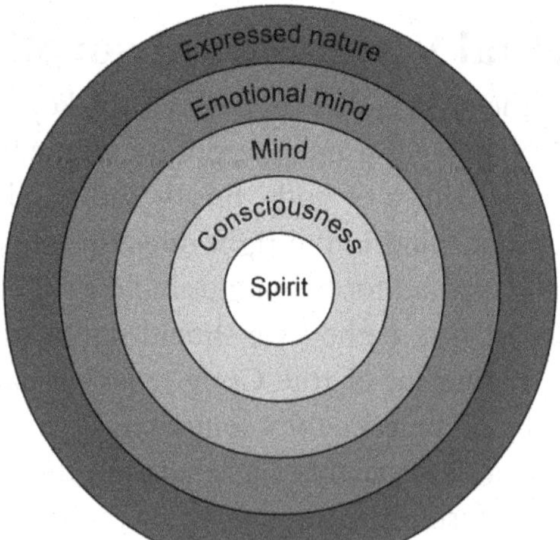

Figure 6.2: Spirit, Consciousness and Mind

The collective name for these three aspects of our being, spirit, consciousness and mind, and how they are expressed into the world, is our Xing (性) or 'nature'. It is said within the classical teachings of Daoism that if we purify and reconsolidate the various components that make up our Xing, then we will regain connection to that original 'spark' that generated who we are; this is an aspect of our deep inner being known as the 'seed consciousness'.

In order to start working towards this end, we must first engage with the outer expressions of who we are – our mind. This is the acquired aspect of ourselves, that part of our inner environment that we associate with mental activities, emotional expression, learnt behaviours and even our personality. It is the part of us that interacts with the outer world and the 'face' that we show to the people we interact with on a daily basis.

Our mind can be taken in many directions, there are countless possibilities. What we do with our mind, how we interact with it and how we decide to train it really decides which direction our mind evolves in. As discussed in Chapter 2, because the mind is the root of our Qi, how we then develop our mind dictates the quality of our Qi. This, in turn, then interfaces with our physical body via the channel system and so our material evolution also begins to take direction.

In order to get the most from our practice, we generally have to learn how to shape the mind in the most effective way for what we do. By 'shaping the mind' I mean training it in a very specific manner. Think of the mind as being no different from your body. As previously stated, if we wish to get the most out of Qi Gong training, we have to build or shape the body in the right way for Qi Gong. This is the same for our mind: it was recognised in Daoism that how we 'build' the mind will dictate just how efficiently we will be able to use it for engagement with the Nei Gong process.

The internally based shaping of the mind comes from understanding the balance between 'focus' and 'release'. We shall return to this at the end of the chapter. First, though, let us look at that shaping that comes from an external origin. These externally originated sources for the mind exist in classical ethical teachings, precepts (yes, Daoism has precepts, no matter what you may have heard), and in psychological qualities that the tradition tried to encourage you to develop. I wish to draw attention to these aspects of Daoism, especially the precepts, since they are an area of the tradition that so rarely appears in contemporary writings on the tradition. Nei Gong as a practice has its roots in Daoism. Of course, other traditions have also been an influence upon its development and there are even Nei Gong systems that are primarily Buddhist in nature, but these are later developments. The source of Nei Gong lay within the Daoist schools.

This is important for two main reasons: first, in order to fully understand any art, you really need to understand the culture it was developed within. Second, these traditions were never 'religions' in the sense we understand the term today; they were systems of practice. The practice was designed to initially change the manner in which your body developed and then to change the quality of your mind. They understood that in order to do this, there would have to be some kind of mental training, guidance on your behaviours that would then influence the way that your mind worked. Essentially, all this comes down to ethical teaching.

Now, I am not saying that you need to follow these guidelines, that is up to you. To give up your free will and blindly obey another's moral compass is always the wrong thing to do; instead, you should explore and question everything to see how it applies to you and your own belief system. The precepts I will discuss here were specifically for those formally initiated into the Daoist tradition and served to guide them and help shape their mind in the right way. They helped to direct a person's actions and outlook on life in a way that was deemed most beneficial to their development. If you look at these and use them as a starting point, what I would suggest is then having a look at your own moral compass and deciding what values and morals are most important to you. The stronger you adhere to your ethical stance, the more your mind is shaped in a very specific manner. That being said, I personally find the basic Daoist precepts to be fairly common sense; I try to apply them to my life as they align very well with my own personal values.

Before we look at them, though, let us explore a little more Daoist philosophy that directly relates to precepts and shaping the mind.

An Introduction to Xing and Ming

Within Daoist teachings, there are two very important factors known as Xing (性) and Ming (命). These two key aspects of human life are vital in understanding the wider scope of Nei Gong practice and progressing your arts beyond the earliest stages. Xing is generally translated to mean 'nature', referring to a person's nature rather than the outside environment. Ming, however, is a little harder to translate; often terms such as 'life', 'destiny' and 'fate' are used.

Ultimately, Daoism and alchemy focused on learning to perfect and then merge Xing and Ming, as it was recognised these two elements formed the 'mechanics' behind the manifestation of human life. Your Xing, or nature, is in simplistic form your mental faculties and, in its essence, the manner in which 'seed consciousness' transforms into your perceptions and connection to existence. This refers to your every psychological aspect from thought processes and cognitions through to your world views and perceptions. Ultimately, the quality of your Xing determines how deeply you can enter into elevated states of consciousness through meditative training. The Ming is more complex, manifesting into the body as your health but also as your process through life on a physical level – it is your connection to the wave of information that passes through into existence from the realm of Dao, as shown in Figure 6.3.

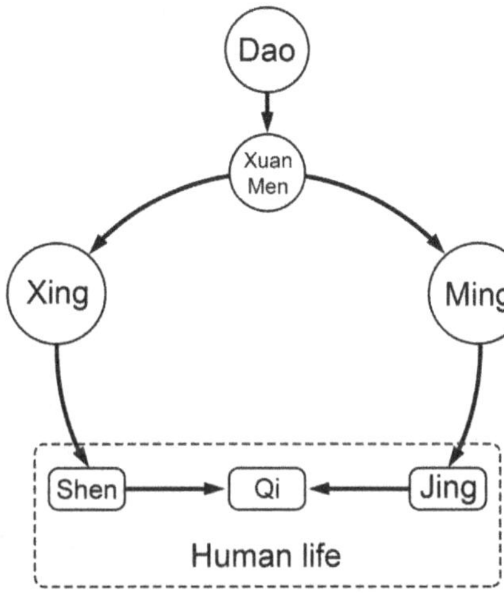

Figure 6.3: The Information of Dao Through to Existence

Xing and Ming are thought to divide from a singular point of origin: the point of creation. This is relevant to those who wish to go deep into Daoism, because by seeking to unify Xing and Ming it is possible to find that original point. This search for union is constantly referred to in Daoist classics, from the Dao De Jing and Zhuang Zi (莊子) through to more obscure, lesser-known writings. These two facets of existence must be brought together in order to create an original point of stillness. When Xing and Ming converge, the opening of Xuan Men (玄門) occurs. Xuan Men is normally translated as 'the mysterious pass' and is perceived through meditation practice as a very literal opening, or gateway, through which information can pass. Rather than having a literal location in the body, the Xuan Men is a pathway through into divine states of being which opens when Xing and Ming move into harmony. This is the result of a very deep layer of Yin and Yang finding union with one another.

An Emphasis on Balance

Within Daoism, both the Xing and the Ming of a person should be worked with for a balanced practice. Some systems, both within Daoism and other traditions, overemphasise one element of the practice over the other. A practice working purely with the Xing would be considered unbalanced as it is understood within Daoism that the body is a manifestation of the Ming and therefore must be engaged with. Conversely, practices focused purely on health, the conditioning of the body and longevity would also be considered unbalanced as the Xing is ignored, and the pursuit of unity is missed. Daoism has a very practical view of unity: if the practice is imbalanced either towards Xing or Ming, the mechanics behind the search for the point of creation are 'faulty' and therefore the practice is redundant. I have personally met teachers who have tried to cultivate one in lieu of the other, and the results are often clear to see. Those who favoured the Xing tend to suffer with poor health; they have a lack of Gong in the body though they may have attained great states of conscious liberation. The second group, those who have favoured Ming over Xing, tend to have great physical health. The efficiency of the way their body functions gives them great power with regard to how they can control and manipulate Qi, and yet, they have a lack of virtuous aspects to their nature. All of their skill does not add up to either happiness or spiritual elevation. Both of these ways of working go against the natural balance of the Daoist ethos.

Daoists Versus Confucianists

Interestingly, the nature of Xing and De (德) (commonly translated as 'virtue[s]') is where you will find the largest divide between Daoism and the other main tradition to come out of China – Confucianism. De is a fundamental aspect of Daoism, its prominence shown in being one of the three characters of one of the most important classics, the Dao De Jing. The De, virtue, is seen to be the purest manner in which a person can interact, perceive and react to the world, which from the outside should appear as wisdom and compassion incarnate. For Daoism, a state of connection to the De is the natural way for a human to express their relationships and interactions; therefore, the more one strips away the acquired self, the more the De should arise – a constant state of original being. The Confucianists, however, viewed humans very differently – within their tradition, humans don't inherently have De, but rather the virtues ought to be trained and maintained through external tools. It is a similar divide in thought as the more Western 'nature versus nurture' argument, and I believe it is this fundamental difference in philosophical thought that created a strong divide between the two schools of thought.

Virtues, Qualities and Precepts

The virtue that a person brings out through their practice is very functional within Daoism. Daoism is not inherently interested in the 'morality' behind being a compassionate and wise human; however, this state helpfully brings about in a person exactly the right internal environment for internal advancement. Therefore, attaining a state of true compassion and wisdom is to be strived for, so as to find this internal point within the body. Another element within Daoism is the Xin (心), often translated as 'Heart' or 'Heart Mind', as the two are interchangeable. It is through the Xin that the purest expression of information can be expressed: the De. If a person manages to sustain and express this level of purity, their expression of pure consciousness shines through in their speech and actions. As a by-product of the generation of De a person is said to begin eroding the influence of cause and effect upon their being, a process simply termed Ye (業) – the Daoist approach to the concept of Karma.

For most people, the De generally becomes distorted into emotion. This is why within Chinese medicine textbooks the emotions are treated as pathogens rather than positive states of being. Whilst that's not to say people shouldn't experience emotions, pragmatically, within Daoism, each emotion experienced and attached to by the mind merely adds layers to the acquired self. This addition of layers moves people away from a heightened state of being, increasing the difficulty in finding and working with the mechanics behind more advanced practices. This process of virtues being transformed into emotions is summarised in Figure 6.4.

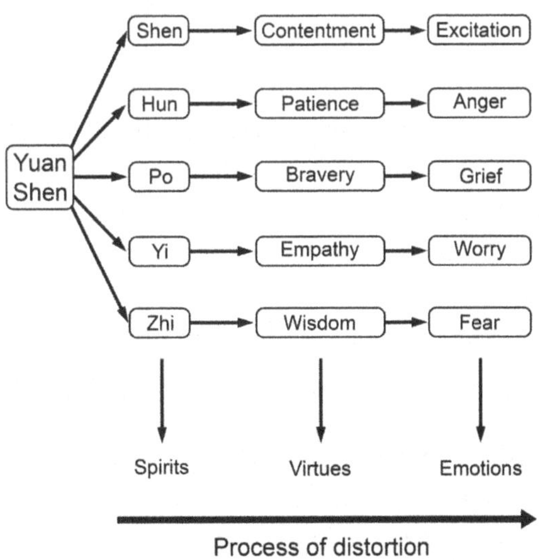

Figure 6.4: Virtues to Emotions

In order to change your Xing, there are two major categories of methods: internal and external. Generally, different traditions place varying levels of importance on one method or the other – for example, Confucianism would place greater importance on external methods of transformation, as discussed in their key text, the Analects. An internal method would be attempting to adjust, through a practice such as Nei Gong or meditation, the way in which information is expressed through the Heart Mind; this generates spontaneous change from internal practice out into your external nature. Therefore, if a person can engage with a practice for a length of time, they should generally become more centred, inwardly balanced and more content.

Whilst nowadays systems such as Daoism often have a preference towards either internal or external transformation, if you take Daoism back to its basis in classical texts, you will find a very even split of internal and external practices. This is mainly because practice at this time was centred on 'sitting and allowing the muddy waters to settle', a phrase essentially referring to the conversion process that takes place within the Xing.

The reason behind using external tools to change the Xing is very little to do with ethics and morality in a classical sense – that would be a Confucian approach. Within Daoism, every one of your thought processes and actions has an energetic mechanic behind it, so one way to change your internal landscape is to change your external actions. Therefore, the external rules in Daoism are designed to retrain your mind through consciously changing your behaviour, to eventually change your Xing. Once this is accomplished, the energetic mechanics behind your thought processes and actions will more efficiently lead you towards higher states within your practice. This directly affects the quality of your Jing, Qi and Shen. This is absolutely key and the basis for many understandings when people first encounter Daoism. Daoism does indeed have teachings on how you should be, how to act and how to deal with others. As with other traditions, the basis of this is to do others no harm and to live in accordance with a humble and compassionate view of life. *But*, the main reason for this was because it set up a certain resonance within the centre of a person's consciousness that would help bring them closer to Dao.

This is why some other schools of thought were against Daoism as a tradition and opposed to its lack of obvious morality at its core. Though the outer result was the same – compassion towards all – the inner rationale was quite clearly 'practice-based'. For those who have problems with this, I would put it to you that perhaps the other traditions we are familiar with had similar reasons in the beginning. Perhaps their rationale for *why* we cultivate certain qualities inside of us was changed in a kind of 'public relations' exercise?

Changing yourself using external methods relies on several things – first and foremost, your intention. This is something that is utilised and worked on from the very start of your training in any spiritual tradition, and often it's easiest to think of it as something that needs to be controlled to settle the mind or carry out a particular function (energetic or physical). However, another aspect to your intention is its governance over how quickly it is possible for you to progress through your chosen system. It sounds simplistic, but creating or 'shaping' your intention correctly towards certain behavioural patterns aids that change to occur naturally within your Xing.

Precepts in Daoism

Precepts in Daoism are classically divided into two main categories, those that are 'rules' and those that are 'qualities'. Both categories of these precepts are designed to help align a person's internal state so that they may resonate directly with the frequency of the Daoist tradition. Below are listed the key rules and qualities that are adhered to and developed within alchemical Daoist traditions.

In modern times, it is actually now little known that Daoism even had precepts of any sort. The generally held view is that a person should simply 'do what is natural', with no regards to curtailing or adjusting their behaviour. This is a very dangerous course to take, as the difficulty lies in the fact that nobody operates according to what is truly 'natural' for their Xing. The layers of acquired mind distort your inner perception so that 'acting natural' with no restraint often leads to imbalanced and damaging behaviour focused largely on self-gratification. To 'act naturally' within Daoism should actually be to 'act in accordance with Ziran (自然)'. In this context, 'Ziran' refers to an inherently natural and unified state of being that is only achieved once the distortions of the mind have been smoothed out, something that only occurs through long periods of deep internal cultivation. The question arises: if we are to act naturally, are we acting according to our mind or our consciousness? This, of course, would depend upon our level of personal cultivation. Precepts were one way of safeguarding people's behaviour when still at the 'mind' stage.

Each Daoist tradition generally had its own take on the precepts, but generally they were all a variation of the following key themes. The examples below are taken from the Zhi Hui Ding Xin Jing (智慧定心經) or Classical Text of Aligning the Will with Wisdom, a series of teachings that form part of the more recently discovered Dunhuang (敦煌) manuscripts.

Rule-type precepts

- Be mindful of the cause and effect of dealing with people
- Do not commit any sexual misconduct
- Do not steal nor deal with those who do
- Tell only truth and do not mislead others with your speech
- Avoid intoxication and conduct yourself with purity
- Honour your family, hereditary line and ancestors
- Carry out kind actions and support those who do
- Assist those who are less fortunate in regaining their dignity and fortune
- Carry out your actions in accordance with the Dao, yet don't expect the same of others
- Place others' attainment of Dao above your own

Quality-type precepts

- Cultivate humility
- Cultivate humour
- Live with simplicity
- Adhere to and develop Wu Wei
- Cultivate compassionate qualities

In understanding precepts within any spiritual tradition, we should understand that they have two levels of usefulness. The first level is the external, often known as 'outer door' understanding of the precepts. In this case, if we look at both the 'rule-type' and 'quality-type' precepts, we can see that they are clearly useful on an external level as a code of ethical guidance. This is the level of understanding that the 'uninitiated' students would classically have had. When the traditions became more widely spread and the general public had access to Daoist teachings, it was the 'outer door' understandings which people were given, and this helped to support harmony within cultures and groups of people.

Daoism as a Frequency

The internal or 'inner door' understanding of precepts is more esoteric and based upon the concept of harmonisation with a divine frequency. According to this way of thinking, Daoism itself is a frequency. Rather than a set of external teachings it is, at its heart, a largely intangible source of information which a person may tap into if they are able to adjust their mind to such a state that their inner mental frequency is in resonance with Dao itself. Any external teachings and methods were largely to help take 'inner door' students closer to this state of mental resonance and, alongside this, skilled masters would use spiritual transmissions known as Xin Yin (心印) or 'mind stamps' and lineage inductions known as Bai Shi (拜師). The principle is that once a person can embody the principles of the tradition on a deep, experiential level, then they will be drawn into line with Dao and thus the teachings of the lineages would pour into their being. This is known as the 'miraculous learning' or sometimes the 'magical knowing'.

Let us look at each of the two categories of precepts individually, beginning with the rule-type precepts.

The Precepts in More Detail

Rule-Type Precepts

Be Mindful of the Cause and Effect of Dealing with People

One of the key concerns within the Daoist tradition was to cause as little change to other people's lives as possible. They viewed the average human as being something of a 'bull in a china shop', trampling their way through life, sending Karmic ripples out into the world around them. With little in the way of self-awareness or awareness of others, every little action generated shifts, some subtle and some large, outwards to change the life paths of those around them.

Cause and effect is a major component of existence and one of the major threads which binds the whole human race together. The Daoist view is that life is like one large cobweb with unfathomable amounts of threads connecting everything and everybody together. The aim is to 'leave no footprints' during your life. This saying has been spread through Daoist literature for some time now; in many cases it has been completely misunderstood. The commonly held view is that a Daoist should be anonymous all of the time; they should not tell you their name nor allow anybody to know they exist. This is a huge confusion; this is not 'leaving no footprints', this is hiding in the shadows. 'Leaving no footprints' means to live without causing any disturbances in the lives of those around you. This can only happen with constant and unwavering awareness of those around you as well as of your thoughts, perceptions and actions. This is something that is very hard to achieve and means that active mindfulness has to permeate through into everything you do.

Interestingly, there is also a second meaning in this phrase that has to do with inner awareness. In the Daoist classics, the term 'people' is often used to refer to the emotional movements of the mind. In this case, the body is viewed metaphorically as a 'country' and its 'inhabitants' the movements of mind. Here, the hidden meaning of the precept is to maintain 'mindful listening' – known as Ting (聽) in Chinese – when dealing with your emotions.

Do Not Commit Any Sexual Misconduct

The strongest way in which two human beings can connect with each other is through sexual intercourse. For humans, the act of having sex is mixed with our deepest emotional layers as well as our ideas of love and intimacy. Clearly, the spiritual nature of sex goes much deeper than simply a bodily act which leads to the production of new life. Even those who are in the greatest amount of denial concerning the emotional nature of sexual intercourse do not get off scot-free when they engage in intercourse. The by-products of sex run from emotional connection through to a change in the nature of Yin and Yang within both participants' bodies. Each time we sleep with another person of either gender, we radically change our own internal frequency so that it moves closer to our partner's. Even with this understanding, we can immediately see how this would be an issue for those who wish to align themselves fully with a spiritual tradition such as Daoism.

It is for these reasons that the Daoist tradition had a great many teachings on sex. Known originally as 'dual-cultivation' methods, they were an attempt to work with the shifting energies involved in having sex. These teachings included instruction on finding the correct partner, how to harmonise your own auric field with that of the other person, and how to maximise the usefulness of energetic release during orgasm. Within many modern schools, these teachings have been twisted and given a great deal more emphasis within Daoism than they originally would have had. Originally, they were always seen as secondary practices that supported the rest of a person's cultivation. It should also be noted that Daoism was never a system which demanded celibacy, though it did support the taking of one sexual partner, as continued work with one person was seen as an easier way to develop a harmonious energetic relationship. Once again, these teachings were clearly for practical energetic reasons rather than coming from any particular ethical standpoint.

Those who have experienced unfair treatment either emotionally or sexually invariably carry the deepest scars. In an effort to extend the principles of doing no harm to others, it was seen that ethical and decent behaviour when dealing with sexual and romantic affairs was of paramount importance.

Do Not Steal nor Deal with Those Who Do

Theft was long recognised as one of the greatest forms of misconduct within the Eastern traditions. Energetically, this was due to the nature of attachment. Mental and emotional attachment to a belonging means that taking another person's property directly takes away from them. The Qi of an object is, in part, made up of the Qi of the owner. For this reason, items taken into a Daoist practitioner's possession or home had to first be cleaned energetically by 'smudging' them with either the herb mugwort or incense. To take the Qi of another person into your living or practice space would mean to distort your own frequency with theirs; this would serve to take you away from the mind-state required for resonance with Dao. At the same time, the Daoist practitioner would seek to develop no attachments to material possessions. Whilst wrong to steal from another, it should be no problem to be stolen from. At work here energetically is the difference between what happens on the level of Qi when something is freely given versus what happens on this level when something is taken without being given. In the case of an item taken, there is a malevolent form of Qi involved that takes away from the owner's sense of self; something which is never tolerated within the Daoist tradition.

Tell Only Truth and Do Not Mislead Others with Your Speech

Practising only truth within the Daoist tradition means essentially to:

- speak the truth
- know the truth concerning self and intention
- act honestly upon this truth.

The resonance of dishonesty brings back to a person more dishonesty, as communication based upon untruth generates distortions. The way in which Daoists view the human mind means that, in many cases in life, dishonesty is the basis for people's communication. This is further complicated by people's ability to lie to themselves about their own motives. The search for 'truth' must begin within, as this is the basis of true speech and true actions. According to the Daoist tradition, the search for contact with Dao is made more complicated if there are excessive distortions in the world of the practitioner. 'Truth attracts truth', and in this way the distortions can begin to clear.

Avoid Intoxication and Conduct Yourself with Purity

Daoism was never a tradition that outwardly banned the use of alcohol or psychotropic drugs. There are classical teachings on the cultivation and harvesting of various types of interesting mushrooms. These teachings showed the best times and manners in which to pick these mushrooms in order to 'cultivate' Shen. On top of this, there are several immortals within Daoist mythology who drink alcohol heavily, the most famous of which undoubtedly being the 'drunken immortal', Li Tie Guai (李鐵拐) – though some say his bottle actually contains medicine and not alcohol!

The basic rule within Daoism was that drugs such as alcohol could be consumed, providing that the practitioner did not consume enough to be intoxicated. Once again, this was not an ethical rule but a practical one. The guidance states that the consuming of intoxicants becomes a problem once it begins to 'erode the will'. To succeed in the Daiost arts, it is highly important that the willpower of the practitioner is developed to a very high level. Without willpower, it was guaranteed that a practitioner would fail in their endeavours to attain Dao. A little high-quality alcohol was not a problem to the Daoists, who supported diligent practice but also indulging a little in the finer things in life. Saying this, though, a practitioner should never become tipsy or even drunk, as this erodes the will.

Linked to this, it was also recognised that habits and addictions eroded the energy of a person's willpower, and so these were constantly sought out and eradicated. Addictions and habits can come in many forms, and so diligent self-analysis was a constant part of Daoist Xing cultivation.

In later manifestations of the Daoist traditions, all intoxicants were banned; this especially happened when Daoism was codified into a more religious tradition.

Honour Your Family, Hereditary Line and Ancestors

Ancestor worship has long been a part of Eastern traditions. The boundary between the realm of the living and the departed is not so clear-cut as it often is in the West. The circular nature of existence states that whilst a large percentage of human spirit goes on into an endless cycle of rebirth, a shadow of this spirit remains connected to its living relatives. Honour must always be given to these ancestors, who often were held in esteem upon a family shrine, and certain holidays according to the Daoist calendar are kept as special dates for giving recognition to your family tree stretching as far back as is known.

This respect is not simply because of a belief in the existence of life after death but also because of a major factor in the way that human life works. When any change is carried out energetically or spiritually within a person, either good or bad, it actually causes a similar (though lesser) change to those in your family. This is why in ancient China, shame to one family member often meant that you yourself were shamed, as were your descendants. It was believed that negative influence on the level of Qi and Blood had been caused upon the entire line, and so in many cases an honourable son or daughter would enter monastic life or the equivalent in order to clear the spiritual debt from the family line. This is also the reason why many families offered up their children to monasteries at a very young age. It was the view that if the child attained a high level of spiritual cultivation, then this would bring good fortune and growth to the rest of the family too.

Another interesting place in which we see these kinds of beliefs is in the concept of a 'blood oath'. Within the Daoist tradition, these kinds of oaths often took place when a student became the disciple of a great master, especially in the Nei Gong or more esoteric martial arts lineages. In these cases, a sample of the student's blood was given, often in the form of a signature. The teacher would store this signature and transmit spiritual energy into it. The idea is that if one part of the student's blood is transformed spiritually, then all of their blood would be, and this would help elevate the student in their practice. In the same way, if a student had broken their oaths, they would have their blood negatively affected and, according to legend, a teacher could even end the life of their student in this manner. We see these kinds of practices also being a part of tradition around the world associated with voodoo or black magic. Honour to your family, especially your parents, in ancient China was especially important, as this kind of transmission also took place through the 'bloodline'.

Carry out Kind Actions and Support Those Who Do

It is an interesting paradox within the Daoist tradition that we are not supposed to affect the lives of others (see above precepts) and yet at the same time we are supposed to carry out kind actions and support those that do. By being generous and carrying out kind acts, we are, no doubt, having an often major effect upon another person. I had it explained to me by one of my own teachers that though we are told to 'leave no footprints', this is actually pretty much impossible. Since we are aiming for something that is never going to happen, we may as well ensure that the 'footprints' we leave are positive in quality: a principle which makes sense to me.

Positive actions generate positive mental states in those around us. This then changes the manner in which De exists and so creates a better world that is beneficial to cultivation of the Dao in general.

It is interesting to note that the basic concept of balancing 'leaving no footprints' with acting kindly generally happens in three stages, described below.

First, the Daoist neophyte does not understand anything about the nature of cause and effect, so they should seek to minimise their contact with others. This is why new students were often taken into the mountains to study away from society.

Second, the student now understood the nature of cause and effect a lot better, so they could now 'come down from the mountain' and live amongst society. At this stage, they should seek to carry out kind deeds and at least leave positive 'footprints'.

The third stage of inner evolution is being able to comprehend the wider nature of cause and effect. At this stage, concepts such as 'kind' and 'unkind' started to fade away. The law of Yin and Yang states that a positive event does not necessarily generate a positive result much further down the line. Whilst somebody of a lower level of cultivation would not be able to see how the 'butterfly effect' of an action may unfold, an advanced practitioner will. This is the reason why there are tales of Daoist sages in the past acting seemingly very badly; though they may have upset people and caused them harm in the short term, it was generally for the greater good. The danger comes when practitioners believe themselves to be at this stage, when they are not.

Regarding those around them, the Daoists should always seek to align themselves with and promote the actions of those who also are kind. In this manner, they are once again contributing to leaving 'positive footprints'.

Assist Those Who Are Less Fortunate in Regaining Their Dignity and Fortune

Daoism always recognised that it was every human being's right to have help moving in the direction of Dao. Whilst they may call this process something different according to their own religious beliefs, spiritual elevation is always a part of their practice. Life is not fair and people are not born on an equal footing; this is the nature of existence, whether we wish to believe it or not. We are not born with the same level of wealth, physical health or potential psychological qualities. Despite this, we are all living our lives and are all a part of the connected web of existence produced by the actions (non-actions) of Dao. As cause and effect takes a hold of our lives we develop in different ways and life unfolds in an infinite number of possibilities. In reality, we are in control of very little of this process, and though we may make our own mistakes in life, it is generally the case that the wider cause and effect on a socio-political level is a major factor in our current state of being. Whilst in many cases it is easier to start pointing the finger and looking to blame a person for their situation, it is in fact as much the state of our own mind and actions which is the collective cause of the world's injustices.

Taking on a part of the collective responsibility for the way in which people's lives turn out, it became important to the Daoists to be charitable and help those in need. The Daoists have a long history of providing help to the needy; in many instances throughout history, the Daoists, like the Buddhists, have provided a kind of social welfare network for those in difficult situations. This assistance may take the form of medical help (in the case of healers), spiritual guidance, practical help or any number of other forms. This extension of kindness to those who are less fortunate results in many Buddhists, Daoists and followers of similar traditions seeking work in areas like social work or community outreach, something I saw quite clearly when I myself worked in drug and alcohol services in the UK.

Carry Out Your Actions in Accordance with the Dao, yet Don't Expect the Same of Others

It is always important to recognise that everybody operates according to their own set of values. Just because you believe something to be ethically acceptable, that does not mean others do. Each of us has our own idea of personal beliefs, and people projecting these expected standards on others have caused no end of conflict. In the same way, dropping your ethical beliefs in a kind of 'revenge' for the actions of others is also not acceptable. We all operate according to the experiences and beliefs we have; the moral standards we hold should be independent of others, and so we should show kindness even in the face of unkindness. Qualities spread, and the world can only be changed through resonance on a spiritual level. The Daoists understood this, and so they sought to establish the kind of resonance they were after, even in the face of adversity. This is an idea acknowledged by many spiritual traditions and most succinctly put by Mahatma Gandhi when he stated, 'We should be the change we wish to see in the world.' If we operate according to our principles only when we seek to have these principles returned to us, then we are only acting out of selfish need for gain; this only adds to the acquired layers.

Place Others' Attainment of Dao Above Your Own

A belief in the concept of there being a 'self' that operates as an independent entity is the root for many of the illusions of mind. One of the first steps to breaking free of this illusion is to place your own 'self' beneath others in terms of its importance. Service and selfless action was seen as a way to change the perceptions of mind in order to shed this illusion. It should be noted, though, that in the case of those with low self-esteem, this kind of idea can be very damaging. It can develop an almost self-destructive mindset which is unhealthy. For this reason, be cautious with this precept as an idea. Strengthen your sense of self-worth prior to raising others above you.

In my experience, this is one of the most difficult concepts for many modern people to accept. Many in the alternative community have come across the idea that they are 'a perfect being of infinite importance'. This kind of idea comes directly from the new-age scene which was essentially a Western creation derived from poorly understood Eastern concepts, mixed with Christian-type ideals, plus our pervading societal idea that we should all strive to be 'special'. On top of this, the idea of simply being a 'drop in the ocean' has been equated with the much-demonised ideas of communism. Sadly, this search in the West for being unique and special often leads to huge holes in a person's self-esteem when they realise that they are unlikely to live up to the glamorous levels of celebrities or whoever society is currently telling them has made it to the magical level of being 'special'. It is a hard and long fall which many people take emotionally when they fail to live up to what they were told they could be. The Daoist concept is that we are all a part of a much wider picture and that none of us is more important than any other. Liberation from ideas of becoming 'special' is the first step on the way to moving towards union with Dao. 'Union' (a key concept within traditions such as Daoism and Yoga) can never be attained if we keep seeking separation from others by being 'more' than they are with regard to our skills, importance or even beauty. By shedding our own importance, we enable the 'self' to fade and thus Ming shines through.

Quality-Type Precepts

Cultivate Humility

This is the first 'quality-type' precept of Daoism, on which a great deal of importance was placed within the teachings of Laozi and the Dao De Jing. Humility originally referred to an opening of space in the centre of one's Heart Mind to the wider nature of existence, rather than to a specific person (e.g. one's teacher). True humility creates a space within your Heart Mind that creates a vacuum within the centre of your being for divine information to flood in and fill. Therefore, if a person can master the mechanics behind humility, they can access spontaneous teachings which pass directly into the centre of their being; in other words, they receive wisdom. Wisdom, within Daoism, is the ability to create enough space internally that you can receive information from the cosmos, giving a pure perception of everything that takes place around you.

Humility is an extremely Yin state of being. To be able to place yourself behind others is a difficult thing but important in Daoism. Energetically, this serves to create a powerful vacuum within your Xing (nature), which draws spiritual learning towards you. When humbling yourself before a true master (or a deity in religious Daoism), you are manifesting the potential to draw teachings into the centre of your being. This is why so many practitioners in the past have had deep spiritual experiences when prostrating themselves before statues of Daoist immortals. In Daoist teachings, it should be one of your aims to be humble beneath the entire universe and understand humility before all beings. In this way the power of Dao, which flows through the cosmos, can enter you and make every aspect of life your teacher.

There are various difficulties here, though. First, you cannot force humility upon yourself. If you try to be humble, you just create false humility, which is a very common facet of human nature. False humility is often a mask for arrogance, hidden by a verbal expression of humility.

To become humble, you must understand that being humble is a very scary thing. Humility opens up the core of your being to the outside world, which leaves the acquired mind feeling extremely vulnerable. This feeling of insecurity then causes the acquired mind to try to strengthen itself through building more layers, more pieces of projected, emotionally based untruth, behind which the true self hides. Each and every time you have been hurt, made to feel small or stepped on by another, you have probably moved yourself further from a state of humility. It is for this reason that the early stages of any internal practice should really be to free yourself from as many tethers to the acquired mind as you can. By purging these emotional imbalances, your mind begins to feel more secure and therefore humility does not seem so scary a state of being. The vacuum opens and then the 'cup has been emptied'. Only at this stage can true teachings be realised.

Cultivate Humour

Surprisingly, humour is a 'quality-type' precept within Daoism. This is a key state of mind you are trying to achieve, and very specifically humour rather than joy. These teachings are characterised by the writings of Zhuang Zi.

Whilst obviously feeling good-humoured is a pleasant state to be in, like everything within Daoism there is an energetic mechanic behind humour that is vital for your practice.

Energetically, humour creates a pulse within the centre of the body. As the body temperature begins to rise, everything begins to open up inside the body, and energy moves from the centre of the body, then dissolves. This is absolutely vital because within Daoism any interaction or experience, either within your own or someone else's Ming around you, adds layers onto your own Ming. To begin to shed these layers, humour sets up a pulse that dissolves everything out from the centre. Zhuang Zi's tradition is based in allowing you to stay as natural and spontaneous as possible by using the energetic mechanism of humour to dissolve potential attachments before they fully form. It is for this reason that much of the humour within Daoist stories can often appear quite 'dark'. This is a reflection of the dissolving nature of the energy of humour and how it can be used to stop difficult emotional layers from anchoring into your Heart Mind.

Live with Simplicity

Simplicity within Daoism is more accurately entitled 'Pu' (樸). Within Confucianism, to encapsulate Pu was to start your life as a block that someone can chisel into to create perfection. Within Daoism, however, perfection of Pu was to be a block that had not been carved. Nothing has been chipped away from the block at all. A state of Pu, or simplicity, was equated with a state of wisdom, as it is through simplicity that you can encounter universal information perceived in purity – or, in other words, wisdom. The way of Laozi to Pu was wisdom; for Zhuang Zi, it was humour. Zhuang Zi used the pulsing/dissolving nature of humour to remove all those things that may attach to the body and cause increased acquired layers that move you away from purity.

Adhere to and Develop Wu Wei

If Pu is attained fully, it is possible to achieve Wu Wei, translated most commonly as 'non-doing'. Whilst this is a correct, literal translation, it is perhaps more useful to think of Wu Wei as 'non-governing' or 'non-controlling', otherwise it is easy to fall into the trap of laziness – particularly in the early years of practice. It is only possible to achieve Wu Wei through simplicity – through Pu – as then enough layers have been dissolved and wisdom through humility and humour is achieved. Wu Wei is a state of mind that is reached after rigorous, daily practice over a number of years, rather than something it is possible to 'do'. A person with Wu Wei can act without building layers onto themselves; they can remain separate whilst still able to function in their daily lives. This can only be achieved through an alchemical and energetic conversion process. Such phrases as 'stay in the shadows, act in the light' and 'stay in the back yet lead from the front' all refer to this state of Wu Wei.

This is required within study and transformation of the Xing, because it is this state that allows the muddy waters to settle, in doing so allowing the virtues to arise; these are the five congenital roots of the emotions and they can be roughly translated into English as empathy, wisdom, compassion, conviction and patience. These were said to be the five virtues that would naturally grow out of a person who could cultivate their Xing until they hit a state of Wu Wei. They are the purest expression of Xing, which can only exist when the acquired layers of 'self' have been eroded.

Cultivate Compassionate Qualities

Ultimately, the path to Daoism was based in 'union'. This union was ultimately with the non-entity of Dao, but in earlier stages it was recognised that the illusion of 'separateness' was a hurdle to our personal development. On a practical level, this helped the Daoists to dictate how they looked and acted; the concept was that a Daoist should not seek to 'stand out' in any way. A practitioner should blend into society with regard to their appearance and actions so as not to draw any attention to themselves which may set them apart from others. Though they would never seek to 'conform' in any way with a society which was detrimental to their practice, a Daoist would also seek to become largely invisible within society. Later, this idea was forgotten and the Daoist 'uniform' of robes and topknot was added. This was a distortion of the original teachings; in essence, a modern-day Daoist would seek to wear whatever clothes are relevant to where they are and never show off for the sake of feeding their ego, as these are things that lead a person further from union.

On a practical and 'action' level, acts of kindness bring people together, whilst acts of cruelty divide. Those seeking union on any level must not develop divisions between themselves and others. The practitioner's 'energy' must seamlessly flow through and within the community they find themselves in and not develop any 'breaks' or divisions. At the same time, accepting gratitude for acts of compassion is also divisive as this raises the practitioner above the level of the people they are seeking to help. It is for this reason that the Daoists sought little in the way of thanks. The fewer acts of gratitude, the less they would run the risk of developing layers onto the acquired mind.

Daoism and Service

It was always understood that 'providing service' was an important aspect of Daoist practice. This serves a number of important purposes within your training and personal development. First, internal training is essentially a somewhat selfish path. This may sound odd, but generally we are training to benefit ourselves in some way: either we are trying to improve our health, elevate our consciousness, or whatever our reason may be. Even though this kind of practice which focuses on our own needs is not inherently wrong in any way – self-development is important – always looking inwards and becoming introspective in this way can be a little imbalanced, especially for those students who make this the sole thing they do with their lives.

Second, giving some kind of service and working for the benefit of others helps to adjust our own nature from the 'outside in'. Whilst our internal work should start to give us a way to work with our nature through practice, the act of giving service to others actually begins to change us from the outside. Our actions will be reflected within our nature.

Third, what is the point of spiritual growth and the development of skill if it cannot be used for the benefit of others? This was a realisation that many past martial arts masters came to; they spent their whole lives developing skill in combat, but in the end, you cannot keep hurting people. They found that many of their skills with regard to body and energy work were transferable to the field of healing, and so they then evolved into this being their main focus.

The classical Daoist path of 'beneficial expression' or 'giving service' is most clearly expressed through the art of healing. Healing may take the form of medicine, spiritual guidance or practical teachings. Human need exists on many levels. These levels can be summarised as benefiting from the following interventions:

- The practical level of the physical realm – charity, kindness and generosity are expressions of virtue for this level
- Medicinal assistance on a physical level – the arts of Chinese medicine, nutrition and internal practice are aimed at this level
- The spiritual freedom of consciousness elevation – the arts of alchemy, meditation and Nei Gong are aimed primarily here

- The spiritual and philosophical guidance of the spiritual path – the ancient ways of the spiritual path are as relevant today as they were in ancient times

Through engaging in such actions, we work with the 'magnetism' of Ming to assist all beings on the path towards Dao. At first, these are external expressions, but with time, such expressions become something deeper, an intangible spiritual ripple which moves out from our centre to affect those around us on a second-to-second basis. When this state has been reached, then the ripples of our actions are a true expression of virtuous being. Intriguingly, the only thing that was seen as higher than attaining spiritual immortality within the Daoist tradition was to work purely for the benefit of others.

The Xing

Changing the Xing or 'nature' within this tradition is first about observation of self in your practice. This is perhaps the simplest yet most vital part of the process before you progress deeper. Observation of your behavioural patterns is an important part of the tradition, relying on continual self-analysis. Often, this would have incorporated focused discussions of the student's behaviour with their teacher, analysing this behaviour from a Daoist perspective – something I myself have gone through during my own training. I consider it a real shame this element of Daoism is missed in the modern day, particularly for younger students; however, it generally requires a considerable age gap between student and teacher. This is why I may not be the best teacher myself for this kind of thing; in the majority of cases my students are older than me!

Observation of self, however, can (and should) be undertaken by all serious students of Daoism. For this to be done effectively, analysis should also be focused on your reaction to events. For example, whilst I am observing myself, I ask myself three questions:

- How did I react?
- Why did I react that way?
- What is the root influence that caused me to act that way in the first place?

The third question in particular is important, because it begins to question your very nature itself. Within Daoism, every facet of your personality is learned – or in other words, it has no relationship with your original nature. All layers of your acquired self are learned from your experiences within your family, society, religious influence, education and social influences. Therefore, the skill of self-observation lies in assessing your reaction to an event or stimulus and trying to spot where within your acquired nature that particular negative reaction came from. It is relatively easy to spot a simple negative pattern (such as fear or anger in reaction to a particular event), yet you must investigate deeper into why such situations occur in the first place – what aspect of your acquired self is attracted to such situations? This observational process relies on intention, and is absolutely fundamental in the serious practice of Daoist alchemy. If you don't engage with this process, you cannot develop awareness of the movements of Shen, or spirit.

Don't underestimate the skill contained within this practice – it is hard work! Other stages are relatively straightforward within our practice. Many people can, for example, learn to tune into their Qi through the exercises in a matter of months. Similarly, developing awareness of Qi's actions is, after consistent practice, quite simple – tuning into the mind, however, requires considerable work. This is predominantly because there is no specific mechanic or exercise to use, merely the intention to develop awareness of these internal movements. Gradually, over time, this awareness will start to unfold, and you will begin to spot patterns and occurrences that pull you off the still, central point you require for your practice.

Understanding the Nature of Mind

Some of you may have read the previous sections on precepts, the Xing, development of the De and so on and be asking exactly what this has to do with practice. The answer to this is typically Daoist, as 'it has everything and nothing to do with your practice at the same time'. What I mean by this is that Nei Gong can be practised as a purely mechanical art form, with no regard for the teachings of Daoism, or it can be an embodiment of an ancient wisdom tradition – the choice is completely yours. If you wish to treat Nei Gong as a purely mechanical art form, then all of the discussion of precepts and virtues can pretty much be ignored; simply focus upon how we work with the body and our Qi. If, however, we wish to use it to understand the tradition of Daoism and perhaps use it as a tool for developing our consciousness, then this is where the above teaching comes in.

One of the greatest tools for shaping our mind in this way is the vast collection of classical texts we can access. What we read and what we watch really has a profound influence upon us. By spending time going through the great classics of Daoism, there is a gradual shaping of the mind that begins to take place…if this is what we want, of course.

The Application of Wei Wu Wei

The concept of 'doing' or 'governing' versus 'non-doing' or 'non-governing' was discussed in Chapter 1. Understanding how this principle is applied to our training is simple enough, but actually applying it is a lot trickier. What generally happens is that you find the 'doing' part much more tempting, and simply letting things run their course is more difficult. I see this in some of the students I teach; they always want another 'method', another thing to 'do', when in fact they should simply 'be' with whatever process is unfolding.

In a similar vein, I will teach a class, and some of this class will involve quite complex instruction. There is a method to follow and a clear exercise to be done. The students find this satisfying enough, they have instruction and so they have an active process to become involved in. In other sections of the class, I won't give a great deal of instruction, I just leave them to it. This is sometimes followed by the simple enough instruction of 'Just stand there and listen to your body.' When I enter this section of the class, I am not really asking them to 'do' anything. This is where many people, especially newcomers, have the most difficulty. It is, inevitably, where the most questions come up, and most of the questions revolve around 'What am I supposed to be doing now?' This is because the 'non-doing' aspect of the practice is so much more difficult than the 'doing'.

Wu Wei is a difficult thing! This is especially so for people of modern society who always want a clear-cut method that will produce clear results. We have that method and we know those results, the cause-and-effect relationship of the exercises serves to fill that void; but we need the 'non-doing' aspect of the practice too. This is where the real evolution takes place.

You cannot 'really' teach a student the correct balance of 'doing' and 'non-doing' in their practice. A teacher can show the methods, but they cannot teach the 'art' of the practice; this has to be found by each student of their own accord. Whether they do or not will really make a difference as to how well the teachings of Daoism will unfold within them.

If we look to the example of the three regulations, we have clear places to apply the balance of 'doing' and 'non-doing'. When we regulate the body, there is a process of making sure we have all of the body principles and alignments in place, but it is when we simply hold them there and allow our awareness to absorb into the body, doing nothing in particular, that the changes really take a hold. When we regulate the breath, it is the same: the changes to our breathing come when we do very little but allow it to unfold in the right way. Regulating the mind also relies on a little 'doing' – we have a method – but a whole lot of 'non-doing', simply allowing the evolution to take place as a natural process we are simply an observer to.

Herein lies the quality of practice that will dictate how well you transform the Fa to Gong.

Between Sleeping and Waking

A final note on regulation of the mind should really address the matter of balancing your 'focus' with your 'process of release'.

The aim of the practices so far is to help the body and mind enter a state whereby they can 'Song' or 'let go' of emotional and energetic pathogens: those acquired energies that are weighing us down. We wish to become uninhibited and lighter with what we are doing. This process is alchemically prevented from happening if we use too much focus. This is another key error for many beginners. I myself had this problem for a very long time. I am, by nature, a fairly intense person and so to ease off my level of focus in my practice was very difficult. I wanted to 'blast' myself through the process with a laser-like level of focus that would penetrate through to the heart of my imbalances! Needless to say, it didn't work. Intense levels of focus and 'letting go' are in direct conflict with one another.

As we will learn more about in Chapter 11, the mind has an energetic 'density' to it. The stronger a thought, the more 'dense' in nature it is. If we wish for something to leave the body, we must 'lighten' it. This is why we have to learn how to relax and work with our level of focus in the right manner; we could almost plot the level of focus we require for our practice onto a simple graph, as shown in Figure 6.5. Although a horribly mathematical way of interpreting something with such complexity as our mind, it does enable us to understand the concept.

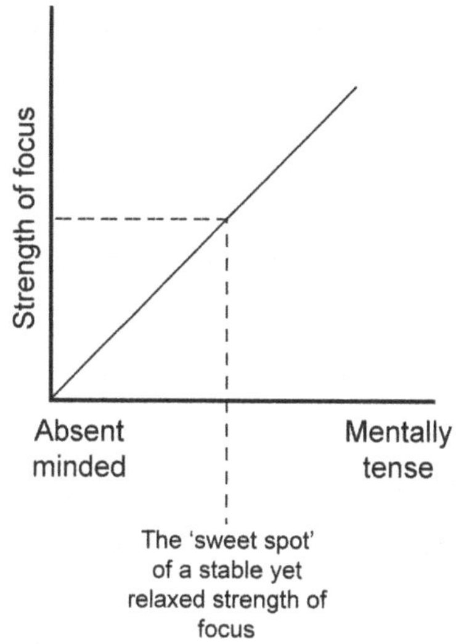

Figure 6.5: The Graph of Focus

If the mind has too much strength in its level of focus, then it will create too much pressure, a type of mental tension, and this tension will prevent us from being able to let go. In short, it stops the important quality of release.

If, however, we use too little focus, we are too far towards the end of the graph labelled as 'Absent minded'. Here, there is too little focus, too little stability of the mind, and so we are no longer absorbed into the process. With no absorption, the mechanism of the practice is no longer there. We are daydreaming, and so there is no release and no development.

Somewhere right between these two ends of the spectrum is the 'sweet spot' of perfect focal strength. It is here, on that exact point, that we will have regulated the strength of the mind so that it reaches the most effective place for our practice. We are focused enough that our mind does not waver, and yet not so focused that we are creating mental tension.

This idea of balancing the level of one's focus was so important that almost every Eastern tradition talks of it very clearly in their teachings. One of the most common ways you will hear it discussed is as the 'state of being between awake and asleep'. I remember hearing this phrase over and over from numerous meditation teachers, and I am sure some of you reading this will have heard it too. As with many other profound teachings in these arts, it often gets badly misunderstood. Generally, this means that it is taken too literally. I was guilty of this error too; it took a long time in my practice before I understood what the phrase meant. It means, quite simply, exactly what was discussed above: finding that 'sweet spot' on the spectrum between having too little focus (being asleep) and having too much (being fully awake).

What I mean by this phrase having been taken too literally is that we have large numbers of people mistakenly believing that they are supposed to enter the experience of hypnagogia in their practice. This is the literal transitional phase that the mind goes through when we are at the onset of sleep; we are not yet fully asleep and neither are we fully awake. The result is a bunch of people trying to meditate by falling to the point of almost being asleep: a practice that never works because you will eventually fall asleep. Cue the Japanese Zen master coming along and hitting you with a wooden stick to wake you up! It is easy to see the reasons why people misunderstand this phrase: language barriers and modern people's tendency to take everything literally. This is compounded by the fact that a state of hypnagogia often brings with it lucid thoughts, dreams and visual phenomena. Whilst these experiences may be fun, they have little to do with actual meditative practice.

On a practical level, to help beginners, I generally tell them that their mind should be 'casually observing' the process they are going through. If they are to have their mind on a specific region of the body, the lower Dan Tian for example, they should be 'casually observing' what is going on. Their mind should still be involved and absorbed into what they are doing, but they are only 'half interested'. If they can follow these kinds of guidelines, it will help them to ease off their focal strength.

Of course, the instruction of 'casually observing' is just a stop-gap, a temporary measure to help beginners until they reach the right state of mind in a deeper way, until they attain Gong in this region of their practice. How do they achieve this level of skill? Through the exact process I have outlined in this and the previous chapter. If you can evolve the breath and the mind through allowing the five keyword qualities to unfold, then it will lead you to the correct level of focus: the balance point between being awake and asleep. If you are led to this point, then the mind will quieten, relax and suffuse itself through your entire body; this is all an aspect of 'regulation of the mind'.

Chapter 7

THE NATURE OF JING

Daoism is primarily an alchemical tradition. What this means is that it utilises a series of practices that work by locating, refining and transforming various energetic 'substances' within the body. The three most important of these substances are Jing, Qi and Shen; collectively, these are known as the San Bao (三寶) or 'three treasures'. If we look into any basic-level book on arts such as Qi Gong or Chinese medicine, we will see that these three 'treasures' are referred to time and time again; they are the basis of transforming the body and mind with regard to both health and development of consciousness.

Rather than being tangible substances, as in the case of blood or body fluids, the San Bao sit within the energetic aspect of our being. Though they are intangible, they can still be experienced through practice, and much of our work at the beginning is around learning how to 'adjust the frequency of our awareness' so that we can contact and thus work with them. We shall return to this as a concept later, but first, let us look at what the San Bao actually are; how are they defined within the Daoist tradition?

A Simple Definition

If we look at how the San Bao are usually defined, we will see that Jing is generally translated as meaning our 'essence', Qi as our 'energy' and Shen as our 'spirit'. These three are then said to inter-transform into one another over the course of our lives. These transformations affect our physical health and mental faculties as well as how we evolve and age. Though this is not really a detailed enough definition to help us fully comprehend what Jing, Qi and Shen really are all about, it is enough to get us in the rough area of understanding.

The thing to understand about Jing, Qi and Shen is that, ultimately, they are one and the same. They are three 'states' of the same creative source. They are just existing in different formats. We can use the simple analogy of ice, water and steam to understand how this is the case. Jing would be like ice, it is the densest form of the San Bao; as it is 'heated', it transforms into the 'water' of Qi, and then, finally, it converts into the most ethereal and 'steam-like' of the substances – Shen.

On a basic level, our Jing is being used up throughout the duration of our lives; it is like an energetic form of fuel that burns up according to our physical and mental activity; when it is gone, we die. Much of the guidance on extending the length of your life and the quality of your health within Daoist literature was based around preservation of the Jing. Your Qi is your 'energy', it is derived from the food you eat and the air you breathe; the quality of your Qi dictates how much vitality you have. Your Shen is the quality of your spiritual nature. It relies, in part, on the quality of your Qi and Shen for strength.

This simple definition of the San Bao is pretty much how many people understand them. Whilst this may be enough for a basic-level Qi Gong practice, we need a lot more detail on these three substances if we are ever going to get to the bottom of Daoism as a tradition. In order to do this, we need to look at some of the background theory that underpins the San Bao. We will focus here particularly on the theory and teachings of Jing and Qi; Shen will be looked at in greater detail in Chapter 12.

What Is Ming?

The concept of Ming was introduced in the previous chapter when it was discussed briefly in relation to Xing or your 'nature'. It was mentioned that it was a difficult term to define, as it is a combination of your 'fate' and your 'destiny'. If we wish to begin to understand any term within the Daoist tradition, it is always best to begin with a breakdown of the Chinese character. This character is shown in Figure 7.1.

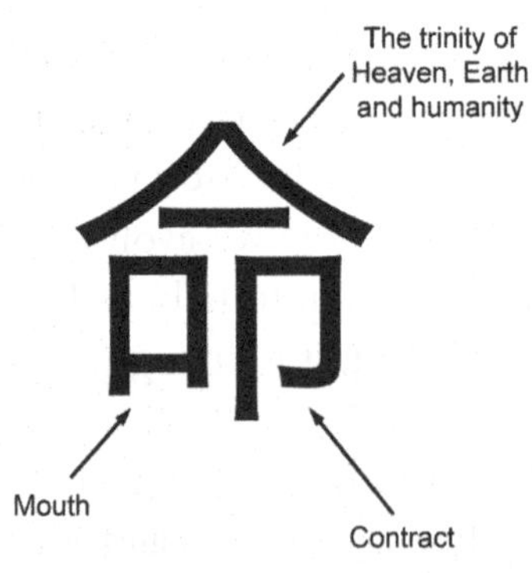

Figure 7.1: Ming

The upper part of the character shows a symbol generated by three lines. These three lines show a relating trinity between the power of Heaven, humanity and Earth. On the left-hand side of the lower half of the character we have a symbol indicating a mouth that is speaking, and on the right is a symbol meaning 'contract'. When we put this all together, it suggests that our Ming is an understood contract that exists between human beings and their wider position between Heaven and Earth.

To the Daoists, Ming was like a wave of information that moved between the two realms of Heaven and Earth like some kind of energetic air current. Ming then interacts with humankind to generate the unfolding events, changes and personal transformations that take place over the course of a lifetime. As human beings, we then travel along these lines of Ming; they serve as the spiritual 'roadmaps' that we take through life. The nature of Ming is to act according to two rules:

- The rule of cause and effect
- The rule of resonance

As we move through our lives, the influence of Ming is unavoidable. It is the reason for the manner in which our lives unfold, as well as the basis for our false sense of linear-based time. Within alchemical Daoism, the unwitting journey along the line of Ming was named Shun (順), and it was understanding Shun that was required for mastery of the Ming.

The Rule of Cause and Effect

The Daoist view of life was that it is based in the simple rule of cause and effect. Every action generated a series of unfolding events like so many ripples spreading out upon the surface of a pond. As these 'ripples' spread out through the Ming of humanity, it served to establish the seed for countless other events. Like some kind of spiritual butterfly effect, no living creature upon this Earth was free from the rule of cause and effect.

When people hear of this rule, they often mistake it for some kind of judgement. They translate this rule within their mind into 'If I do bad things, bad things will happen to me.' Whilst there is a certain satisfaction to this kind of Karmic justice, it is really not what the Daoists were discussing. There is a saying within Daoism that originated in the Dao De Jing – 'Heaven treats humanity like so many straw dogs.' The 'straw dogs' referred to are a kind of piñata coming from rural parts of ancient China. The 'straw dog' piñata were celebrated as deities during a yearly festival as they were paraded around the villages and venerated by the locals. Then they were smashed up and burnt in a demonstration of impermanence when nightfall came. Heaven treats humankind like so many 'straw dogs' by ultimately viewing us as disposable. Though it is more comforting to think of ourselves as being wildly valued by those that may reside in the heavenly realm, this was not how the Daoists viewed human existence. Instead, they saw Ming as extending down into the realm of existence and influencing the events taking place there; these events are free from any kind of justice and so can, at any time, bring you calamity or even end your life.

This lack of any kind of idea of 'justice' then extends out into the way that the rule of cause and effect plays out in the world. This means that the fruits of your actions are highly likely to cause effects in other people's lives, not just, or even necessarily, your own. In the same way, you may have generated very little in the way of 'seeds' for calamitous events, but the actions of others around you may result in these calamities befalling you all the same. Such is the interconnected nature of Ming as it expands out like a great web that joins all life together as one.

On a simple level, we can see how this view is applied to the world at large. The overconsumption of resources and wealth by some parts of the planet has a detrimental effect upon the wealth and resources of other parts of the planet. Some countries have more than enough, whilst others starve as a result of the plentiful countries' actions. This takes place on a societal level as well, and then continues down on a holographic level into the microcosm of family and social groups. In this way, the cause-and-effect nature of Ming is shared between us. Like throwing a handful of pebbles into a pond, the ripples all travel outwards and influence one another.

The Rule of Resonance

Aside from the rule of cause and effect, there is also the rule of resonance. Unlike the previous rule, this does have an influence upon our lives in a very individualistic manner. This rule is based around the fact that every experience we have and every movement of our mind has an energetic quality to it. This energy serves as a kind of information and then, in turn, this information has a very specific 'frequency' to it. The result of this is that 'like attracts like'. This means that anything we 'hold on to' within our energetic system will change this frequency and thus change the nature of the resonance we have with life. Again, this concept is free from any concept of justice or fairness; it simply 'is what it is'.

The built-up sources of information that we store are held in the acquired aspect of our being. They then draw towards us similar experiences that can feel as if they are repeating over and over. Many of us will have experienced this in our lives: the same repeated events that seem to keep coming up time and time again. Perhaps the same problems keep befalling you, or maybe many people you meet end up betraying you in the same manner? It is as if the line of Ming is stuck and can't seem to move beyond repeating itself.

Many call this kind of repeating event 'life lessons'. There are things you need to learn from this kind of event so that you can move on. Whilst there is a degree of truth to this, it is not always healthiest to see it this way; to the Daoists, this would be far too much like giving a 'higher-level' quality to the events than they deserve. They are not 'lessons' so much as repeating 'qualities of Ming' that you keep experiencing as the rule of resonance is drawing them towards you. To change the nature of how you experience Ming, we need to shed those layers of the acquired mind that are generating the potential for this resonance to take place. This is a process free from any kind of judgement or lessons to be learnt.

The Divisions of Ming

As with pretty much anything in the Daoist tradition, Ming is divided up into three constituent parts – Yang Ming (陽命), Yin Ming (陰命) and Ren Ming (人命). These are three 'levels' of Ming, and they work upon us in very different ways.

Yang Ming

The Yang Ming is the 'higher Ming of Heaven'. We could liken this to 'destiny' or 'higher purpose'. To have a connection to Yang Ming would mean that there is a great meaning behind your life and a distinct role that you have to play in the grand scheme of existence. Sadly, it was said that you could 'lose your connection to Yang Ming with every breath'. This implies that though we may all have had the potential for higher purpose at some stage, the development of the acquired mind, over time, separates us from this purpose.

Yin Ming

The Yin Ming is the 'lower Ming of Heaven'. We can liken this to the concept of 'fate'. It is the origin of those events that are out of our hands. Note that there is a clear distinction between the nature of 'destiny' and 'fate' here. 'Destiny' implies a higher purpose, a function behind a series of events, whereas 'fate' does not carry this same higher-level quality. Ultimately, the fate of all of us is to die and continue the process of transmigration; an end point that we shall all, no doubt, achieve! It is here, in the expression of Yin Ming, that the rules of resonance and cause and effect largely play out.

Ren Ming

Ren Ming is the Ming of 'humanity'. Here are the seeds of our own, personal connection to Ming that is established at our time of birth. Whilst we will always have a connection to the fluctuations of Yin Ming, they may shift and change. We may have fleeting glimpses of Yang Ming, but ultimately, this level of Ming is not really ours, it is something we can reach if the circumstances are just right. Ren Ming, on the other hand, is fixed. It is beyond our control and 'gifted' to us as a result of three main sources: our previous resonances from past incarnations, our family line, and the astrological timing of our birth.

These three aspects of Ming interplay with one another and generate the potential for those things that occur within our lives as well as the potential for our level of innate health, our constitutional being. These interrelationships are summarised in Figure 7.2.

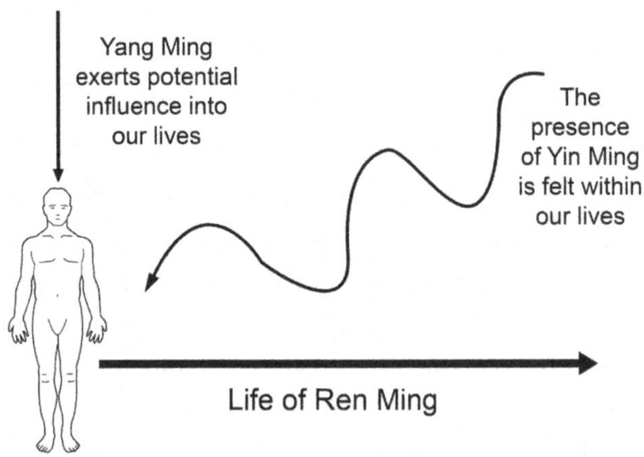

Figure 7.2: Interplays of Ming

Another key tenet of the Daoist tradition is that everything that exists on a spiritual level is also manifest on an energetic level, and then this is either rooted into or reflected in the physical realm as well. In the case of Ming, it is manifest into the quality of our Jing. It is primarily the Ren Ming that influences the nature of our Jing, but then our Jing is also subject to changes according to how our connection to Yin and Yang Ming develops. So, we could say that when we are born, the potential contained within our Ren Ming manifests through the level of our potential Jing.

The Building of Our Personal Ming

The Ren Ming is our personal Ming. We can think of the nature of Ren Ming as being like a database of information about our mental and physical health that is already established for us before we are born. It is a sad fact of life that we are not born equal with regard to our personal Ming. The Ren Ming we are granted is dependent upon factors that are beyond our control. As discussed above, it is to do with three factors.

Resonance of Past Lives

Not everybody reading this will have belief in the idea of past lives. That does not matter. I am not trying to sell you a new belief system; I am simply writing about the belief system of those who formulated the practices of Daoism. Understanding this will help with understanding the tradition, and thus the theory behind the practices. If it does not sit within your own personal belief system, then don't worry about it.

The theory of past lives dictates that a specific aspect of the Hun (魂), an element of human consciousness that continues to move between lives, carries with it energetic information from our previous incarnations. This means that certain qualities have already been established within our nature and health by the events we have experienced prior to our birth into this life. Once again, these ideas are free from any idea of judgement in Daoism – you are not born into a better life because you were a nicer person or vice versa; you are simply born into a life that has the potential for similar resonances to those that were previously established. It is a 'mechanic' of energetics rather than a spiritual aspect of reincarnation within esoteric Daoist thought.

I would also like to add a note here that, in my opinion, an over-concern with accumulated trauma from past lives is an unhealthy thing. I have known several people who looked to understand all of their ailments as purely a result of what had happened in their past lives. This is a greatly disempowering place to view your life from. There are enough problems in this life already, without having to worry too much about what has already been and gone. I am only including this brief section on past-life resonances for purposes of completion.

Our Family Line

It is understood that the health of our parents and grandparents, along with their innate psychological traits, are passed down to us through the Ren Ming. This is the root for everything from our physical family traits through to our innate temperament and, of course, our constitutional health. Inherited genetic disorders would fall under this aspect of the Ming as well. To go into a full exploration of this aspect of our being could take volumes; if you are interested in looking into this in more detail, then go and explore the teachings of Chinese medicine – there are many books that explore this area of your health and nature in greater detail.

Astrological Timing

When we discuss the Heavens in Daoist teachings, we are not usually talking about a realm where the immortals live. Though religious Daoism does explore this aspect of reality, esoteric or alchemical Daoist teachings are usually referring to the stars and planets and how they influence us upon the Earth. It is understood that as the Qi of the Heavens moves, it directs a powerful influence upon all life. These influences change from hour to hour, and there is a strong tradition of astrology coming from Daoism that aims to understand this aspect of life. A Ba Zi (八字) reading is a chart that Daoist astrologers use to understand the Qi of the Heavens at your time of birth and how these have had an influence upon you.

What these three aspects of Ren Ming put into your Ming is a starting point for who you are and how you are going to take shape. These things are largely out of our control, but we still work towards harmonising them through our practice. Figure 7.3 shows the formation and influences of the Ren Ming in greater detail.

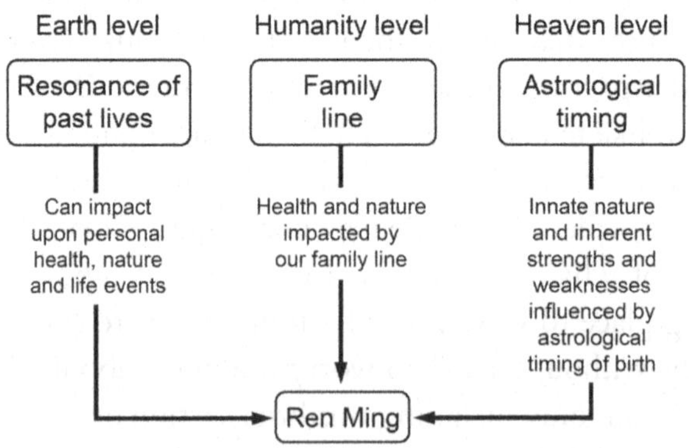

Figure 7.3: The Formation of Ren Ming

So, now we have a basic understanding of the nature of Ming, let us look at how this manifests within our body. To do this, we need to look to the alchemical process of Jing production within the body.

The Alchemical Process of Jing Production

There are several steps involved in the manifestation of Jing, as well as how our Ming is involved in this process. It involves the further division of the 'treasures' into more parts. These parts include Yuan Jing (元精), Yuan Xi (元息) and Yuan Shen (元神). This process is shown in Figure 7.4.

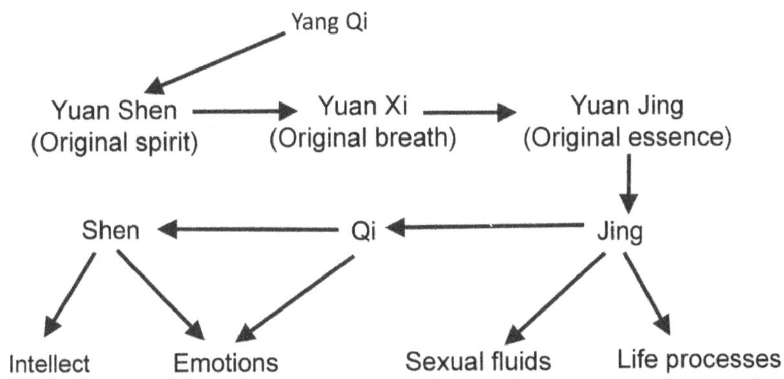

Figure 7.4: Alchemical San Bao Development

At the top of the chart sits a type of Qi known as 'original Qi'. It is often also called Yang Qi, but it is a different form of Yang Qi from the type we will aim to use for our Nei Gong practice further down the line. To avoid confusion, I will refer to it from now on simply as 'original Qi'. Original Qi is the prime energy born from the space of Wuji through the motivating force of Taiji. It is the very 'substance' of Heaven and the seed which was born from the potential for existence. Those seeking divinity within the Daoist traditions understood that this Qi should be sought out, as this was the true way to unite the consciousness with Heaven.

Since this 'original Qi' is the energy of pure Heaven, it is also the energy of original consciousness, and once this 'slows' in frequency to the level of manifestation, it becomes Yuan Shen or 'original spirit' as shown in Figure 7.4. Yuan Shen is the undifferentiated light of illumination that exists before the fragmented aspects of spirit, consciousness and mind come into being.

When original spirit begins to stir into movement it becomes Yuan Xi or 'original breath'. This is the movement of Yuan Shen as it flows through the space between Heaven and Earth. Sometimes called the 'breath of life', this is the 'magical' animating spirit which brings life to everything within the cosmos. If Yuan Xi did not move through us, then we would not live, and it is this breath which leaves the body upon our death, thus freeing our spirit from its tether into the physical realm. This is the original form of 'human Qi' within Daoist teachings.

Gradually, Yuan Xi begins to 'condense', and this forms Yuan Jing or 'original essence'. This is the Jing we are gifted upon our birth. It is here, in this stage of the alchemical process of Jing development, that our Ren Ming anchors into our being. Profoundly, the Yuan Jing also contains the potential for Yuan Xi and Yuan Shen if it can be refined, and herein lie many of the principles of alchemical transformation once we move beyond the foundation and intermediate stages.

The 'Yuan' stages of being are still not manifest within human existence, instead they sit in the background behind the various mechanisms of life, ensuring that all the world can come into being. Once Yuan Jing condenses downwards once more, it becomes Jing, the basis for our well-being, constitution and health. This Jing governs our life processes and functions of the body. For men in particular it is also closely linked to their sexual fluids, which is why so much guidance on regulating sexual activity is given within Daoist scripture.

The Jing is then converted upwards within the body into Qi and then further into the Shen, which is now refracted into the various components of the human psyche. These all work to govern our body's activities and our mind as we progress through our lives.

Once this process has been played out, we come into physical being. This development of the Jing is taking place all the way through gestation and only fully completes as we are ready to be born.

Jing and the Ming Men

It is an interesting aspect of the Daoists' tradition that their entire philosophical teachings also have to have a basis in the realm of manifestation. Ultimately, the Daoists were 'explorers of the nature of life', and the system they developed reflected this. If we look at the above process, the formation of Jing, we then need to see where this process actually connects with our physical lives. The answer to this is: in our body, at the acupuncture point known as Ming Men (命門). This point is shown in Figure 7.5. It sits in the centre of the back, beneath the spinous process of the second lumbar vertebra.

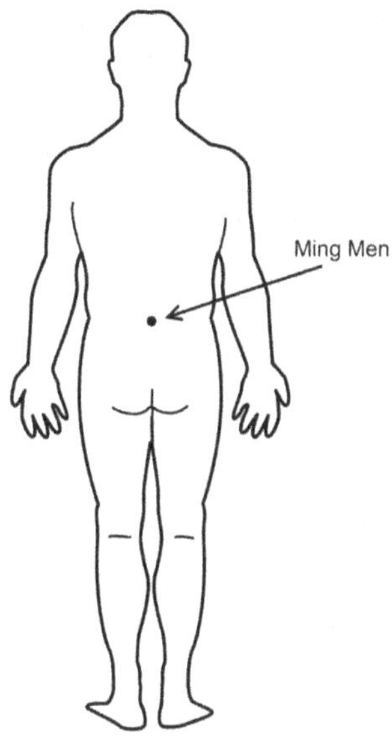

Figure 7.5: The Ming Men Point

We can translate the name of the point 'Ming Men' as the 'gateway to your Ming'.

Within Daoism, the term 'gateway' is used as a metaphorical reference to a boundary which exists between the Xian Tian (先天) – the congenital – and the Hou Tian (後天) or the acquired. Within the nature of energetics, these two can be thought of as the difference between the potential for something to manifest and its actual manifestation. In the case of Ming Men, it is referring primarily to the manifestation of the acquired Jing from the stillness of the Yuan Jing; it is the point whereby the 'blueprints' of the Yuan Jing become the 'fuel' of the Jing.

According to traditional Chinese medical teachings, it is here, at the Ming Men point, that our acquired Jing is stored. It is still, in this state, intangible in nature. From here, there is a second process that the Jing goes through in order to form the basis for both our health and our developmental stages. We shall explore this shortly.

Just next to the Ming Men region are the two Kidneys. It is the Kidneys which Chinese medicine classically associates with the Jing, and so when the Kidneys are treated, it is ultimately the Jing stored around the region of Ming Men that the therapists are generally trying to influence.

The reason that the name of the point is 'Ming Men' and not 'Jing Men' is that it is here that our Ming starts to manifest into our body – primarily the Ren Ming aspect of Ming, our own personal Ming. It does this through the 'vehicle' of the Jing. In this way, and this is of prime importance, our

Jing is a reflection of the quality of our Ming and nothing else. How we then treat our Jing over the course of our lives will influence our personal Ming as well. It was stated that the Daoist transformational arts work by consolidating both our Xing and our Ming; the Ming aspect must be worked on through developing and mastering the cycles and qualities of Jing.

The Movements of Jing

Once we reach the stage of our acquired Jing, the Jing that resides in the region of the Ming Men, near the Kidneys, we have a process we can actually become involved in through our training. The Jing that sits here is the 'finite fuel' that is discussed at length in Chinese medical texts. This fuel then goes through a series of movements as it generates certain other substances within the body. This is summarised in Figure 7.6.

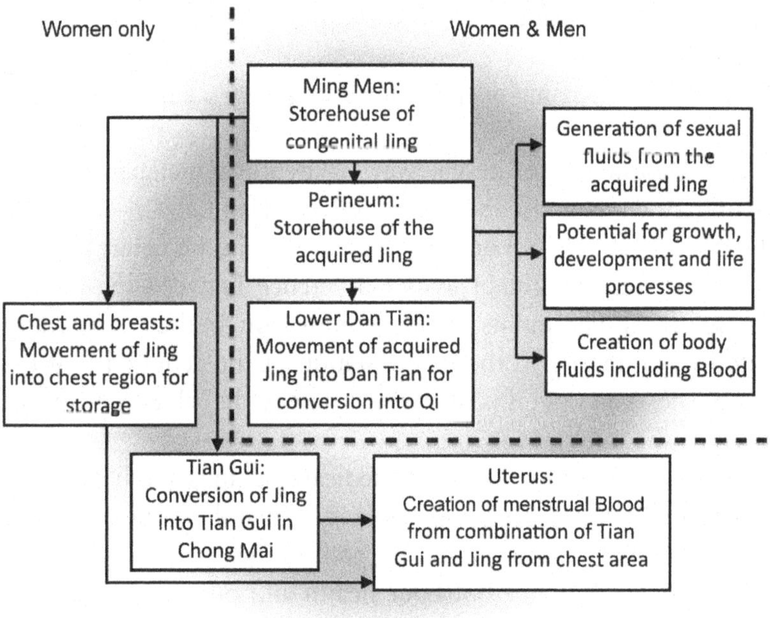

Figure 7.6: The Actions and Movement of Jing

The natural movement of acquired Jing is to form into various bodily substances and fluids. In men this includes semen, and in women it is linked to the creation of the menstrual Blood. As men ejaculate and women menstruate, the Jing moves deeper into a state of decline. It is here that we are fully removed from the 'congenital' state of Yuan Jing and fully connected to the 'acquired' state of our own bodily Jing. This is because, as the acquired Jing begins to convert into various elements within the body, it is in movement; the nature of 'congenital' is stillness, and so 'movement' takes us away from this state of being.

Men tend to use up their acquired Jing faster than women due to it being lost primarily through male orgasm. According to Daoist medical teachings this is one of the key reasons why women tend to live longer than men.

As well as its conversion into fluid substances, Jing also governs the developmental processes which cause us to age and gradually decline. Figure 7.7 summarises these aspects of Jing.

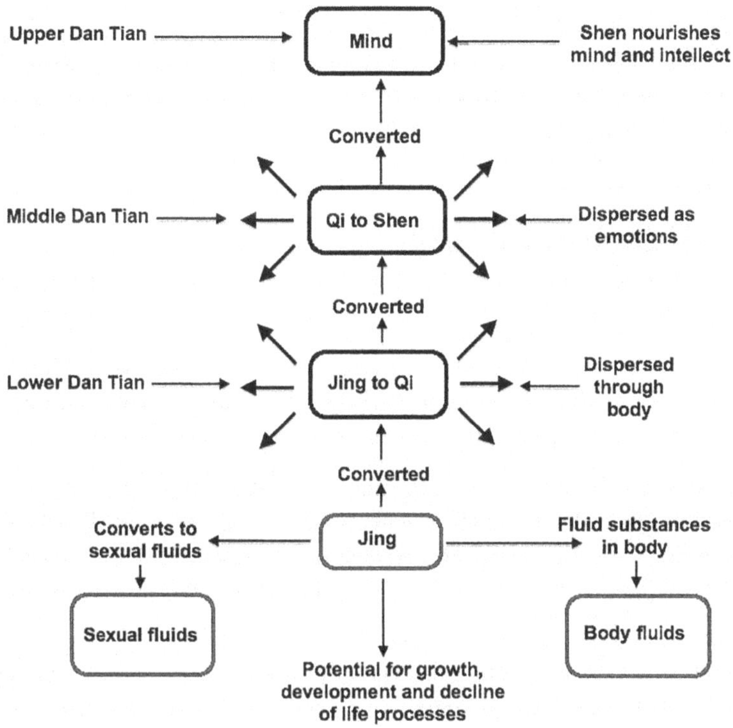

Figure 7.7: The Movements of Jing

From its base around the region of the Kidneys, your Jing travels down to the perineum area of the body where it is metaphorically referred to as 'Kidney Water' within classical texts. It is from this location that Jing then moves into the sexual organs, and from here that it rises gradually up into the lower Dan Tian for steady conversion into Qi. This is the formation of acquired Qi from acquired Jing. This acquired form of Qi is then passed out into the rest of the body via the channel system. The Qi then carries out all of the activities of functional life. Chinese medicine is essentially a study of this process, and the work of practitioners is based upon the theory that poor health is due to either stagnation, deficiency or excess of this form of Qi as it moves through your energetic matrix. The nature of your health dictates how smoothly this energy moves through the body and how much is used up. Poor health results in a greater dispersion of this Qi which, in turn, requires that more Jing is used up to replenish these energetic reserves.

Some of the Qi which passes up into the middle Dan Tian is then converted into acquired Shen, which nourishes the mind and stimulates your intellect. All activities of mind use up some of the acquired Shen, especially if that activity is very emotionally driven. All of this dispersal of Qi and Shen from the various energetic centres of your body leads to a decline of the acquired Jing which is supplying support to the two other aspects of the San Bao. The decline in the state of your Jing then results in poorer health and a speeding up of the ageing process; this was all classically said to be a reflection of 'speeding up your Ming'.

Consolidation of Jing

The actual mechanism of how Jing moves and functions within the body is very closely linked to the action of Yin Qi. We shall return to the concept of Yin Qi in greater detail in Chapter 9 when we will break apart what both Yin and Yang Qi actually are, as well as how they interact with one another in the body. For now, it is enough to understand that Yin Qi works as a kind of magnetic field with regard to how it is formulated and influences your body. This means that it moves in spherical patterns within the body and does not move in a linear fashion through the channel system as in the case of Yang Qi.

The influence of Yin Qi upon the lower Dan Tian and your abdominal cavity is a major aspect of both the foundation and more advanced aspects of Nei Gong training. Essentially, the Yin Qi within the region of the lower abdomen can be very dispersed in nature or very condensed; there is then a whole spectrum that exists between these two poles. How developed and condensed this field is will dictate just how efficiently various energetic mechanisms within the lower Dan Tian are taking place. One of these mechanisms is the consolidation of the Jing.

We can condense the Yin Qi field of the lower abdomen in various ways; some methods are simple and some are more advanced. We could summarise these as follows.

First, we can begin to look at some practical uses around the nature of Jing's functions. Rather than 'exercises' as such, these are simply guidelines on lifestyle behaviours that can be taken into account to help the way in which Jing moves.

Yin and quietude have long been associated with one another in the Daoist arts. There is good reason for this. Mental activity and constantly being on the go causes a dispersion of the Yin Qi field within the lower abdomen. As the field is weakened, it causes the Jing to start dispersing as well. This means that it starts to move through the body and generates larger amounts of Qi; this Qi serves to feed your mental activities. By making the mind quiet, we can start to bring the Yin Qi field into a stronger state; this begins to have a strong effect upon the actions of Jing in the lower abdomen.

Absorption of the mind into the lower abdominal region will also help with the consolidation of the Yin Qi field down there. This will help the Jing to change its behavioural patterns. There is a fine balance between having a light awareness there and focusing your mind onto the region of the lower Dan Tian. The former is essentially an application on Wu Wei or 'non-doing', the perfect state for enabling change to start taking place.

More complex stages involve sinking your mass into the region of the lower abdomen so that the Di Qi of the planet can start to build the lower Dan Tian under the influence of resonance. This is discussed in the next chapter in great detail.

Beyond this point in our practice, we have directed work involving reshaping the conductive Huang within the abdomen so that it can direct the spherical 'container' of the lower Dan Tian. This will massively strengthen the lower Dan Tian which will help a great deal in preservation and consolidation of the Jing.

The methods introduced above are all explored within this book. They are to be carried out over a fair length of time; do not expect to be able to manage the more advanced stages of Dan Tian development and Jing 'reprogramming' in the first few years. There is always a lot of work to do within the foundation stages if you are very serious about your practice. Racing ahead is a bit of a false economy with these arts anyway, as you will always hit a point that you cannot proceed beyond. Inevitably, you will have to return to your foundations and look for the reason you have stopped progressing. In the long run, building the foundations and moving slowly and steadily through these practices is more efficient.

Jing and Overwork

On a very simple level, one major aspect of your Jing is that it has to convert into Qi in order to help you carry out your daily activities. If you overwork, then you will be burning up your Jing. Be aware of this, especially as, even without looking at the repercussions on your long-term health, you require a healthy amount of Jing for much of the Nei Gong process.

It is a facet of modern society that we often consider productivity, always being active and being useful as the most important things. I know, I am very guilty of this and find it easy to neglect those 'down times' where I just rest. Learning to rest is very important. Relaxation and simply 'being' is one of the most important ways we can look after our long-term health and help rest our Jing.

I would advise those starting out in Nei Gong practices to try to time your work on these foundation stages with a period of your life that is not too busy. Don't pick up a new interest or pursuit at a time when you are extremely hectic with work and your lifestyle. You need to strike a healthy balance in order to get the most out of all this.

Jing and Sexual Desire/Fluids

It is a major facet of Daoism that your mind and body are one and the same. This means that pretty much every facet of your emotional makeup and psyche has a direct reflection within a physical region of your body. One major connection between your mind and your body exists in the region of the perineum. When the Jing from the Ming Men area moves down into the perineum, it begins to go through a series of processes. One of these is to begin establishing the potential for conversion into sexual fluids. As these fluids are produced, they also start to fuel the part of your mind that reacts to sexual desires.

The body is generating sexual desires so that you are driven to breed. The human sex drive is a little extreme though, and for many people far too much of their mental energy is taken up with this aspect of their nature. There are so many acquired layers built up around sexuality, confusion around the subject, awkwardness and obsession with sex that it is one of the most difficult aspects of our acquired self to deal with. On top of this, media-driven imagery bombards our mind on a daily basis with images of the most 'perfect' and 'sexually attractive' people to make society feel both inadequate as well as to keep people focused upon their most base desires.

Whilst both genders suffer the difficulties of mental layering attached to sexuality, it is primarily men who suffer a loss of Jing through the sexual act. Women's energy is seen as moving inwards and upwards during orgasm, meaning that there is no major (but still a slight) loss of Jing during sex. Men, on the other hand, lose Jing as their energy goes downwards and outwards when they ejaculate.

It is for this reason that many of the classical teachings around sexuality stated very clear guidelines on how often a man should allow himself to have sex. These guidelines varied a great deal and so I always tell my students to follow their bodies instead. If, after having sex, you feel like your back and knees are weaker and you need to rest afterwards or sleep, then you are using up too much Jing. You need to regulate your sexual activity to a higher degree.

There is a curious pattern that can be seen with sexual activity. The more we have sex, the more it drives us. This means that though we are temporarily satisfied, the urge for sex comes back stronger afterwards. It is like a form of learnt behaviour for the mind, meaning that your sex drive enters a kind of addiction pattern. This is why, if you ever enter into a period of celibacy, it is easy at first, then it becomes difficult after a week or so, and then, after a few weeks, your sex drive actually diminishes. This is due to the behavioural patterns of Jing. When the Jing moves, it stirs our desires; when it grows still, our desires are no longer at the forefront of our mind. This does not mean we can no longer have sex or that we become impotent in any way, it is just that there is a direct choice in the matter rather than a drive that takes control of our thought patterns and behaviours. It is here that we should aim to be if we are hoping to consolidate the Jing for internal training. This kind of stage will be the result of the stilling of the Jing once you move beyond the foundation stages of practice.

Many people, when I have explained this, have been uneasy about this process; it is not something they wish to happen. This is especially true of male students. We are socially programmed to believe that being driven by our sexual desires is what gives us some kind of power – it makes us more 'manly' or a more 'powerful' woman – so when we are told that there is a way to change this aspect of our nature, it seems unappealing. The truth is that when you gain control of your sexual drive through adjusting the nature of the Jing's behaviour, there is a major change that takes place in your nature. It is the first time you realise how many relationships you have with people are hugely distorted by this issue, and, on top of this, how many of your insecurities are based in this area. When sexual activity becomes a choice rather than an uncontrollable urge, then the Jing has reached a more balanced state for our practice. For many, this may sound off, but if we look at Eastern traditions that discussed a series of changes that needed to be made for spiritual development to unfold, our base desires were generally the first hurdle.

The 'Right' Amount of Sex

As stated above, the best way to understand if you are having too much sexual activity is to look at how your body is feeling. If sex is draining or weakening in any way, then it is too much for your body. As a general rule for physical health, this is easy enough to follow. Generally, men will find that less sex is needed to take them to this point than women.

For guidelines of practice, the classical teachings varied in the amounts they recommended, but as an approximate and rough guide, they averaged at around one ejaculation every four days for men in their twenties, every eight days for men in their thirties, every sixteen days for men in their forties, and every twenty-one days for men in their fifties and beyond. These are guidelines for people who practise the internal arts, so that the Jing is not overused. For some, this will sound like it is not very much, which is why the mental stilling of sexual desires needs to take place as well if you wish to go down this route. Note also that it refers to men here and not women. Women were not given such stringent guidelines, as sex was not seen as such a destructive force for female essence. Instead, they were to follow the healthy guidelines above of listening to their body.

Many reading this will spot an obvious issue with regard to different amounts of sex for the two genders. How do men and women have a healthy sexual relationship when they have unequal amounts of sexual activity suggested? The answer to this is that men were advised to have sex without orgasm in order for the woman to be satisfied without the male partner losing excess Jing. It is suggested that 'no orgasm' is aimed for, not just no ejaculation. There are many contemporary schools that have trained men to orgasm without ejaculating. This is considered a major misunderstanding within the classical Daoist school, as there is the same, if not more, damage done to the Jing and Qi of the practitioner through these so-called 'in-gasms' as there is through ejaculation. They can lead to a very specific condition known as 'poison fire tainting the Heart'. This is a condition we shall look at in the appendix.

It was stated within the classics that having sex with no orgasm for the male, but orgasm for the female, would have several health benefits. These are as follows:

- Once will make the Qi stronger
- Twice makes the hearing stronger and the eyes brighter
- Three times grants the strength to stave off illness
- Four times and the mind becomes stronger

- Five times strengthens the heart
- Six times strengthens the waist and back
- Seven times toughens the buttocks, thighs and legs
- Eight times causes the Qi to expand and radiate
- Nine times leads to a tonification of the Jing
- Ten times and you are on the way to immortality

Okay, so the last one may be a slight exaggeration. The Daoists always had a little humour in their writings, but you get the idea. The reason that sex without ejaculation for the male is so helpful is due to a principle known as He Qi (合氣) or 'conjoining energy'. When two people have intercourse with one another, there is a sharing of frequencies between the Yin and Yang Qi of both bodies. Women benefit from this energy, provided the emotional content of the sex is healthy, but men lose out on it, as their body is kind of short-circuited temporarily by the act of orgasm. Without the orgasm, the energy is absorbed into the male body and it has beneficial effects for them.

After sex, if the male partner is not going to orgasm, then there is a process of 'stilling the Jing' that must be practised. This will avoid any form of sexual frustration from developing. It can be difficult at first, but, with practice, it is very useful for governing the Jing. Note here, though, that not enough ejaculation can be negative as well. To completely end all sexual activity for good is against what is natural for the body. It is all about balance and striking the right level of activity versus rest – as per usual.

I do not wish to go into too much detail concerning sex and sexuality according to Daoism as it is a long subject and quite complex. I just wish to point out some guidelines and teachings concerning sex in relation to Jing that are relevant to the practices. Almost every alchemy or Nei Gong teacher I have met has had their own guidelines on sex and, whilst they vary a little from person to person, they are all roughly describing the information above.

Sex was never a way to enlightenment or even self-development within the Daoist tradition. It was simply an aspect of life that was inevitable, and so the Daoists found ways to understand the energetic and alchemical nature of it. It was understood that it could be healing in nature or destructive; they sought to harness the positive sides of it, without ever denying a natural part of human life. But it was never seen as a spiritual practice in its own right; this was a later development by contemporary teachers who found that sex as a form of spirituality was easy to sell to the new-age crowd.

Jing and Menstruation

Though women do not lose their Jing through sexual activity to anywhere the same degree that men do, their monthly cycles still have an impact upon their Jing. One of the major aspects of Jing development within the female body is that it converts into menstrual Blood. When women go through their monthly bleed, they lose some of their Jing. If a woman has a healthy quality to her menstrual cycle, then she loses the 'right' amount of Jing and menstruation is also a psychologically balancing event. If, however, she has imbalances in her menstrual cycle, then this can mean that her Jing is negatively impacted. Much of regulation of the menstrual cycle is related to how a woman's cycles of Jing are established, as well as how she relates to environmental elements such as the moon.

Since menstruation and the cycles of female Jing are fairly intricate, I would like to point those interested to a previous book written by myself and my wife, Roni Edlund, entitled *Daoist Nei Gong for Women: The Art of the Lotus and the Moon*, published by Singing Dragon in 2016. It has a great deal of information on female-specific practices, and is highly relevant both to female practitioners of Nei Gong and teachers of these arts.

Jing and Qi Inter-Relations

When the Jing enters into the lower Dan Tian, it also begins to be used up in the process of developing Qi. Though we derive a large part of our energy for Qi production from the air we breathe and the food we eat, we also require the catalysing agent of the Jing. If we look at the characters for Jing and Qi next to one another, we can see how this is alluded to. Figure 7.8 shows these two characters.

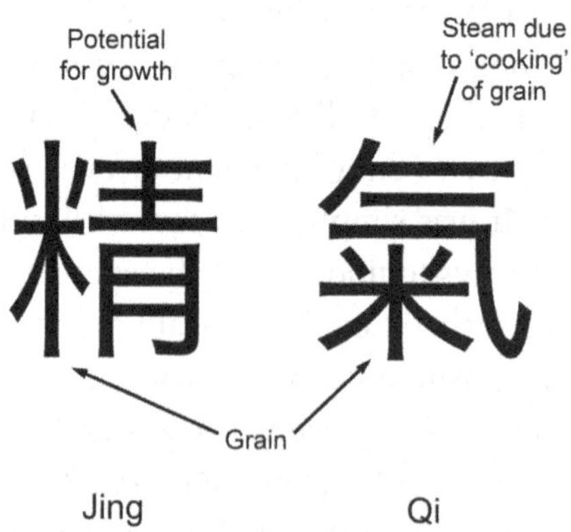

Figure 7.8: Jing and Qi

Looking first at the character for Jing, we can see that the first part of the character shows 'grain', or sometimes people will say it means 'rice'. The second part of the character shows that the 'grain' has potential for growth. This is important to understand: Jing has potential for growth, the potential for life, but only potential.

Like Jing, Qi also contains the character for 'grain' or 'rice', but this time, the image of 'potential' is replaced with 'steam' coming off the rice. It is showing the 'grain' being cooked. What is being indicated here is that the potential of Jing is now going through a process under the action of Qi. In this way, Jing requires Qi in order to manifest any kind of life process, and Qi requires Jing in order to either exist or to have any potential essence to move into action. If we look at the body and how this can be applied on a basic level, we can see that Jing is also initially responsible for the formation of a physical organ itself, whilst the functional activities (the usefulness) of that organ are dependent upon the actions of Qi. If somebody is congenitally weak in Jing, there is the possibility of underdevelopment of the physical body or organs, whereas if a person is congenitally weak in Qi, then these organs will not function as efficiently.

When Jing is moved into action under the influence of Qi, it generates one very important process for us: the process of physical development. This process begins with development of our physical body in the womb and continues throughout our life to take us through the ageing process and, eventually, death. It is here, at the point of leaving the mortal coil, that our Jing exhausts its function; it has completed its job, and so it ceases to be.

The process of Qi is to dictate just how smoothly and healthily we move through the developmental path laid out by our Jing. So, if we have healthy Qi, then we will have a high level of well-being, and so our Jing will carry us through the ageing process in a state free of disease, right into our final years. This is obviously highly oversimplified, but if we break down how Jing and Qi work into their absolute basics, then this is the underlying model we are left with.

The inter-relationship of these two 'treasures' means that they work as one unit, but we very clearly need a 'stilling of the Jing' to help us efficiently generate Qi for the body. This means that, even on a very simple level, the heathier we eat and the better we breathe, the more effective our Jing's actions will be.

Jing, the Zhi and Habits

As stated previously, the Jing is an expression and 'vehicle' that we can use to travel along the path of Ming. Your Jing is a physiological component of Ming, as every aspect of existence, spirituality and consciousness has to be rooted into physicality through the body; this is the key to understanding Daoist mind/body training.

It is said that the key to mastering your Ming is to harmonise the Zhi (志). Zhi is often translated as meaning 'willpower', though this is a slightly inadequate way of understanding the concept. We shall return to the meaning of the Zhi in Chapter 12 when we look at the nature of spirit in greater detail. For now, it is enough to understand that the Zhi acts as a kind of driving force for your consciousness and that it is that part of your psyche which determines how well you will contact the various aspects of your Ming. Part of the reason why I do not favour the direct translation of Zhi as 'willpower' is that it suggests that it is a very 'forceful' aspect of your mind. In the West, we would associate using willpower with using a lot of mental tension. Conversely, in the Daoist arts, we actually build the strength of our Zhi by taking away those factors which prevent it from developing, not through the use of adding mental tension. In essence, we 'take away', instead of 'adding'. The things we take away are primarily our unconscious habits. By relaxing and releasing our habitual mental patterns, the Zhi begins to shine through. Let us look at the mechanics of using mental force to develop 'willpower' as opposed to 'taking away'.

When we try to consciously develop our willpower through using mental force, we do stimulate the Zhi, but we harm it. We do this because mental effort causes the Qi to be used up; this, in turn, starts to deplete the Jing through the reciprocal relationship between Jing and Qi discussed above. The Jing being drained damages the health of the Kidneys which, in turn, are said to be the home of the Zhi. So, in this way, by focusing hard and trying to 'use' our Zhi, we are actually damaging it. This is a common error for many who come into Nei Gong and alchemy; they tend to be those overly obsessive people who wish to race through the process using as much determination as they can.

The quality of the various components of our conscious makeup is determined largely by our mental behaviours. One of the major obstacles to the development of Zhi are our habits; these are unconscious behaviours that we go through as a result of acquired layering. Rid yourself of unnecessary layers to allow the willpower to naturally arise.

Daoism clearly points out that the enemy of the Zhi is habit: common, automatic behavioural patterns that unconsciously add layers to the acquired self and lessen the strength of the Zhi. This ranges from small daily rituals such as always having a cup of tea at a certain time of day, through to more serious addictions. It also concerns thought processes and emotional patterns that are triggered subconsciously – mental habits. Operating according to habits, even helpful ones, becomes a problem that must be challenged at some point if you want to move more deeply into understanding the Zhi, Jing and Ming. It is for this reason that spontaneity of thought and behaviour became a valued quality within Daoist teachings, even if this spontaneity can seem a little mad at first. If you wish to see just how ingrained habitual patterning is in many people, then watch how uncomfortable they are around spontaneity! Those acquired layers don't like it when they are challenged.

If we look at the most extreme of habitual patterns, what we end up with are addictions. Yes, I am aware that there are a whole number of other reasons why addictions develop within us; there are layers of complex psychology involved in why we have them, but in their most simple sense, they share the same internal mechanics as all other habits with regard to how they affect the Zhi. What we have in an addiction is an ingrained habit, often combined with a strong base desire. Both of these combined attack the health of the Zhi and the Jing. Consequently, they will also impact heavily upon the Ming. This gives us an interesting 'health dynamic' when we look at afflictions such as alcoholism or smoking. Not only do these behaviours affect the liver and lungs, they also damage the Zhi and Jing; not simply because of the toxic nature of alcohol or nicotine, but because of the psychological root of these kinds of behaviours. This is why all of our addictions must be looked at and let go of, from obvious addictions such as the ones mentioned above, through to addictive mental states, television, phones, biting your nails, and an infinite number of other issues. What are your habits? Identify them and change them – seek spontaneity and freedom from your mental patterning; this will help strengthen the Jing.

Retraining of Jing Movement

If we look at Figure 7.9, we can see the rough sequence of movement that our Jing goes through. As you can see, there is a little variation between men and women.

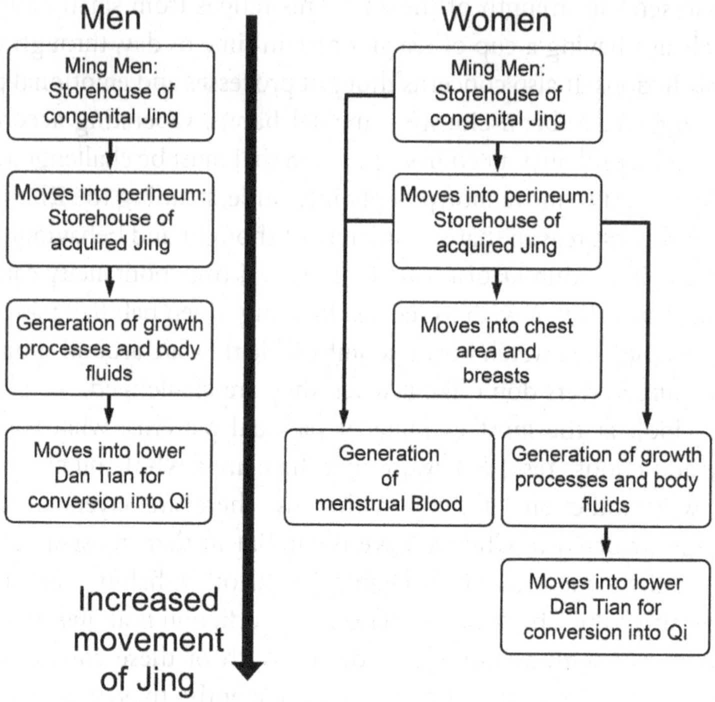

Figure 7.9: Jing Movement in Men and Women

In men, the Jing moves from the region of the Ming Men and Kidneys through into the perineum, and then from here, it goes through a series of transformative processes. Much of it is used up in the generation of body fluids as well as for any physical 'creation' processes within the body, such as skin and cell reproduction. Some of this Jing then also moves into the lower Dan Tian for conversion upwards into Qi. This takes place under the action of the Dan Tian's ability to convert the San Bao from state to state.

In women, this is the same at the beginning, but then varies around the region of the perineum. In the female version of the Jing cycle, there is still the production of body fluids and other physical matter, but there is also the generation of the menstrual Blood in the years prior to menopause. As well as this, some of the Jing travels up the front of the woman's body through the Conception channel to the area of the chest and breasts where it is stored. The Jing in the region of the chest helps to strengthen the emotional centre of the middle Dan Tian as well as producing breast milk when a child is born.

Though there are variations on how the Jing is moved, we wish for similar changes in both genders. We wish for there to be less 'leakage' of Jing so that the processes described above take place more efficiently.

The Difference Between Nei Gong and Alchemy

A special note should be made here concerning the differences between how Jing is governed in the practice of Nei Gong and how it is transformed through alchemy. For those not familiar with the term, alchemy is a type of Daoist meditation that aims to lead a practitioner towards developing the 'alchemical pill', a method leading to spiritual growth. Whilst there are many shared principles across both Nei Gong and alchemy, there are differences in the way that they develop the Jing. To keep it simple, alchemy wishes to 'reverse the course' of the Jing creation process and return it to its congenital form. If we look at the alchemical process of Jing that we discussed previously (shown in Figure 7.10), we can see the direction that Jing naturally takes and how alchemy wishes to reverse that process.

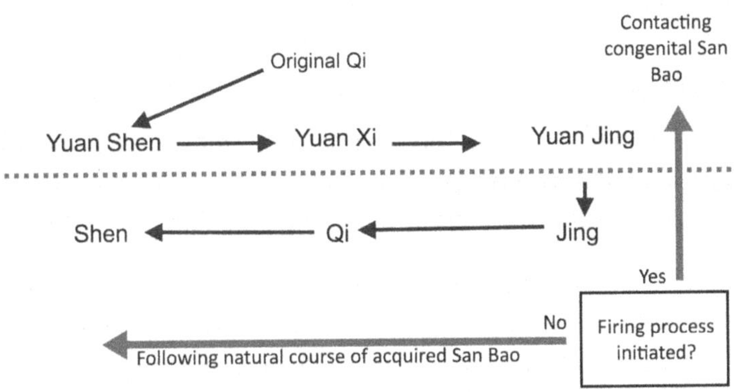

Figure 7.10: The Jing Process of Alchemy

Nei Gong works quite differently. Whilst it is working to change the efficiency of how the Jing functions, it is not going deep enough to contact the congenital forms of Jing. In short, Nei Gong is not so advanced in its approach to the practice. Nei Gong seeks to increase the efficiency of how your body functions, whilst alchemy works to completely 'reprogramme' it. Generally, I advise my students of alchemy to develop a strong foundation in Nei Gong as well; in my opinion, it is almost impossible to approach the alchemical meditation method without prior and parallel Nei Gong training.

The Improved Movement of Jing in Nei Gong

Within Nei Gong, we work to improve the efficiency of the lower Dan Tian region and thus the way in which our Jing is processed. On top of this, we work to change certain psychological aspects as discussed above. These can be summarised as:

- Look at the amount of work and rest we have in our lives; we must try to get this balance as harmonised as we can within the realms of what is possible for us. This is obviously a lifestyle adjustment we may need to make.
- Look at the nature of our sexuality and how it drives us. This is a combination of external changes we can make to our behaviour, as well as a change that will naturally start to evolve for us as the Jing grows more still.
- Look to balance the menstrual cycle for female practitioners. The healthier the quality of a woman's menstrual cycle, the more regulated the Jing's actions can be.
- Look to harmonise the relationship between Jing and Qi through healthy living (for the Qi) and 'stilling the Jing' practice as outlined below.
- Look to explore our habits and help bolster the Jing and Zhi in this way. This is a combination of self-awareness, lifestyle changes, and an aspect of transformation that is helped along by stilling the Jing.

The result of these changes is that our Jing will still carry out the same functions as it has done previously, but at a far more efficient rate. Nei Gong, remember, is all about improving the efficiency of the body's functioning. The more efficient the Jing, the higher our level of health. On top of this, when we build the lower Dan Tian, as described in Chapter 8, the level of Jing efficiency within our body's functioning will help with this process.

Controlling the Lower Basin Practice

Now we are armed with the above information, it is time to actually look at how we can work with the Jing to change the way it functions. We need to help it grow more still, as it is the movement of Jing that leads to its dispersal; we then need to harness the results of this practice. When we can understand both of these elements, then we are said to have governed the lower basin within alchemical teachings. The 'lower basin' is a collective term for the lower abdomen, lower Dan Tian and various mechanisms of the Jing. Note that the term is often used in a slightly different context within martial arts circles, but when the lower basin is referred to within Nei Gong, it matches the alchemical usage of the expression.

Stilling the Jing

Stilling the Jing is, in part, an extension of the exercises outlined in previous chapters. It is all to do with the location and quality of your awareness. In essence, each of the previous chapters and their exercises have been building on one another. The changing of your breathing pattern according to the five keyword qualities then feeds into the regulation of the mind. This then, in turn, starts to lead into the 'stilling of the Jing' practice.

The reason I have split the stages up like this into three chapters, with associated theory, is to make clear just how much importance can be placed upon this aspect of the practice and how long should be spent upon it. In the past, I have written the process out very briefly and given people the wrong impression either that it can be completed quickly or that it is very simple. It is a lengthy process which serves to build a solid foundation. The associated theory should help to show why it is important and why we spend such a length of time on it. Also, as with many aspects of Daoist practice, the theory is quite complex, and yet the practice is quite simple. Curiously, though, we need the practice to 'shape the mind' in the right way, so that the practice unfolds as it should. The 'uninformed' are generally held back in their results.

To still the Jing we simply sit, or stand, and allow the mind to sink down within our body. Allow the absorption of awareness into the breath to lead you to the attained quality of 'deep', and your mind will reach the region of the lower Dan Tian. Note here the importance of this process. Your mind *must* sink to the lower Dan Tian as a result of your absorption into the breath and, so, the body. The natural place for your awareness will be in your head; the cerebral location of the mind. When we enable the quality of 'deep' to develop within us, then our awareness will naturally sink down towards the lower Dan Tian and root itself there. This is in direct contrast to placing your mind on the lower Dan Tian: a common error which many, including myself for a long time, are unaware of. Figure 7.11 outlines this process.

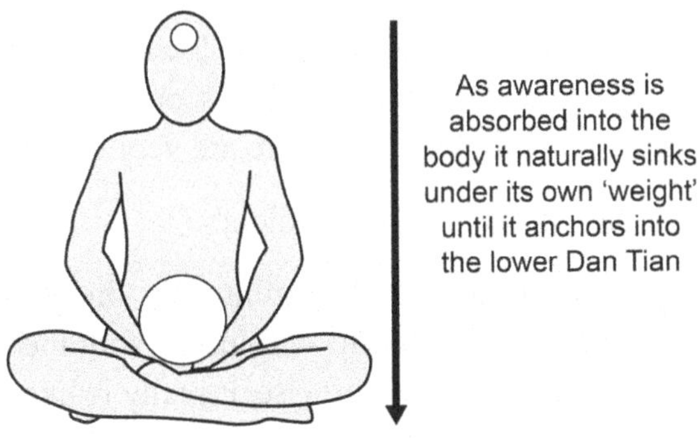

Figure 7.11: Sinking the Awareness Through Absorption

Placing the mind on the lower Dan Tian, or indeed any part of your body, generates a form of mental tension. It is a clear 'action' and as such does not adhere to the power of Wu Wei. 'Actions' are based upon 'adding', and allowing something to take place as a naturally unfolding process 'takes away'. Though the placement of the mind into the lower Dan Tian won't cause problems as such, it will slow down your development and make the process less efficient.

As the mind learns to sink to the lower Dan Tian and anchor itself to this location, we just have to stay there and give the lower Dan Tian some attention. We don't have to 'do' anything as such, we just wait and leave our awareness here on this region of the body. Turn this into a daily practice; spend maybe twenty to thirty minutes each day simply sinking your awareness down to the lower Dan Tian and absorbing it into the body. Allow your awareness to do the work for you. Remember, do not use too much focus, work on the strength of your mind so that it is just right for the practice. 'Casually observe' what is unfolding for you.

You will know when the Jing begins to consolidate or 'still', as there will be a change to the temperature within your lower abdomen. This change in temperature is quite clear. It is quite different from the warmth you feel as a result of an increase in blood circulation; this is more akin to a warm fluid that starts to fill up your abdominal cavity. It is around the same temperature as a warm bath.

The brain registers every experience you have and processes it in a way that you can understand it. So, on a wider scale, much of the information you perceive of the outside world through your senses is translated by your brain into a format that you can interact with. This is also the case inside your body. In general, we can say that the San Bao are experienced in three very clear and distinct ways:

- Jing is generally experienced as heat or a warm fluid that feels as though it is moving somehow.
- Qi is experienced as movement, vibration or sensory changes. Qi is more complex and varied in its possible manifestations, but movement and 'feelings' of pressure are very common.
- Shen is experienced as light or colour.

When the brain starts to process the stilling of the Jing, then the very distinct warmth will start to build up within the abdomen. It is very clear and not easy to mistake for something else; it really is like warm liquid that is flowing around within the abdomen.

If the Jing is in the early stages of stilling, then it will remain within the abdominal cavity, but if it reaches a higher level of development, then it can begin to flow into the lower back, hip joints and groin region of the body. As it moves through these regions of the body, it can be very relaxing and the tissues will unwind as a result of the Jing's presence.

For women, this Jing will often move up the front of the body and into the region of the chest. I have been reliably informed that it causes the breasts and nipples to become warm as well.

If this starts to unfold for you, simply let it be. Allow it to do its work and stay with your practice of absorbing the awareness into the breath and body.

You will know when the Jing has consolidated to a fairly high level, as the heat will move into the perineum itself and start to build there. This time, the heat you experience can be quite different. It will move beyond warmth into a very hot feeling; it can feel as if it should burn you, but it never does. I remember being quite confused and concerned over the level of heat that builds here at the base of the body but you should not worry. As with all tangible experiences, it will manifest and then, after a few weeks, start to fade away. The mind and body normalise experiences very quickly and then they are no longer perceivable by your mind. What will remain, however, is the feeling of warmth in your abdomen and lower back. These areas will always stay warm as a result of the work you are doing with your Jing. I have had both complaints and thanks from partners of students who share a bed with their now very warm lovers. It is like sleeping next to a radiator – something some people like and others don't! It is a good sign, though; your Jing is functioning well for you. If you feel the abdomen of a young child, they are generally warm to the touch; at this age, their bodies are functioning healthily and so the Jing is acting as it should. As we age, most of us lose this quality of Jing and this is what we are trying to return to.

By-Product of Sexual Energy

There is a common issue that many people experience with these kinds of practices, and this is a temporary increase in sexual energy. This is particularly prevalent for male students who then struggle to not give in to sexual temptation. If we wish to develop this practice, then it is no good if every session ends with an orgasm!

Your sexual desire is rooted in the Jing and becomes particularly active when the Jing first starts to still through these kinds of practices. The Jing then moves into the length of the penis, in the case of men, and the increase in energy here generates the reaction of an erection.

In order to reverse this process, there is a simple practice for men which causes their erection to vanish and the acquired Jing to move back into the lower Dan Tian region. Upon having an erection and a feeling of sexual arousal, male practitioners should sit quietly as if beginning meditation practice. With a long slow inhalation, first gently contract the muscles at the base of the penis and then, once they have raised a little, contract the muscles around the perineum until it lifts upwards. On the exhalation, allow both points to relax and release. These two points are shown in Figure 7.12.

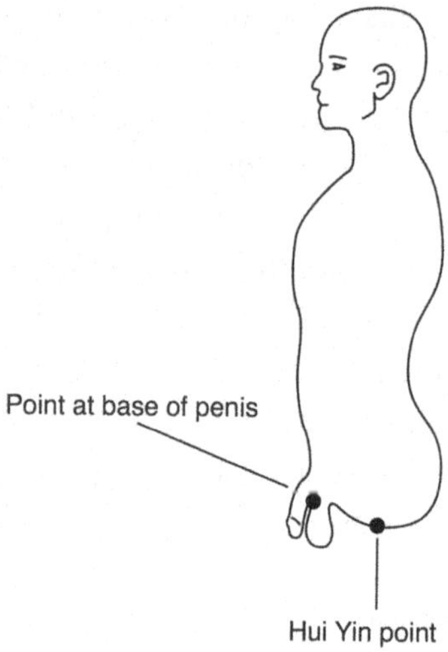

Figure 7.12: Ending an Erection

Throughout this practice, you should gently rest your awareness on the region of the kidneys. You do not have to be too exact, as your mind will understand where to lead the acquired Jing, providing you are roughly within the kidney region of the lower back. Continue with this practice for a few breaths, and the erection should begin to go away. After you have become used to this technique, you will find that you can feel a strong movement of warmth that travels from the shaft of the penis back into the perineum, and then deep inside your body, up into the Kidneys. With practice, this exercise becomes very quick, and then even a simple mental command will be enough to move the acquired Jing.

Women should not worry too much about sexual desires that arise, other than to try to place their mind on another subject. There is less risk for them, as the body is not moving their acquired Jing into a position where it is going to be ejected from the body.

These experiences are generally fleeting and happen as a result of the Jing changing. With time and practice, they will become less; your body will process the Jing in a different way, and so the mind won't register it as a sexual urge.

The Foundations of Jing Stilling

Stilling the Jing should be worked on by new students until the warmth has begun to develop. For those seeking practices to simply help in improving their health, then this is enough; there is no need to go further into Nei Gong. If the breath can be regulated, the mind harmonised and the Jing stilled, then you already have all the ingredients you need for helping to rejuvenate your mind and body. There is enough here for you to adopt as a daily practice and enjoy the benefits of.

If, however, you wish to proceed beyond the foundations of these arts into the more intricate aspects of Nei Gong training, then it is here that you should make sure your foundations are of a high enough standard. We are not after perfection, none of us ever achieve that, but we should try our best to ensure we have the following:

- We need correct bodily alignments when we are standing. Ideally, we should have practised these enough that they are starting to become built into the soft tissue structure of our body. It should almost be difficult for you to stand without these principles being in place.
- Your breathing should have begun to change through the various qualities discussed and be moving towards a healthy level of 'release'. We wish for our breath to become a tool for letting go within our practice.
- The level and quality of your awareness and how you use your mind should have been adjusted according to the teachings in Chapter 6. Once you have managed these three points, then you will have built a foundation in the three regulations of these arts: the body, the breath and the mind.
- Finally, you want to adjust the Jing, its actions and its quality as discussed in this chapter. Ideally, before moving on to the awakening of the energetic system, you should have built up a certain degree of warmth in the lower abdomen. We want our Jing to support our development, and so it is worth spending some time on this exercise. Once we have managed this, then the foundations of our practice are at a satisfactory enough level to build upon with more complex internal work.

Marrow Washing

A more advanced aspect of Jing development lies within the teachings of the Xi Sui Jing (洗髓經) or 'Marrow-Washing Classic'. This was originally a paired scripture, along with the Yi Jin Jing, the Sinew-Changing Classic, which is purported to have been left behind by Bodhidharma at the Shaolin monastery. As discussed in Chapter 3, there are some controversies regarding the accuracy of this historical account, but it does not matter. What is important is that the sinew-changing methods went on to influence bodywork and energetic development within the internal arts of China and that the 'marrow-washing' teachings then had a great impact upon higher-level inner development. Sadly, although the sinew-changing teachings were preserved (if only to a small degree) in written format, the marrow-washing teachings were not so fortunate. Instead, the concepts of marrow washing have been passed on orally within the Daoist tradition. On top of this, a great deal of the marrow-washing teachings were integrated into Daoist alchemical meditation and so many of the teachings from this lost scripture have been integrated into high-level Daoist practice.

The marrow-washing teachings were always saved for those more senior within a tradition and were not generally seen as beginner practices. The aim of the teachings was to help a practitioner understand how their bone marrow, brain tissue and Jing were to be used and developed within the internal arts. Rather than a set of practices or exercises, the marrow-washing principles were a layout of the path that your body transformation would go through at a certain point on the road of your inner development. You will find that many of the Daoist classical texts are like this: they are written to show you where you will go, they are 'confirmational' in nature and not a set of instructions as such. The instructions come from your teacher and the tradition you are in; the classical texts serve to double-check that what is happening for you has been experienced by those masters who came before you through these arts.

Within Daoist practices, one way of categorising people's skill level was according to the 'five depths'. These depths are:

- skin depth
- sinew depth
- channel depth
- viscera depth
- marrow depth.

Though this is not a way of looking at a skill level that is commonly used any more within the arts, mythology said that Bodhidharma only had one student who had attained the Gong of reaching marrow depth. Essentially, this was a metaphorical story to show just how difficult it is to reach the level of marrow depth within these arts.

Skin Depth

Essentially, those who enter into the foundation stages of Qi Gong will have experiences related to various sensations around the body. The nervous system will 'read' and process the information contained within moving Qi to give you the experience of the Ba Chu or 'eight experiences'. Most practitioners of Qi Gong reach this stage within a relatively short space of time. It was known as the 'skin depth' skill within these arts.

Sinew Depth

When a person enters the 'skin depth' level of these arts, it means that they are starting to change the nature of their physical body according to the teachings of the Sinew-Changing Classic. The sinews and the Huang will transform as a result of the practice.

Channel Depth

At channel depth, the physical body has transformed to such a level that the Qi is conducting powerfully along the length of the soft tissues. The result is that the channels begin to open. This is the stage of achieving the various circulations and orbits of Qi Gong as well as having developed the efficiency of the body's functioning to a high level.

Viscera Depth

Beyond the channels come the viscera. At this depth of attainment, the Qi and Shen of the organ systems begin to move into harmony with one another. More than simply implying a high level of 'organ health', attainment of this level of skill means that the 'houses' of the spirits are in order. The result of this is that the Shen is being worked on through your training. It is a high level to reach.

Marrow Depth

When your training reaches the level of marrow depth, then it means the results of the marrow washing will start to take place within your body. This will generally start to happen as an automatic by-product of your training and not as something you particularly need to 'do'. There may be some practices that help this process along its way, of course, but in general, it should start to take place as a natural result of your internal cultivation. This is the deepest stage of work with the body; the stage of transforming the Jing and the marrow.

No Marrow-Washing Practice

Often, classical teachings and scripture are misunderstood and turned into 'exercise systems'. This happened with the sinew-changing teachings, which essentially looked at how the body was formed and how to change it according to internal methods. The result of the sinew changing was that practitioners of these arts would then start to open their channel system. What this was turned into was a number of different exercise systems that involve a lot of stretching and visualisation. Whilst these exercises may indeed utilise some of the teachings from the Sinew-Changing Classic, they are not what the teachings were about in the first place. Instead, they were a series of guidelines that were absorbed into many of the Chinese arts.

This has also happened with the marrow-washing teachings. Though this was actually a discussion of how the Jing and marrow will convert at higher stages in the practice, it has been falsely interpreted as a practice that you 'do'. The results of this are systems of exercise ranging from hitting yourself with steel rods through to massaging and even hanging weights off your testicles if you're a man! Whilst it is true that, in men, testicles are involved in marrow washing, there is no need to start tying any weights to them. Instead, most of the results and benefits of the practice will arise out of your Nei Gong or alchemical meditation.

What Is Marrow Washing?

Marrow washing is based upon the conversion of the Sui (髓). 'Sui' is translated as 'bone marrow' within Chinese medical thought; it has crossovers with the bone marrow as it is understood in Western science, but then has its own unique properties as well. These general properties are:

- It assists in the production of blood

- It nourishes the brain
- It fills the hollows of the bones

When the Qi of the body can conduct deep enough into the Huang, then it will start to reach the bones. This takes place as the level of conduction of Qi reaches a state where it connects into the bones' surface. After this, there is a conduction of Qi, primarily Yang Qi, through to the centre of the bones where it starts to affect the marrow that is filling the hollows of the bones. Some people have tried to assist in this process by 'beating' the Qi in, towards the bones, through the use of steel rods and similar tools; although this may work on a superficial level, it is the full conduction of Qi deep into the body that is needed. This will happen as the soft tissues of the body convert under the process outlined within the Sinew-Changing Classic. Thus, the marrow-washing changes will take place in the correct way as a natural advancement of the sinew-changing process.

Many modern Western theorists have linked the marrow washing to the production of red and white blood cells. Whilst this may be true – as the 'marrow factory' functions at a higher level, the cell production rate will be higher – this was not actually the original aim of marrow washing. Do not misunderstand me, I am not saying that I disagree with the theories of red and white blood cell production being improved as a result of these practices; this may well be the case. I am just saying that this was not the original aim of the methods and so, if this takes place, that is a happy bonus for your health!

Within classical Chinese thought, the Jing produces your marrow. It is as if the marrow grows out of the Jing, and this then goes on further to produce the physical matter of the brain. The original development of the bones, marrow and brain was set out in the earliest stages of your physical development. This is why, within Chinese medical thought, congenital defects involving the brain, bones or their developmental process are considered a sign of inherent Jing imbalance. In the vast majority of cases, this is as a result of deficiency in the Jing.

Over the course of your life, one of the draws on your Jing reserves is the maintenance of the energetic health of the marrow and brain. One developmental pathway of the Jing takes place through the bones, especially along the vertebrae upwards into the brain where it is then converted into energy that helps to nourish the brain. In this way, the physical matter of the brain receives Jing, whilst the energetics of the brain's functioning receives Qi.

So, there are several functions of the marrow-washing process:

- To lead Qi into the marrow of the bones
- To consolidate the Jing to a higher level
- To purify the Jing
- To lead the Jing to the brain
- To generate more Jing

Let us look at each of these in turn. There are very specific reasons for, mechanics and results of each of these processes.

To Lead Qi into the Marrow of the Bones

As the Qi can conduct deeper into the body, it will start to travel into the bones. From here, it will move into the marrow, as shown in Figure 7.13.

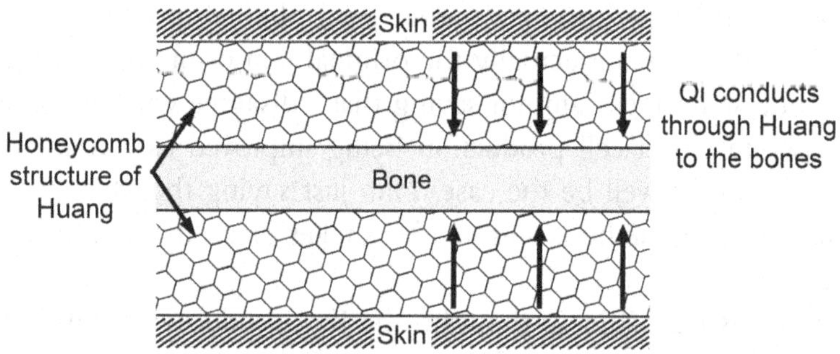

Figure 7.13: Leading Qi to the Marrow

As the Qi begins to interact with the marrow, it will impact upon the production of Blood within the centre of the bones. As discussed above, there is, no doubt, an impact upon Blood cell production involved, but this was not the desired effects of the Qi reaching the bones for the Daoists. Their aim was to strengthen the Blood, as it was understood that the Blood was an anchor for the spirit as it travelled around one's body. This is why there are quite a few psychological symptoms attached to chronic imbalances with the Blood in Chinese medicine. When the Blood starts to move into a deeper state of harmony, then the spirit is affected, and this helps to bring the mind closer to a state of inner stillness. The Daoists worked to strengthen the Blood to calm the spirit. This was important for the later part of the process which involved moving refined Jing into the physical matter of the brain itself.

To Consolidate the Jing to a Higher Level

The Jing can be stilled through cultivation, as described in this chapter, but there is a further level of consolidation that arises naturally out of the practice; this takes place at the seat of your 'lower Jing', the perineum. When the Jing reaches this stage, it is a later advancement of the experiences outlined in this chapter. The deep warmth around the lower back and groin will begin to move into a very fine point that sits in the region of the perineum. It is as if there is a hot point around the size of a marble that sits at the Hui Yin region. This is a common experience to have in periods of deep alchemical practice, but it can also arise here, in Nei Gong, when you begin to move into the stage of the Jing wanting to move into the marrow-washing phase.

If this experience arises, then you should work to maximise the effects. Continue to practise and end all sexual activity for a period of time. You do not want to disperse the Jing at this point, as otherwise this will end its evolution into the marrow-washing phase. If you continue with your practice, then the Jing at this area will begin to purify. This is where the clearest signs of the process are to be had.

To Purify the Jing

Purification of the Jing takes place on two levels, physically and mentally. The Jing is linked to the base-desires aspect of your being – in particular, your sex drive. When the Jing starts to heat up and focus to a very fine point, it goes through a period of purification. As per usual, with many of these processes, it is not all that pleasant! But don't worry, it is a very temporary stage and should only arise a few times at most in your practice. As far as I am aware, the purification of the Jing, the 'cleaning', takes place as a result of the level of energetic compression the Jing has gone through. The feeling of heat at a very fine point happens as the Jing is 'squeezed' by your perineum and the Hui Yin region of the body. Once again, this should be very natural; do not add to it in any way. There is no need for any physical assistance in this, simply allow it to run its course.

On a psychological level, the Jing being processed will start to release a lot of mental imagery. It is as if every sexual image you have ever seen is suddenly replayed to you as a series of fast-moving pictures inside your head. This can be sexual experiences you have had, images you have seen in movies or any other source. They can be pleasant or unpleasant, it does not matter, it is almost like a purging process for your mind, as it wishes to remove attachments to sexual stimuli that you have received. These images will move very fast and it is quite amazing just how many there are stored within your brain, anchored into the 'substance' of the Jing. It can last for several days, a hyperactivity of the mind as it is saturated with your sexual connections. When you try to sleep, the images will still be there, so expect some insomnia during this time!

It is very important that, even though your sexual drive will be incredibly high (for obvious reasons), you do not have sex whilst this visual process is unfolding. You want to allow the purging process to continue, so that the Jing can go through its purification process. Orgasm will cause the Jing to move, and this will end the process. Just let it run its course and, with time, it will be over. Afterwards, many will find that past sexual trauma is released. It is quite amazing just how many human hang-ups are associated with our sexual attachments and imbalances, so this is a healthy process to go through.

The physiological side of the Jing purifying can happen alongside or, often, separate from the psychological side of the process. It will vary from student to student, with some having a very strong mental connection to the process whilst others will experience it in a more bodily fashion. When the Jing starts to react with you on a physiological level, it will hyper-stimulate the energy of your sexual organs. The result of this is a very high level of sexual arousal and a hypersensitivity of feeling around the genitals.

Though, to some, this may sound pleasant, students and practitioners I know who have gone through this do not enjoy the process. It essentially leaves you on the verge of orgasm (and ejaculation in men) for several days, sometimes up to a couple of weeks. It is best, at this stage, to shut yourself away from society and be on your own, as even the most innocent of physical contacts with another person can send your arousal level spiralling out of control. As the Jing starts to end this process, your sex drive returns to normal and the sensations around the sexual organs will fade away. For male practitioners, this will happen as a result of moving deeper towards the stage of marrow washing. For women, curiously, it can also come at different stages in their practices, though to a lesser degree and for a shorter period of time. Many women will find that the Jing begins to purify when they engage with practices such as 'moon gazing', a common Nei Gong method that is specific to female practitioners. It is normal for the Jing to react to the practice and for sexual arousal to take place; it is even not uncommon for women to reach orgasm through Qi Gong methods like this. It is nothing to worry about; though many people have an embarrassment around discussing sex and their sex drive, these are all just aspects of the Jing – more bodily processes to unfold through the practice.

To Lead the Jing to the Brain

The Nao (腦) is the 'brain' in Chinese. It is said to govern our level of intelligence as well as the nature of our sensory connection to the outside world. As well as this, it is a kind of translator for the world around us. Within Daoist thought, the world is made up of a series of energies, frequencies, that are held in place by a spiritual energy known as the Ling Zi (靈子) or 'spiritual particles'. You can think of the Ling Zi as the smallest possible particles of matter held together by a divine form of consciousness through which flows Dao. The job of the brain is to receive information (via the senses) and then interpret it into a format that you can understand. Some of this information is filtered out and so most people do not perceive this level of reality, whilst other information is processed to give us the sense of reality that we live within.

At the centre of this process is the upper Dan Tian, anchored into the pineal gland, which works to receive the same type of information – Ling Zi – but from 'higher' places. Within Daoist thought, when the brain has been nourished in the right way, the 'marrow' of the brain will be cleaned and this will then impact upon the upper Dan Tian and how it functions. The result is an opening of the Tian Mu (天目) or 'spiritual eye'; you could equate this with 'opening the third eye' as it is commonly known within most alternative circles. When the Tian Mu is opened, then the 'bandwidth' at which your brain can interpret the Ling Zi of 'reality' widens and so more information can be received. This information can often come in the form of 'spiritual information' and it was understood as a way to heighten the efficiency of the mind's functioning.

There are many signs of the Tian Mu opening as a result of the Jing reaching the 'marrow' of the brain. These generally come in the way of an increased level of visual awareness that begins with the ability to perceive the frequency of Qi and then develops further in other ways.

To Generate More Jing

The final and most important aspect of the marrow-washing process is that it helps to actually build Jing. This is a controversial aspect of the Daoist internal arts. Can we replace Jing or can we not? The debate rages on amongst practitioners! Part of this debate is because Chinese medical teachings state that it is not possible. Daoist alchemical teachings, however, assert that it is indeed possible.

More Jing can be generated within the body if you have reached the stage of full marrow washing within your practice. Since you are generating more Jing, the body will be able to restore itself to a high level of health and youthfulness. It is at this stage of the practice that many of the famed longevity aspects of the Daoist arts have their root. As you go through your practice, more Jing is generated within the body and it moves down into the usual storage locations for your Jing. It is a long process, though; the extra Jing is produced in the equivalent of very small drops and so, if a person wanted to fully restore their Jing, it would take many hours of continuous practice after reaching the marrow-washing state.

It was made very clear to me by my teachers that, even though we can experience some of the benefits of this process, to really focus on rebuilding the Jing would require removal from society into seclusion in order to minimise distraction. This is where many of the Daoist myths arise of very ancient masters living in the caves of China. It is also where the youthful face of the Daoist master came from. It is understood that although the masters may have white hair and be very advanced in their age, they have youthful faces. Indeed, some of the high-level masters I have met have youthful physiques and faces despite their advanced ages; it can give them a somewhat ageless appearance.

For those who, like me, live a normal life as a part of society, there are still signs of the Jing going through this process that can be experienced through the marrow-washing process. The first of these is the production of the 'jade fluid' as a result of the Jing's cycling into the 'brain marrow'. The second is the regenerative effects of the practice; these are obviously more subjective experiences as it will depend upon our personal feeling, but certainly, the more I practise these arts, the more open, supple and strong my body becomes.

The Jade Fluid

If you have previously managed to open the Conception channel of the body and your Jing is starting to reach the brain, then the Yu Ye (玉液), or 'jade fluid', will start to manifest. This is a very strong, thick, sugary-tasting substance that fills the mouth during your practice. Do not underestimate just how strong-tasting this fluid is. It is as if the mouth has suddenly been filled with a substance that is a mixture of honey and cola; you cannot mistake it. It is also slightly thick and viscous in nature, like slightly watery molasses. In my experience, it starts to form on the roof of the mouth, where your tongue naturally rests if you let it relax, and then it starts to drip into your mouth.

This fluid is said to be the result of the production of pure Jing within the region of your 'brain marrow'. In this way, the marrow of the bone serves to build Blood, whilst the marrow of the brain has the potential to form Jing; this is very rare, though. Some traditions will actually cause this substance to manifest out of the crown of the head as a visible fluid, whilst others will seek to generate it through mantra and ritual cleansing of the body. Within Daoist alchemical practice, this fluid forms on the roof of the mouth, an area known as the 'magpie bridge', as a result of the Jing moving into the brain via the congenital circulation of the microcosmic orbit. It is considered a high-level attainment that arises out of progression from sinew changing to marrow washing.

Interestingly, if you ever have the chance to experience it, it can also be scraped off your tongue and sniffed. Yes, I know that sounds gross, but I am curious by nature. If you smell it then it is very sweet smelling too; almost like a natural perfume. This is because 'pure' Jing, Jing in its congenital state, is supposed to be sweet tasting and sweet smelling; it is the basis for what they call the 'golden fragrance' in Daoism. Essentially, this is the pleasant-smelling scent that a Daoist master's body should give off if you ever deem it appropriate to give them a sniff!

This fluid must be swallowed down to the lower Dan Tian in order to complete the marrow-washing congenital aspect of the microcosmic orbit. There is a very clear method which ensures that the essence of the jade fluid is extracted and ready for absorption into your body's system. Within Daoist metaphorical language, the rising of the energy along the Governing channel is often referred to as 'clouds' rising from the 'water' of the perineum. From here, the clouds condense back into 'rain' – the jade fluid – which then falls back to the base of the body once more.

When the fluid appears in your mouth, you should gently stretch up your head to extend your neck as shown in Figure 7.14. This opens up the top of the Conception channel which runs down the length of your neck.

With your neck stretched like this, press your tongue with a little force against the roof of the mouth to reinforce the connection between the two main channels of the microcosmic orbit. Now, swallow the fluid in your mouth whilst resting your awareness along the length of your Conception channel. If you manage to do this correctly, then, as you swallow the contents of your mouth, there will be a wave of warmth that travels down the length of your Conception channel all the way to the lower Dan Tian. Some of my students and peers have reported that this also feels like a small electrical current.

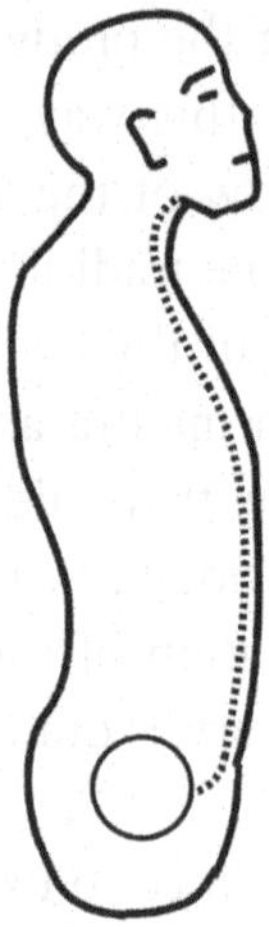

Figure 7.14: Extending the Neck and Conception Channel

When the movement of the jade fluid reaches the lower Dan Tian, you will feel a glow of extreme heat radiating out from the abdomen; it will then begin to shift around quite powerfully. It is as though the Dan Tian was filled with warm, bubbling fluid which begins to rotate around in its core. It is normal for the physical body to begin to follow it to some degree, and sometimes quite violent twisting motions can be experienced in your torso. These are nothing to worry about and will subside on their own after the first few times you experience them. It is also quite common for a light glow to appear to emanate from the lower abdomen when you have your eyes closed. It is as if there was a low light coming up inside your mind's eye whilst you are sat in your practice.

The reason that you can extract essence from the fluid within your mouth is because of the Conception channel which runs from the throat along the front of the body and then via an internal branch to the Dan Tian. When you swallow, the saliva is taken into your stomach. This is the physical, manifested component of the jade fluid which is only the vessel for the essence which you are trying to extract. When you use the above method, you separate the fluid from its energetic essence which then travels directly along the Conception channel and through into the lower Dan Tian. From here, some of the essence also reaches the perineum area and it is common for this to produce a sudden sexual arousal, particularly in male students. If this happens, then simply use the method of extracting Jing from an erection that was discussed earlier in this chapter, and the feelings of arousal will subside.

As with many aspects of Daoism, there have been misunderstandings of this process and so there are now many writings saying that you should look to swallow lots of saliva when you practise Qi Gong. There are 'saliva rinsing methods' for the mouth that many people do and exercises aimed at generating more saliva by moving your tongue around in your mouth. Sadly, although there may be other benefits I am not aware of, this was not what was being discussed in the classical teachings. It was not the saliva that was sought after, but the Yu Ye, the jade fluid. This was because the sweetness of the jade fluid was said to carry with it fresh Jing that had been processed within the marrow of the brain and then led downwards to the lower Dan Tian and perineum region. In this way, our acquired Jing is used to create a more efficiently operating 'marrow factory' and this, in turn, produces healthier Blood, a more harmonious mental state and fresh Jing for the body.

It is my personal experience that the jade fluid will come and go. Perhaps this is different if you live in seclusion and this is the focus of your practice, but currently I live in a house in a town! As the marrow washing is just a part of what I do, I allow the process to develop of its own accord and, when appropriate, swallow down the jade fluid as and when it arises.

If we look to the three instructional words of these practices, they are:

- Yan (嚥) – swallow
- Xi (吸) – inhale
- Bi (閉) – close.

The jade fluid should be allowed to arise, it should then be swallowed as described above, and inhaled by the lower Dan Tian as a natural result of the swallowing process. It should then, finally, be 'closed' or 'sealed shut'.

Closing the Jade Fluid

After your practice of swallowing the jade fluid, you should 'close' the body. As discussed above, as the Jing reaches your lower Dan Tian, it is normal to have several heat-based and often movement-type reactions. Just allow these to conclude of their own accord. Then, when finished, close down the body by gently but firmly patting the lower abdomen and back for a couple of minutes. Follow this by massaging the lower back around the kidney region. This will help to bring Qi to the area. As the Qi reaches this part of the body, it will help the function of the channel system and so the Jing will be stored within the body or else be led back to the Kidneys; in this way, it helps to build up the reserves of your Jing.

Okay, so the process of marrow washing I have outlined here is the foundation of what is taking place within your body. I hope that you can see that marrow washing is a natural evolution of the sinew-changing process and also involves some of the mechanics of the microcosmic orbit. Beyond this, the further teachings of the Xi Sui Jing were concerned with alchemical transformation of substances from their acquired to congenital state. Although there are obviously crossovers here with Nei Gong, this is more relevant to Nei Dan meditation and I will therefore not go into more detail here; you can find this in my other writings around the subject of Daoist meditation.

Chapter 8

AWAKENING THE ENERGY BODY

Once we have established a solid enough foundation with our bodywork, we can begin to look in more detail at the process of waking up the energetic system. This is a process of developing the Dan Tian, in particular the lower Dan Tian, and utilising it in order to move Qi to a higher degree through our body. We can think of waking up the lower Dan Tian as being like putting the keys in the ignition of our car; without this, the car will not drive. Once the engine is running, though, we will have access to a whole other layer of our body's functioning; it is here that the real 'internal' journey begins.

I should remind you here that before you enter into the realm of working with the Dan Tian in this manner, you should have really established a healthy pattern of breathing, as well as a certain degree of stilling of the Jing. We want the body to be as prepared as we can make it prior to entering this phase of our training. The initial stages of waking up the Dan Tian can be very 'active' stages of the process for many people and so we wish to buffer this step in our development by having a very deep, calming quality to our breathwork, along with a consolidated nature to the Yin essence of our Jing.

Before we look at the processes involved in working with the body in this way, let us return to and explore the Dan Tian in more detail. In previous chapters, there were brief discussions of the Dan Tian, but now we wish to look closer at exactly what we mean when we use this term.

The Dan Tian

The first thing to look at when defining the term 'Dan Tian' is the Chinese characters. They can often give us a more in-depth understanding of the term. Figure 8.1 shows the characters for Dan Tian.

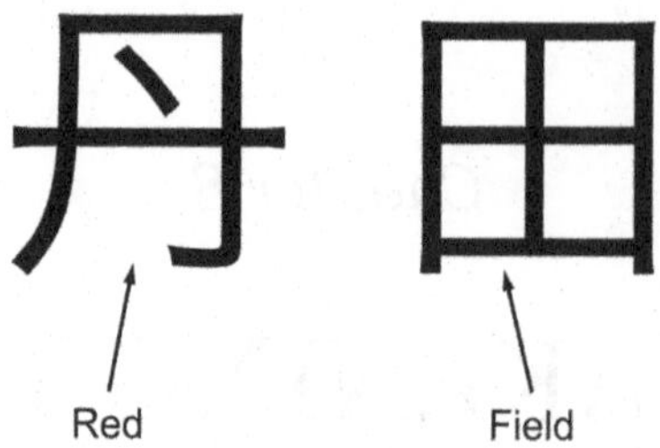

Figure 8.1: Dan Tian

The first character means 'red' or 'cinnabar' – the ore of mercury – which in internal alchemy refers metaphorically to the divine substance that is produced within the consciousness of the practitioner through diligent and correct practice. This substance is processed by and stored within the Dan Tian region of the body at very late stages in the alchemical process. Interestingly, the character can mean a 'refined medical substance' as well. So, the first character is showing us that the Dan Tian are the regions of the body used in very late stages of our practice to store the refined spiritual substances that we can form through our practice; it is also showing us that here, in the Dan Tian, is the potential for inner health. As with other Chinese terms, though, it is showing us the highest possible attainments of the Dan Tian, not where we are right now. We currently, at this stage, do not yet have 'Dan' in our lower abdomen!

The second character means 'field' or 'farmland'. It is showing us that we need to 'plant the seeds' of a practice here to develop the 'crops' of a developed Dan Tian. There is work to be done. Interestingly, as well as this meaning, there is also an added clue as to the location of the lower Dan Tian. The character of 'Tian' shows 'cross-hairs'. This is an allusion to the process of locating the Dan Tian, as discussed in Chapter 4, whereby we draw a line between certain acupuncture points to find its centre.

The higher-level function of storing the 'Dan' indicated within its name is more relevant to its function in Daoist alchemical meditation; within Nei Gong training, we actually use the Dan Tian for other processes. These are primarily to do with driving, directing and transforming energetic substances within the body. At later stages, we also store Qi within the Dan Tian, but this really should not be your first concern. For the early to intermediate stages of practice you really are better off forgetting any notion of storing Qi in the Dan Tian, as it can actually cause you problems if the body is not properly prepared for it.

Dan Tian Location Controversy

As with many things in the world of the internal arts, there are differences of opinion between teachers on the nature and location of the Dan Tian. Most (but not all) teachers would agree that there are three main Dan Tian within the body that we use for our practice, but then they are often placed in different regions of the body. I have had different teachers myself who have worked with different Dan Tian, but generally they fall into one of two models with regard to where they sit in the body.

Figure 8.2 shows the first and arguably most common model for the location of the three Dan Tian.

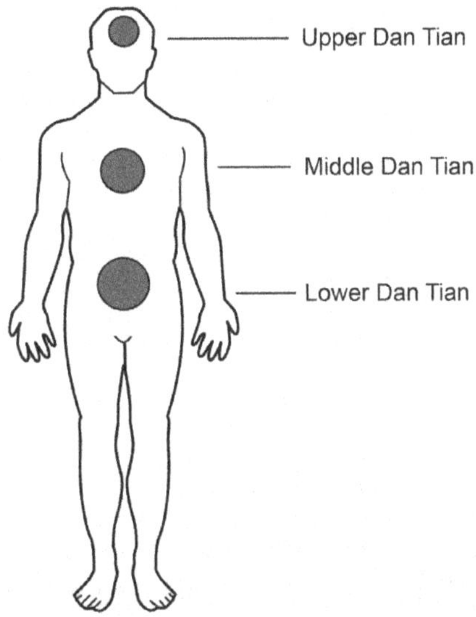

Figure 8.2: The Energetic Model

Here, we have the lower Dan Tian situated, as stated above, within the lower abdomen. Its location will vary from person to person for various reasons, such as individual body shape, size and age, but generally it is located within the lower abdomen behind the Qi Hai acupuncture point, as discussed in Chapter 4.

The middle Dan Tian sits within the centre of the chest at the height of your heart. This is the emotional centre as well as the place in which the mind and our Qi interact with one another.

The upper Dan Tian sits within the centre of the head, with the pineal gland being the physical anchor by which this energetic sphere attaches itself to the realm of manifestation.

I tend to refer to this common model of the three Dan Tian as the 'energetic model', as it tends to be used by Qi Gong and Nei Gong methods concerned with energetic movement, rotation and refinement. Commonly, practitioners are aiming to nourish the body with an increase of Qi, circulate it more effectively through the body, and then finally refine it upwards so that it nourishes the consciousness. There may be a number of variations on this theme, but this tends to be the general theory behind those practices which utilise the energetic model. It is common within medical Qi Gong as well as spiritual Qi Gong and many Nei Gong systems.

Figure 8.3 shows the second common model for understanding the location of the three Dan Tian.

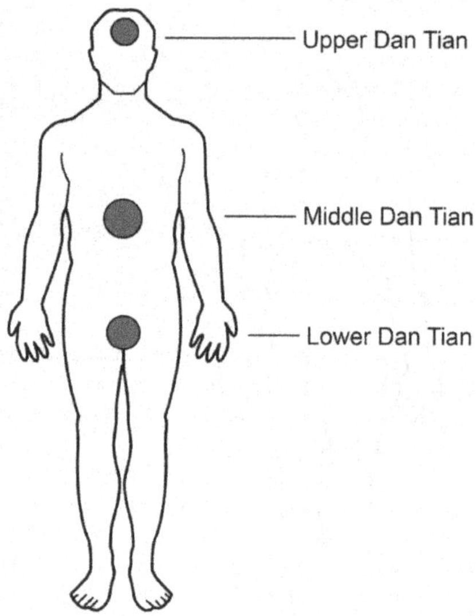

Figure 8.3: The Alchemical Model

In this model, the lower Dan Tian is situated right on the perineum itself. It is much smaller than the lower Dan Tian is seen to be within the energetic model and its location is non-variable from person to person. The middle Dan Tian is situated within the centre of the body. This is a region of the body commonly known as the 'yellow court', and it is around the solar plexus region. If you wish to locate this area on yourself, then measure four fingers' width from the upper border of your navel. This will get you in the rough region; now palpate around a little until you locate a slightly tender region of the body. In many people, there is a slight depression to be found as well. The upper Dan Tian, like the previous model, is located within the centre of the head (though I have seen variations on this where it appears on the crown of the head).

I refer to this as the alchemical model, as it is the view of the energy body commonly used by systems of practice greatly influenced by Daoist alchemical meditation.

Whichever model is being taught, it is common for the teacher to state that theirs is the correct model. The fact is: both are correct, it just depends upon what your aims are in the practice. The confusion comes when both models use the same term, the Dan Tian, to discuss the energetic conversion centres they are focusing upon.

In order to avoid confusion, when I teach, I use the common names of the three Dan Tian when discussing the energy centres shown in the energetic model. I then use the alternative, alchemical names for the centres shown within the alchemical model. When put together, what we have is the combined model shown in Figure 8.4. This is a model used within more esoteric systems of Daoist practice. These systems use a combination of Qi Gong, Nei Gong and alchemy in order to achieve their aims.

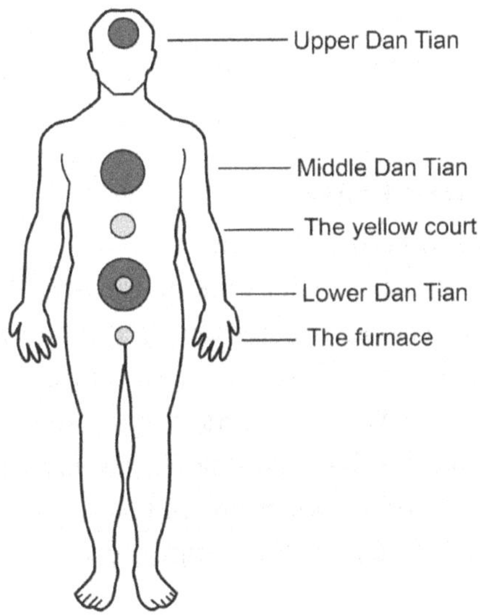

Figure 8.4: The Combined Model

In the combined model, we can see that the lowest energetic centre is the Lu (爐), the furnace. Above this is the lower Dan Tian with the Ding (鼎), the cauldron, at its centre. Above the lower Dan Tian is the yellow court, and above this again is the middle Dan Tian. Situated within the centre of the head is the upper Dan Tian: the energetic centre agreed upon by almost all systems of practice. With this model, we can see how the Ding and the Lu interact with and function alongside the three Dan Tian.

So, the lowest of the centres would be the Lu or furnace. Though some schools would term this a Dan Tian, I would disagree on the basis that no Dan is ever stored here. Instead, this region is used within early stages of alchemical practice as a way to 'ignite' the 'firing process' of alchemy.

This process uses the centre of the lower Dan Tian sat within the abdomen to capture the results of this process; this is called the Ding or cauldron. If you would like more information on these two centres and how they work, then please refer to my previous title, *White Moon on the Mountain Peak: The Alchemical Firing Process of Nei Dan* (published by Singing Dragon in 2016), which details the alchemical processes of Daoist meditation.

The final point worth noting is the yellow court or solar plexus region of the body. This area of the body is sometimes known as a Dan Tian, because it has a strong relationship to the Qi produced through your digestive processes, as well as being linked to an important region of your nervous system. Within the methods I teach, the yellow court is used for merging Fire and Water within alchemical work and, as such, I do not refer to it as a Dan Tian myself. The three locations within the combined model shown in Figure 8.4 are where I place the actual Dan Tian, and it is these that I will be referring to when I discuss the Dan Tian in practice.

The Upper Dan Tian

It was briefly discussed earlier that the upper Dan Tian is the centre of all higher 'spiritual' functions as well as the place where Shen is converted into emptiness. It is also here, in this region of the energetic matrix, that the Ling is developed. We shall return to this concept in Chapter 12. The upper Dan Tian is made up of various layers, each corresponding to a different frequency of existence for your consciousness. Generally, we are shut off from these nine layers of information, but with practice it is possible to contact them. Figure 8.5 depicts these nine layers.

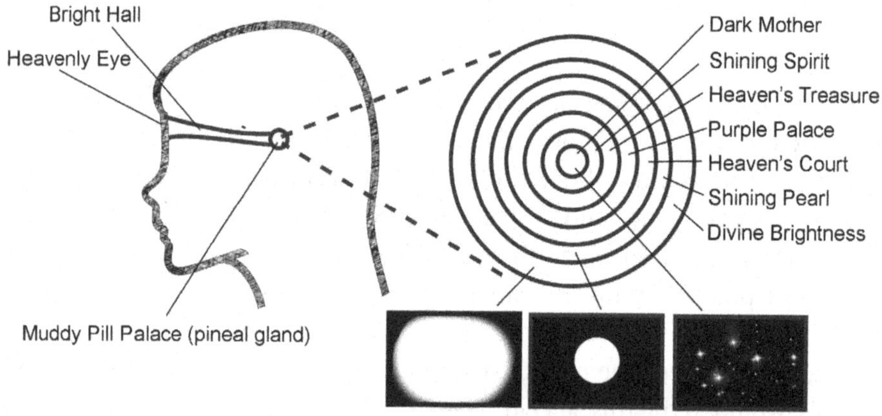

Figure 8.5: Nine Layers of the Upper Dan Tian

Note that layers one and two – the Heavenly Eye and the Bright Hall – exist as forms of Shen that are rooted into the space between your eyebrows, as well as the 'passageway' that runs between this point and the centre of your head, near to where the pineal gland sits. The other seven layers of the upper Dan Tian exist as spherical fields of information that expand outwards from a central point, anchored into the pineal gland itself – a part of the glandular system known as the Muddy Pill Palace in Daoism.

At later stages in your training, you will know when you have touched upon the frequency of the upper Dan Tian layers, as various visual phenomena manifest within your mind's eye. When you reach the layer of Divine Brightness, you will see a white light that fills your vision. It is a very strong light that feels as though it should hurt your eyes but doesn't.

The next layer is known as the Shining Pearl, as the result of touching this layer is that the white light within your mind's eye starts to shrink down and condense into a pearl-like form. This light can either flicker (if the mind is unstable in its movements) or sit there as a stable manifestation as you move deeper through the layers of the upper Dan Tian.

At the absolute, deepest region of the Dan Tian, the Dark Mother region, you will experience a vast ocean of stars; it is as if you are floating out in space. This is a profound place to touch upon in your practice; it sits on the border of the gateway to Dao, the result of passing along the Xuan Men. Some teachers say that the stars are simply movements of the mind, like spiritual versions of the synapses firing off in your brain, whilst other teachers say that these stars are the Ming connections to both past and future existences; whatever the case, it is a very beautiful place to reach in your practice and pretty frustrating when you cannot return there at will!

It is here, within the upper Dan Tian, that many of the mysterious paranormal abilities of Nei Gong myths reside. The upper Dan Tian contains a huge level of spiritual, psychic and evolutionary potential; much of this aspect of human existence is barely understood within even the oldest of the wisdom traditions. It is also here that most connections to regions such as Wuji and Dao are to be had.

The Middle Dan Tian

The middle Dan Tian is a spherical field of energetic information that is anchored into the Heart centre. Note that the Heart centre and the physical organ of the heart are not actually one and the same. The actual Heart centre sits directly behind the sternum, an inch or so back into the chest cavity.

It has a strong relationship to the heart as well as a resonance with the thymus gland. The location of the middle Dan Tian is shown in Figure 8.6.

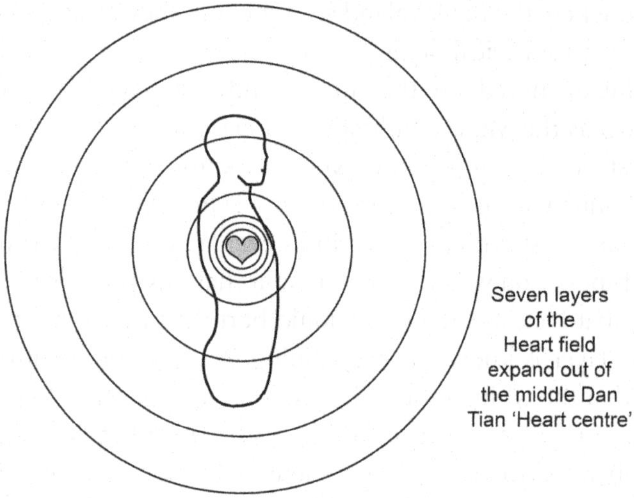

Figure 8.6: The Middle Dan Tian and the Heart Centre

There is a large electromagnetic field that extends out from around the Heart centre, and this essentially makes up the outer field of the middle Dan Tian. As with the upper Dan Tian, there are numerous layers of this field – in this case seven – which correspond to different levels of density of this field. These seven layers are shown in Figure 8.7 along with their names.

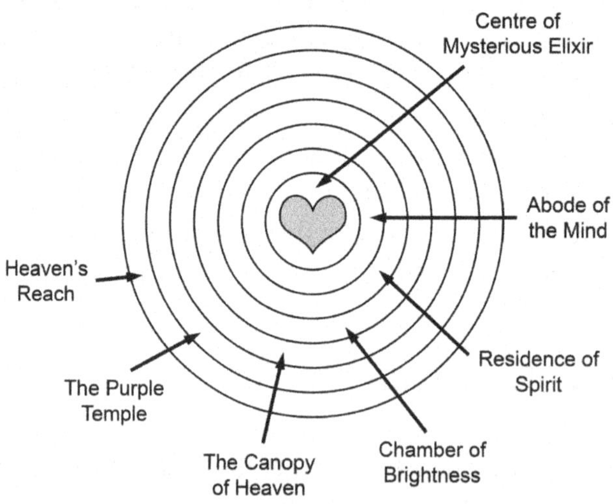

Figure 8.7: The Seven Layers of the Middle Dan Tian

Layers one through to three are the densest of the seven layers. They exist within the 'frequency band' of Qi and are layers that still reside within the chest cavity. The fourth field breaches the physical boundary of the body, whilst layers five through to seven exist outside of the body. Depending upon the strength of a practitioner's middle Dan Tian cultivation, these fields can either remain close to a person or expand out into a very large space. If the field is too close to the body, then a person can feel shut off from others and the chest can even look collapsed inwards, whilst if there is too much space within the outer three layers of the Heartfield, then a person will be too 'open' and absorb emotional information from those that they interact with.

These fields of the Heart centre are essentially expressions of the strength of the middle Dan Tian; it is here that Qi is either converted 'upwards' into Shen or else 'leaked' outwards into emotional expression. If the mind is not stable, if it is filled with thoughts and mental action, then most Qi converted within the region of the middle Dan Tian serves to become emotional energy. This energy then feeds our mental processes to give them an emotional quality. Then, some of the Qi within this region is instead converted into a more ethereal substance so that it may nourish the intellect. If, however, we can still the mind, then the middle Dan Tian is more stable. The result of this is that more Qi moves upwards into the upper Dan Tian region to nourish either consciousness or spirit, depending upon our stage of development. It is for this reason that the Daoists prescribed a healthy practice of stilling the mind in order to move towards spiritual cultivation; it was, in part, so that the middle Dan Tian did not draw away too much Qi for emotional expression.

When we send Qi upwards through the body, it is important that we understand the process of stilling the mind, otherwise we run the risk of sending any excess Qi developed into the region of the Heart centre and so cause emotional swings and sometimes chronic emotional imbalance. We will discuss this more in Chapter 9.

As the middle Dan Tian becomes more 'cultivated', then it is said that the seven spaces of the mind open up. This is essentially a way of saying that we stabilise the seven layers of the middle Dan Tian's field and so can contact our consciousness to a higher degree. When this happens, there is generally a sense of blissful connection to life and others that can develop, though this in itself can be a kind of trap for our practice. Again, we shall discuss this in the next chapter.

The Lower Dan Tian

The lower Dan Tian is the primary centre that we will be working with during these earlier stages of 'waking up' the energy body. It is also the only centre that we spend long periods of time developing directly. This is because it sits at the base of the body, amongst the more 'dense' and less fragile elements of our inner environment. Direct work involving the intention and the upper or middle Dan Tian can actually be a little risky; it is like tinkering with the inner workings of a machine that we don't fully understand. Direct work with the lower Dan Tian is not risky in this way, as it is based in dense, physical components of the body and does not have such a close relationship with the psycho-emotional aspects of our being. Essentially, as we practise, the lower Dan Tian work like a series of cogs. As the lower Dan Tian is developed, it begins to influence the middle Dan Tian and then this, in turn, influences the upper Dan Tian. In this manner, we develop the middle and upper energy centres as a by-product of our work with the lower Dan Tian. This is then combined with mental cultivation, as it is the stillness that we cultivate that causes this relationship to unfold in the correct manner.

The lower Dan Tian is a particularly interesting and complex aspect of our inner workings, as it comprises both energetic and physical material. This is something that is often missed – some schools claim that the Dan Tian is a purely energetic thing, whilst others claim it is purely physical; in truth, it is both. It is an energetic sphere made up of a combination of the body's inherent Yin and Yang Qi combined with various soft tissue and muscular aspects that sit within the region of the lower abdomen. Both the energetic and the physical aspects of the lower Dan Tian require development for it to function properly, but we *must* cultivate the energetic aspects of the lower Dan Tian first for efficient Nei Gong usage. I wish to make this clear, as there are certain schools that work by trying to develop the physical components of the Dan Tian first, and this can actually get in the way of your Dan Tian's most important function of driving the Qi through the channel system. The physical aspect of the Dan Tian must be developed as a result of the energy work taking place at its centre.

Figure 8.8 shows the location of the lower Dan Tian along with some of the physical components it comprises.

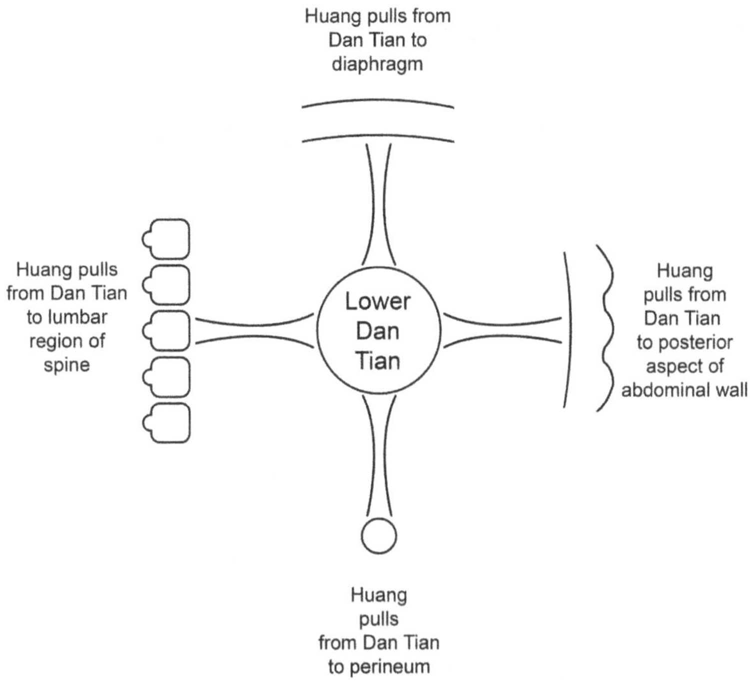

Figure 8.8: The Energetic and Physical Aspects of the Lower Dan Tian

Let us now look at the energetic and physical components of the lower Dan Tian in turn. We shall look in more detail at the lower Dan Tian than we did with the previous two Dan Tian since it forms such a major aspect of our practice at this stage in the Nei Gong process.

Energetic Components of the Lower Dan Tian

The lower Dan Tian is essentially a 'field' of energetic information that resides within the lower abdomen, beneath the diaphragm, and focused largely behind the navel. The Daoists likened it to a 'sea of Qi'. This is how the lower Dan Tian is structured within the abdomen of the majority of people who do not train in any way, once they have gone through puberty. Though there is still a concentration of energy within the abdomen, it is somewhat dispersed and lacking definition, like a cloud of Qi. This Qi moves within the abdomen over the course of a day and is distributed throughout the channel system as well as into the viscera of the body. It is then continuously fed, in part from Qi we receive from our air and food, but also in part by the conversion of the Jing.

This quality of the lower 'field' is quite different from when we are much younger. As children, the Qi within the lower abdomen was much more condensed in nature and formed a defined sphere rather than a 'cloud'. It rotated freely and delivered Qi to a far higher degree through our channel system; this helped with our developmental and physical growth processes, as well as serving to give us an abundance of youthful energy. In essence, one of our first tasks is to return the lower Dan Tian to this quality that we once had: from image A to image B as shown in Figure 8.9.

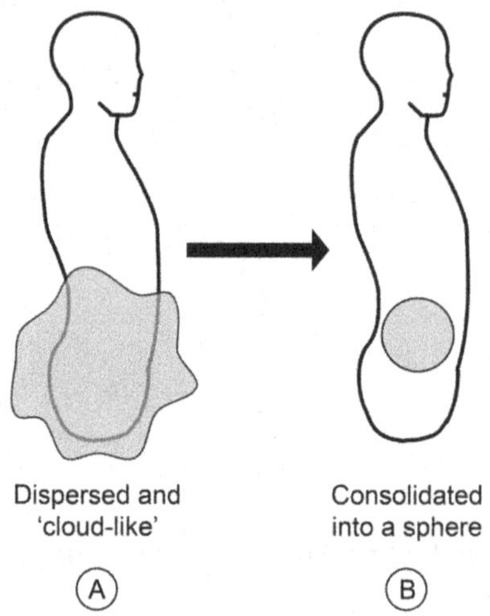

Figure 8.9: Dispersed and Condensed Lower Dan Tian

This is yet another aspect of 'reversing the course' or 'returning to the state of a child', concepts that are very important within the Daoist tradition.

There are several reasons why the lower Dan Tian starts to disperse as we move beyond our childhood, described below.

First is the change of our gait as we walk. As toddlers, we tend to walk in a very sunk-down manner. The centre of our gravity is within the lower abdomen, and this means that there is a strong resonance between our inherent Yin Qi and the Qi of the planet. As we begin to stand more upright and walk with our centre higher, this causes the relationship between the Dan Tian and the Earth to decrease. This begins at a very young age, and here lie the initial stages of the Dan Tian dispersal process.

Consistently standing and walking with our weight focused into our heels is another reason for the Dan Tian dispersing. We tend to learn to stand and walk in the easiest fashion possible, and that is by dropping our mass down through the skeletal system to the floor. This shuts the Yong Quan points on the feet, which prevents a conduction of earthly Qi, as well as closing off the lumbar region which, as we shall discuss shortly, is very important for the lower Dan Tian's functioning.

When we are in the womb, we still receive energetic nutrition via our mother directly into the lower Dan Tian. This means that it is the main source of our energy. All of our Qi is of this 'pre-natal' fashion, and the lower Dan Tian is the prime 'conversion centre' for this energy. Once we are born, the lower Dan Tian is already changing function as we receive our energy from our food and the air we breathe. This shift of importance away from the lower Dan Tian in this regard is another part of the reason why it starts to decrease in quality as we age.

The relationship between our Jing and the lower Dan Tian is a major aspect of why the lower Dan Tian is so negatively impacted by us moving through puberty. In males, once the Jing starts the enlargement of the testes, it begins to move in a new direction, down towards the perineum. Here is the beginning of sexual fluid development. Upon the first ejaculation for boys, a new cycle of the Jing has been set into action, and so the Dan Tian is impacted. Now, instead of all Jing moving into the lower Dan Tian as it did during childhood, it moves into the cycle of our sexual organs instead. The result is that the natural abdominal heat of childhood decreases and instead the Jing's warmth is often felt in the sexual organs during arousal. This begins the final stages of the lower Dan Tian dispersing away from its natural spherical shape.

In the case of women, it is not actually sexual maturity that takes away from the lower Dan Tian, but rather the onset of menstruation. The Jing has to begin the production of menstrual Blood, and this new development of the Jing means that, as in the case of boys, it is no longer solely moving into the lower Dan Tian region.

There is an additional strain upon the lower Dan Tian that can come as a result of sexual experiences at too young an age. I commonly see a kind of 'shock to the Jing' that has taken place in students who were sexually abused as minors. This 'shocks' the Jing's developmental processes as well, as it disperses the lower Dan Tian at too early an age. This can lead to chronic Qi deficiencies developing.

It should be noted here that the dispersal of the Dan Tian that takes place as we age is a completely natural process. It is normal for this to be the case so it is nothing to worry about. I have had new students who misunderstood and thought that the dispersal of the Dan Tian was a sign of sickness and a result of something that they had done wrong in their lives. As there is no need for such a heavy focus of the body's functioning on the lower Dan Tian past childhood, we no longer develop in this manner; it really is that simple. But, within the practice of Nei Gong, we would like to return the Dan Tian to its spherical state of being, so that we may utilise it in our practice. This is done through the main exercise of this chapter – rotating the lower Dan Tian. We shall get to this shortly.

When the lower Dan Tian has been reconsolidated into a sphere, it will then have a number of energetic relationships with surrounding elements of the lower abdominal energetic matrix; these relationships are shown in Figure 8.10.

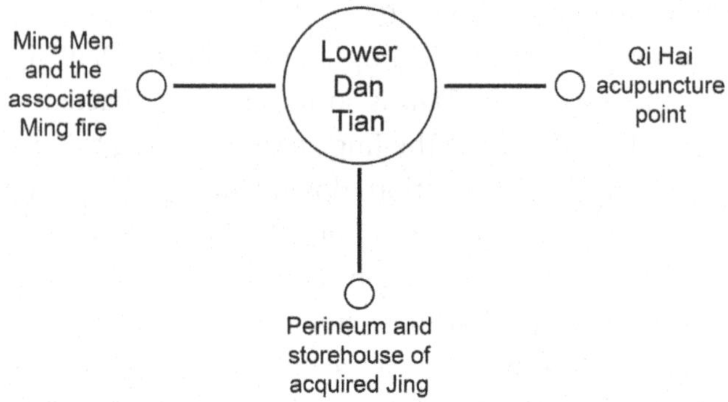

Figure 8.10: Dan Tian and Energetic Relationships

The first of these is its connection to the Qi Hai point on the front of the abdomen. Within Daoism, it is stated that we wish to 'become like a bellows between Heaven and Earth'. Within the body, this is referring to the action of the lower abdomen and the Qi Hai point. When the Qi Hai point is the focal region for abdominal breathing, then we have set up the bellows of the lower abdomen. This was a principle discussed in Chapter 5. In the analogy, 'Heaven' refers to our mind, and the 'Earth' is our physical body. Once the breathing is established in the right way, then the mind and body will begin to merge to a higher degree with the lower Dan Tian at its centre.

The second energetic relationship that is strengthened by the consolidation and awakening of the lower Dan Tian is the connection to the perineum and the Jing that is housed there. As the lower Dan Tian starts to develop, then the process of our Jing's conversion is transformed. This is a continuation of the development of Jing that happens as a result of stilling the Jing, as discussed in the previous chapter.

The third, and most important, of the energetic relationships of the lower Dan Tian is its connection to the Ming Men point on the rear of the body. It is here that we establish the greatest catalyst for the opening of a major circulation of Qi within the Governing and Conception channels. We require this connection for there to be a high enough level of Qi movement within the channel system as a whole.

Note that without reconsolidating the energetic centre of the lower Dan Tian, we will not be able to:

- open the flow of Qi along the length of the Governing channel
- move Qi through the channel system as a whole beyond a very small amount
- move through the Yi Jin Jing process
- develop the more complex aspects of Dan Tian work
- store Qi in the lower abdomen.

Note that the last entry on the list, 'store Qi in the lower abdomen', has been included specifically to correct an issue I see with many people in the Qi Gong world. They are often making the error of attempting to store Qi in a lower Dan Tian that does not yet exist in a very efficient manner. The result of this is that they are largely wasting their time; you can't store water in a cup that does not exist.

In fact, storing Qi in the lower Dan Tian is a much more advanced principle than people often realise. Not only does the energetic nature of the lower Dan Tian need to be established, but the Huang, the physical aspect of the lower Dan Tian, needs to be there too. This level of development is beyond the basics of our practice. This is why even a practitioner of Qi Gong of many years will go to a true Nei Gong master and be told that their Dan Tian is still empty. They have not 'built the cup' yet. It is so far down the line in the Nei Gong process that I always tell my own students to forget about it. We don't store Qi in the lower Dan Tian in any way at all; this is not a concern for us until we are deep into the Nei Gong process.

I have even seen people damage themselves quite badly by trying to store Qi within the lower abdomen using a lot of force. Since they had an awareness of a lack of Dan Tian 'contained', they essentially forced the Qi in using a lot of power, and so developed a lot of energetic stagnation in the body; in some cases, this can lead to very serious illness. Truth be told, I was actually hesitant about saying that Qi can be stored in the Dan Tian and sharing the method for doing so; maybe some things should really be left to verbal tuition from teacher to student on a one-to-one basis, but now there already are so many writings on how to do this out there in the public eye that I feel compelled to. At least if the information is there, it can provide some guidance to practitioners of these arts. Many more traditional teachers will fully deny the possibility of actually storing or filling the Dan Tian with Qi until the student reaches the relevant stage in their development.

Physical Components of the Lower Dan Tian

There are also a series of physical aspects to both the lower Dan Tian's form and functioning. Note that these always exist within the body, regardless of our practice, in the same way that the Dan Tian is there anyway; it is just *how* condensed the lower Dan Tian is and *how* developed its physical connections are that matters. We are always aiming to improve the efficiency of the body's functioning through these practices.

To understand the physical connections of the lower Dan Tian, we need to understand that this takes place within the Huang of the body. These connections are a result of the Huang stretching out and connecting the lower abdominal cavity together like a sort of organic cobweb. The lower Dan Tian sits at the centre of this web, and as it moves and functions, it influences the Huang. These physical connections are shown in Figure 8.11. Remember, though, that the diagram depicts the Huang extending out, as if the abdominal cavity was hollow. This is simply for ease of understanding. In fact, there are the intestines and other organs within the abdominal cavity; the Huang stretches out and surrounds these physical components, meaning that the Huang's 'pulling' of the body is actually taking place around the viscera and not through them.

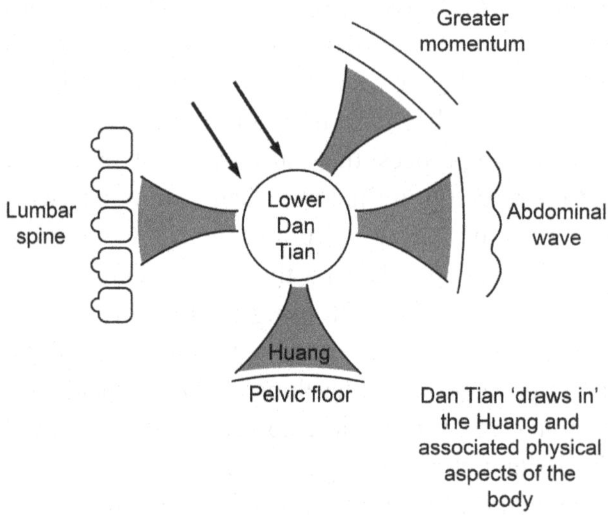

Figure 8.11: The Huang Connection to the Abdominal Cavity

As we can see, the lower Dan Tian connects to several physical components of the body.

The first physical connection is on the front of the lower Dan Tian, and it is here that the Dan Tian connects into and pulls on the posterior aspect of the abdominal wall. As the physical aspect of the lower Dan Tian builds, then the abdominal wall is 'tugged upon' from the insides. The result of this is that there is a great degree of pressure exerted upon the Qi within the abdominal space. When it starts to build, there is a distinct feeling of a physical tightening of the abdominal wall from the inside of your abdominal cavity.

This frontal extension of the lower Dan Tian also pulls on the greater omentum, which is a sheath of membranous tissue that lines most of the abdominal cavity, connecting the internal organs together. As well as serving to connect the viscera together, it also has an important role to play in immune system function and tissue cell regeneration. When this connection begins to form to a high degree, then the greater omentum is stimulated with Qi; this warms it up, and this heat radiates to the abdominal wall. Essentially, this heat is a type of 'resistance' resulting from the Dan Tian Qi moving through the semi-conductive material of the omentum. That being said, it is not a negative heat, though, it is a positive sign of the Dan Tian developing properly. This heat comes when the immune system and body's internal repair mechanisms have been improved by your Dan Tian development.

The lower aspect of the Dan Tian connects into the pelvic floor and associated tissues. As the Dan Tian develops, it draws up the pelvic floor to a certain extent. This helps to apply gentle pressure to the Qi of the lower abdominal space and contributes to the health of the bladder, intestines and, in women, the uterus.

The rear of the lower Dan Tian connects into the Huang running from the lumbar spine. This strengthens the back and anchors the Dan Tian into the lower back – an important principle for later on when we do learn how to store Qi in the lower abdominal cavity. It also starts to develop a connection to the Kidneys and adrenal glands. This connection helps to support and tonify their function.

The sides of the Dan Tian are encapsulated by the tissues of the sides of the abdominal cavity. When they start to develop to a high enough degree, then the soft tissues of the abdomen start to stretch and become more elasticated. It is particularly clear to feel on the sides of your abdomen, just above the hips, as it feels as if the Dan Tian is drawing this region of the body inwards.

Most importantly, when the physical aspect of the Dan Tian builds, the stage is set for the more advanced aspects of Dan Tian work which regard 'building the gourd' shape within your body.

The Yi Jin Jing Revisited

It was stated above that we should build the lower Dan Tian energetically first, and then allow the physical side of the Dan Tian to build as a natural by-product of this. This is the internal way, remember: Qi first, body second. Though we have to establish an initial 'frame' for the body using alignment principles, we then switch to the internal way of working and focus upon the Qi. When the Qi starts to 'overflow' into the physical body, then it will start to develop in the right manner. This adheres to two of the main rules we discussed in Chapter 3 when we looked at the Yi Jin Jing and its teachings. These rules were:

- The body must be built in the sequence of Qi, then Huang and then tendon.
- The Qi must mobilise; the result of this is the engagement of the Huang. This will strengthen the Huang.

One should keep developing the Qi until the Huang fully stretches and the tendons are strong.

The result of this is that the channels will open and the Qi will reach every part of the body.

In the examples above, you could think of the Dan Tian as the source of the Qi, the Huang as starting to connect together and 'stretch' as a result of the Qi moving into it, and then the 'tendons' are actually the denser and thicker aspects of the body, such as the abdominal wall and pelvic floor. This all works because when the Qi reacts with the Huang, then the Huang engages naturally. We don't have to physically pull or stretch it, we simply allow the Qi to flow into its length. The flowing of Qi into the Huang influences its structure. It is much like gently tightening a series of slack cables.

Note here, though, that for the time being we shall be focused solely upon the energetics of the Dan Tian. The physical side of the Dan Tian has been included in order for you to develop an overview in your understanding. We shall return to this in much greater depth in Chapter 11.

Three Ingredients in the Lower Dan Tian

Now that you have established a solid enough foundation, it is time to begin consolidating and waking up the Dan Tian. This is accomplished through combining the location of the lower Dan Tian with your breath, your awareness and your centre of gravity. There is quite a skill involved in accomplishing this, but it is achievable by anybody if they have worked step-by-step on preparing their body for this practice. It should be noted that as soon as you start to wake up the lower Dan Tian, you will immediately start to generate change with regard to the quality and circulation of your Jing and Qi. This means that we should keep the following considerations in mind:

- An internal arts practitioner should be aiming to have a healthy diet anyway, but certainly before trying to wake up the lower Dan Tian you want a good, solid couple of weeks with a healthy diet. If you are not usually a healthy eater, then it is vitally important that you change this for the period building up to direct work with the Dan Tian. Try to cut sugar and spices from your diet, along with any processed food or carbonated, sugary drinks.
- After reaching orgasm, there is a slight tightening of the lower Dan Tian. It is as if it temporarily closes up to help reconsolidate Jing and Qi in this region of the body. This closing up of the Dan Tian makes it difficult to start the process of waking it up, and so you should avoid sex for 24–48 hours prior to these practices.
- Do not engage in this practice if you are feeling very low in energy or unwell in any way. This is because the initial process can be quite energetically demanding. If you are unwell, then there is a chance it can make your condition temporarily worse.
- Do not practise this exercise when under the influence of drugs or alcohol of any kind.
- This practice can develop a lot of internal heat in the early stages of the training due to an increased movement of Qi and Jing. Please be cautious if you have any weakness of the heart or high blood pressure, as this heat can tax the heart. If you are unsure of this, please consult a Chinese medical practitioner for assistance or train under a qualified teacher who can advise you on your development.
- Ensure you have built a solid enough foundation in the prior stages we have already outlined within this book. The better the foundations, the more efficient your practice.

Once these guidelines for the practice have been taken into consideration, it is time to start looking at the awakening of the lower Dan Tian. The first thing we need to do is learn how to consolidate the three required elements into the lower abdominal region. These key elements are shown in Figure 8.12. They are each discussed in detail below.

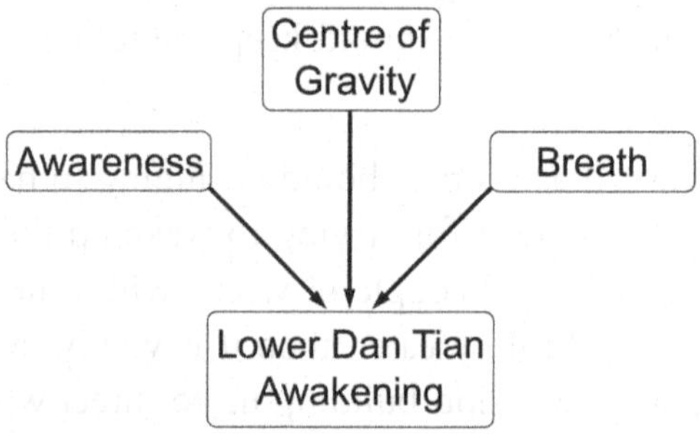

Figure 8.12: The Three Elements of Lower Dan Tian Awakening

If one or more of these elements is not effectively connected into the location of the lower Dan Tian, then the effectiveness of the practice is lessened.

Centre of Gravity to Lower Dan Tian

We should carry out this practice in the Wuji posture. This is because one of the key functions of this posture is to enable you to sink your centre of gravity to the lower Dan Tian in the foundation stages of Nei Gong practice.

Before starting to use the Wuji posture as a practice to bring your centre of gravity down to the lower Dan Tian region, you will first need an internal point of reference. This comes back to the exercise outlined in Chapter 4 for locating the lower Dan Tian; this will be the focal point for our practice.

If you have practised the Wuji posture to a point where it has become comfortable, then your next task is to continue with the refinement of its alignment principles. Stand in Wuji for a short time and use your awareness to tune into and locate your physical centre of gravity. It is a key realisation of anybody who has trained in the internal arts for any length of time that your centre of gravity is actually a relatively fluid thing which can be moved around your body according to how you structure it. It seems that with a fairly high level of skill, it can even be transmitted through the soft tissues of the body according to intention. For our purposes, in Wuji training we don't need to reach this level, though; we simply need to bring our centre of gravity down from the chest into the lower abdomen and then adjust our posture so that our mass is directed downwards to the location of the lower Dan Tian. The pressure of your mass going to the lower Dan Tian is then released down through the legs into the 'surging spring' points as previously discussed.

Awareness on Lower Dan Tian Region

The second ingredient involved in the awakening of the lower Dan Tian is the effective placement of your awareness upon this same point that you have by now located. The awareness should be placed as exactly as you can onto the point where you are directing your centre of gravity through the Wuji posture. The strength of your mind should be balanced according to our principles of regulating the mind, and so you should be 'casually observing' this point.

Once you have practised enough to regulate the strength of your awareness, you should bring it to the point of the lower Dan Tian in your Wuji standing practice and rest it there. Remember that it should sink to this point rather than being forcibly placed there. You should already be familiar with this idea through your practice of stilling the Jing.

Leading the Breath to the Lower Dan Tian

The final ingredient for awakening the lower Dan Tian is the application of your breath. Your breathing should be sunk to the lower Dan Tian in the correct manner, so that it combines with your centre of gravity and your awareness. All of the previous principles for regulating the mind, body and breath will mean that you can do this in the correct fashion. Remember that with these arts, like in life, it is not *what* you do but *how* you do it that matters. The prior work on the three regulations will have put you in good stead for establishing your work with the lower Dan Tian in the best possible way.

How Long to Continue?

Possibly the most important question for any internal practitioner to ask is how long they should continue with any practice. Once the correct principles have been learnt, then timing becomes a major issue. In order to answer this question, we can divide practices into two main categories.

The first category of practice is one which has no defined aim or set limit to the amount of growth it can bring. Many Qi Gong exercises, meditation forms or martial arts practices fall into this category. These practices are a lifelong study which sincere practitioners should only stop doing when they are on their deathbed. The skill with this kind of practice is to understand where it is supposed to be leading you and so, in turn, ensure that it keeps leading you down a continuous path of development. Many practitioners fall down in these kinds of practice, simply because they lose sight of a developmental process and so allow their practice to become stagnant. Once it does not lead to growth, it does not help along the path, and it has become a useless practice.

The second category of practice is one which leads to a very set place. These practices have a very specific goal, a set amount of time they should be practised, and a limit to how far they can take you. It is normal to practise them until you have reached whatever the aim of the practice is and then to leave them and move on. They are stopped when you have attained the correct Gong for the exercise.

Awakening the lower Dan Tian is an aspect of Nei Gong training that falls into the second category. It is a practice which has a definite conclusion, but it should then be returned to every now and then to ensure that you have consolidated your foundations.

When the lower Dan Tian begins to wake up, it generally produces the following results. Some of these experiences you are likely to have had already in the previous stages outlined within this book.

First, your Jing will start to react. You should, by now, be used to the warmth that develops in this area of the body as a reaction to the Jing stilling. This time, though, it can be a little different. The warm fluid feeling will combine with the standing posture and the use of the breath, and will often leave you soaked in sweat. We have had students surprised at just how warm the body becomes. Don't worry, though; your body will grow used to it soon enough, and the sweating will draw to a close. You can expect it for a few weeks at the most.

Beyond this stage, the lower Dan Tian then starts to generate more life and movement within the channel system. This sends more Qi through the body, which then, in turn, stimulates movement within the physical body. A student who has reached this stage will generally begin to shake or vibrate at a very high rate. At first these vibrations will be localised to within the legs, but after some time it is normal for these vibrations to then move through the rest of the body, through the arms, and out to the hands. They are nothing to worry about and simply a sign of increased energetic movement through the body. As they take place they cause a great deal of energetic re-patterning to take place, changes which have a positive effect upon your health. These shakes should come and go in short bursts. As with the experience of heat, once the body has normalised the experience, the shakes will quieten down and become subtler, and you will be left with a gentle feeling of vibration through the body which is practically invisible to any onlooker.

Once the Dan Tian starts to become consolidated to a point of waking up, it will begin to make sudden jerks within your lower abdomen. These jerks come quickly and can take you by surprise. Don't panic when they begin to manifest, as they can be quite strong sometimes. They generally come quite a few minutes apart in your practice, with no observable pattern as to when they appear; they are not linked to either your mindset or your breathing, as far as we can ascertain. They are a clear sign of developmental progress when working towards awakening the lower Dan Tian, though.

As these jerks go off within the lower Dan Tian, they motivate the physical body to follow. Do not be surprised if the sudden twist of the lower Dan Tian causes you to suddenly turn around to either side. We have even had many students who were thrown off their feet by the movement of the lower Dan Tian. The lower Dan Tian is the energy centre of movement, activity and action. It is the driving force for energy and life. As it wakes up, we are simply accessing these aspects of its nature and so we experience these various reactions.

Once you have started to experience these reactions, then the lower Dan Tian is successfully awakened enough for you to move onto 'rotating the lower Dan Tian', which is the next stage in your practice. As a rough timescale, we have had some students achieve this after only a few weeks and yet others take around a year. It is really individual from person to person. There is nothing to worry about, it is not a race, and you should never hurry the process; everything will unfold in its own time.

The Spiritual Mirror

Esoteric Daoism talks of a Ling Jing (靈鏡) or 'spiritual mirror' that resides within the head. It is located in the rear of the head, behind the pineal gland, and is approximately one inch (2.5 cm) across. It sits at a 45-degree angle facing downwards and has the role of receiving light from the third eye and then reflecting it down into the Central channel of the body. Although this 'mirror' is clearly metaphorical – there is no literal reflective object sat in your brain – there is a very important aspect of Nei Gong training involving this aspect of the energetic system. At advanced stages of practice, it is normal for the practitioner of these arts to start perceiving flashes of white light within the mind's eye. These lights will flicker and jump around, but with time they will begin to stabilise within the space just behind the eyes. Beginners may get brief experiences of this light, but only experienced practitioners of the internal arts will generally be able to stabilise this light into a bright glow that appears whenever the eyes are closed. This is the light of spirit and is a good sign of progress.

There are many practices that become available once the light is stabilised. These practices can be used to help move towards the ability of full energetic Nei Guan (內觀) 'inner viewing', or else they are used to build a foundation in either Xin Fen Xi (心分析) 'mind analysis' or the development of the Ling Tai (靈胎) 'spiritual embryo'.

In the case of full 'inner viewing', the light of Shen is 'reflected' off the 'spiritual mirror' and sent downwards through the inside of the body. With time and the correct methods, the light of Shen begins to illuminate the inside of the body and so it can be perceived in a visual sense. This skill then becomes the basis of viewing not just your own channels and organs but also the channels and organs of others; high-level Daoist physicians are said to have been using this skill for many generations.

In the practice of 'mind analysis', the light of Shen is 'reflected' off the 'mirror' and sent into the region of the heart where Shen and Xin can then start to interact with one another. The result of this is that the negative Karma or Nie (孽) can then be 'burnt' from the mind through the use of spiritual energy. Though related to Daoist methods, this kind of training is more prevalent within the Buddhist Nei Gong traditions.

The development of the 'spiritual embryo' is one of the final attainments of alchemical practice whereby your own consciousness has been nurtured to the point of being able to exist independently of the physical anchor of the body. This becomes the basis for spiritual immortality, a very high-level stage of development indeed! In this case, the 'mirror' was used to reflect Shen into the correct regions of the body where it could be developed.

It is interesting to note that the root of the upper Dan Tian is the Ni Wan (泥丸) or Muddy Pill Palace, an ancient name of the pineal gland. This gland is recognised as being able to receive and anchor the light of Shen within alchemical practice. Once this stage has been reached, the 'muddy' pill begins to shine and is often metaphorically known as a diamond or jewel that resides in the centre of the head. This 'jewel' then serves to send the light back onto the 'mirror' so that it can be worked with through esoteric Shen Gong (神功) practice as discussed above.

Rotating the Lower Dan Tian

Now that the lower Dan Tian is starting to react, we can say that it is waking up. It is time to start teaching it how to move through rotating it. This practice is not actually so difficult, providing that you have built a strong enough base in the previous stages outlined.

The correct direction for the initial rotation of the lower Dan Tian is shown in Figure 8.13. Make sure you only go in this direction, as this is the way we connect the Dan Tian function into the Governing channel.

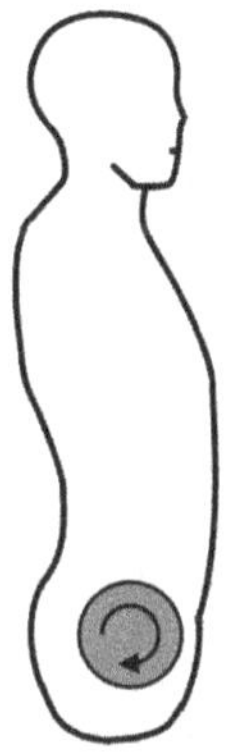

Figure 8.13: Rotating the Lower Dan Tian

In order to rotate the lower Dan Tian, place your mind onto the point which you have already ascertained is the focal point for the lower Dan Tian. In Wuji, combine the three ingredients of breath, gravity and awareness as best you can at this place; now stand in this fashion for a few minutes to half an hour. Ignore any sudden jerks the lower Dan Tian may make, though you should have progressed past that stage by the time you get onto controlled Dan Tian rotations. We wish for a smooth quality to your practice by this stage.

The next stage is to start the rotations. Use your awareness to establish a smooth rotation of the lower Dan Tian in the depicted direction. Most beginner students find it easiest to carry out this rotation in time with their breathing, though it is not vitally important that this is the case.

In order to understand exactly what Dan Tian rotation is, we should clarify one thing – we are not discussing a physical rotation of any muscles or joints within the region of the pelvis or lower abdomen. Neither are we talking about using your imagination to picture a rotating ball in your gut. Instead, we are referring to setting up a forward rotational direction with your awareness within the lower abdomen and then being patient! After some time, the lower Dan Tian will begin to rotate and you will experience a full turning of this energy centre. It is a clear sensation of something turning over deep within your lower abdomen in time with your awareness. This turning has been compared strangely to a 'fish turning over in the guts'. It is a very strange sensation at first, but after some time it becomes normal like anything else. To reiterate, we don't make any physical movements; our awareness just makes small rotations around the point of the lower Dan Tian, within the lower abdomen. The mind is still relaxed, it is simply moving. It is as if you were following a point around within the abdomen rather than leading it.

As the Dan Tian rotational practice becomes easier, you will find that the Huang within the lower abdomen begin to follow its movement. Once again, we wish to underline that you do not *make* any movements with the body yourself, you simply stand in Wuji. As the Dan Tian turns, it will begin to strengthen the connection between the energetic and physical bodies, and this is what starts to generate tangible movement within the lower abdomen.

There are various bodily reactions which often take place when the lower Dan Tian starts to make a full rotation, which are discussed below. They are common and normal reactions to the practice.

As the lower Dan Tian starts to rotate, it is normal for the body to enter into a period of energetic and physical purging. A combination of poor diet and negative emotional debris has left many people's bodies full of stagnant toxins. As the Dan Tian wakes up and begins to move energy through the body, it will aim to naturally reverse this state, and the result can be feelings of nausea or even vomiting. These should only last a day or two at the most, and seem to occur in about a quarter of the students we teach, far more often in male students. In every case, after the temporary sickness has ended, students state that they feel much better for it.

The second 'purging' body reaction which may manifest is a kind of colon cleansing which can result in loose bowels for up to a week. The material which comes out during these spontaneous colon cleanses is not just faecal matter but also the same toxic leftovers that a person will experience leaving the body when completing prolonged fasting and enemas. As with the previously mentioned nausea, this only ever seems to happen once at the beginning of a Nei Gong student's training, and it always improves their health. This reaction is much more common than the nausea and affects roughly half of those starting to rotate the lower Dan Tian.

If, in the case of women, the rotation of the lower Dan Tian causes an increase in heaviness of the flow during menstruation, then stop and wait until you have moved past this part of your monthly cycle before continuing practice. The extra heat generated by the beginning stages of rotating the lower Dan Tian can sometimes increase the expulsion of menstrual Blood by the uterus.

If any of these reactions take place, please don't worry, it is quite normal. You are entering into some of the stronger aspects of internal work, and so bodily reactions like this are common. They should only last for a short space of time. If they last any longer than they should, please visit an experienced Chinese medical practitioner, and they should be able to assist you by correcting any inherent Qi imbalances that the practice has brought to the surface.

So, What Is Actually Happening?

Though the above practice is named 'rotating the lower Dan Tian', it does not actually work quite like that. As discussed prior to this, the basis of your body's energetic functioning comes down to one of two types of Qi – Yin Qi and Yang Qi. These are explored in greater detail in the next chapter, but for now we can understand that Yin Qi moves in fields, spherical energetic structures that serve to shape and contain the other forms of Qi within the body. They act like electromagnetic fields of information that have a consolidating effect upon certain regions of the body when they are functioning to a high level. Yang Qi is quite different from this, it moves within the channel system in a more linear fashion.

The lower Dan Tian is primarily made up of Yin Qi. At first, it sits within the abdomen in a fairly dispersed manner. It is like a weak electromagnetic field that results in a dispersion of vital energetic substances within the abdominal region. When you lower yourself down so that the three ingredients of posture, breath and awareness are in your lower abdomen, there is a reaction that takes place between your 'sea of Qi' and the Yin energetic field of the planet. When the lower Dan Tian point can relate to the Qi of the planet to a more efficient level than it normally does, then the natural effect of the planet's Qi, the Di Qi, is that it begins to cause the Yin field of the lower abdomen to consolidate as well. The more accurately we can place the 'three ingredients' discussed previously into the lower Dan Tian 'point', then the more we can locate the centre of this field, and this also helps it to develop. In this way, we are using one of the classical Daoist rules of macrocosm and microcosm directly reflecting one another to bring us on in our practice. This is depicted in Figure 8.14.

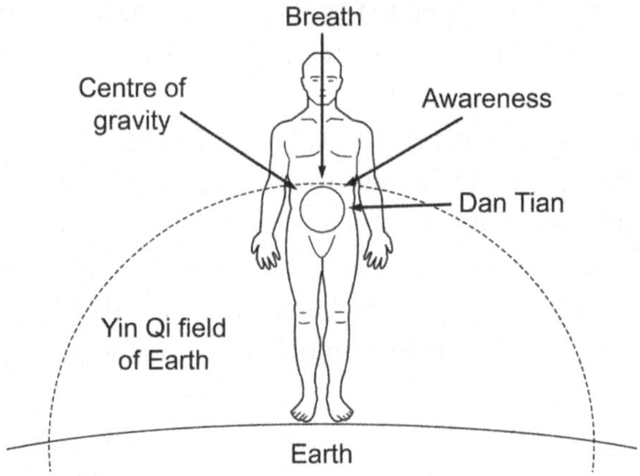

Figure 8.14: Macrocosm and Microcosm of Yin Qi and Dan Tian

Remaining here, with this connection, and refining the principles of our practice will help the lower field of the abdomen to begin to consolidate. As discussed above, this can result in the Jing being affected (the feelings of heat) and a certain degree of erratic movement from the abdominal Qi field. This will result in a period of twitches and jerking movements coming from inside of the abdomen; don't worry about it, let them do their thing, and then it will begin to subside after a while. These twitches are starting to take place because the 'magnetic' qualities of the Yin Qi are pulling upon the Huang of the lower abdomen. Where there are adhesions or blockages in the Huang that need releasing, the Qi will tug them and the result is that your body twitches a little. It is an interesting phenomenon but nothing to concern yourself about. It will pass, and when it does, you are ready to move onto the rotations.

When you begin the 'rotating the Dan Tian' exercise, you are actually using your awareness to establish a little movement of the Qi within your abdominal region. It is not the Dan Tian per se that you are moving but actually just the Qi beneath your diaphragm region. This disturbance of the Qi can happen because your mind has a direct influence upon the quality of your body's Qi. You can think of it like stirring the Qi in your abdominal region. This helps to bring more change to the Qi there.

Because of the focal point of your centre of gravity to the lower Dan Tian, as well as the sinking of the Dan Tian into the field of the planet's Qi, there is a central point that this stirred Qi will move towards. This will begin the rotational consolidation of the lower Dan Tian. This is depicted in Figure 8.15.

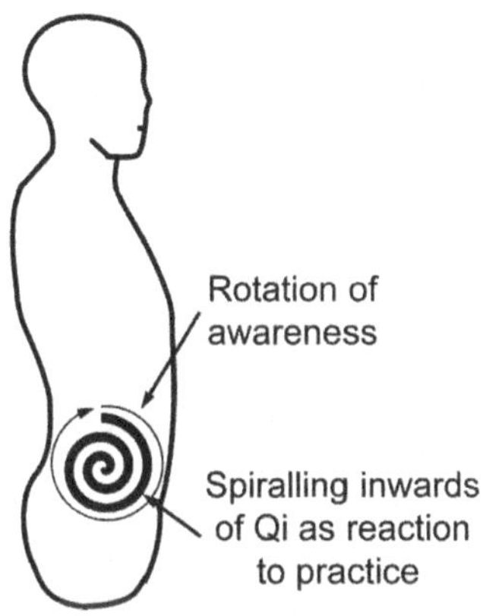

Figure 8.15: Rotational Consolidation of the Lower Dan Tian Field

As the field starts to move inwards, it will reach a point whereby the Yin Qi field of the lower Dan Tian is strong enough to exert an influence upon the rest of the body's Qi, and so this will result in an increase of energetic flow within the channel system of the body. This is where we wish to get to within our practice. It is a sign that the lower Dan Tian is ready to move on.

Lower Dan Tian Consolidation Reactions

If you can think of your energetic system as having two key movements of Qi – the linear flowing of Qi through the channel system, and the spherical fields of Qi that are anchored into a number of energetic centres within your body – then you are able to understand the next part of the process. How does the lower Dan Tian consolidating influence the body? Figure 8.16 shows the energy body according to these two key movements of Qi.

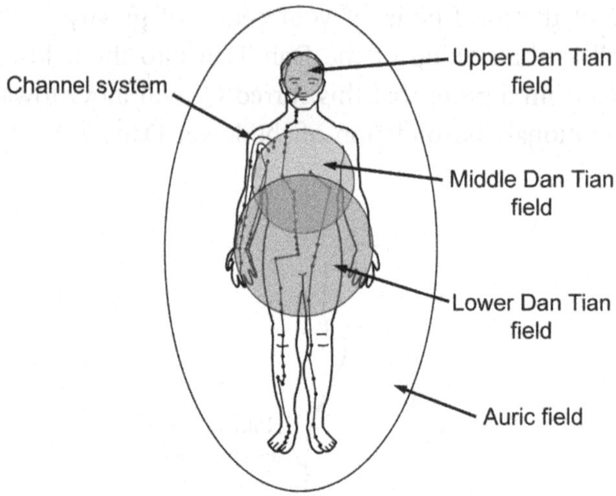

Figure 8.16: Two Key Movements of Qi

Note that only a small percentage of the various channels and fields are shown on the above diagram; it is simply to give you an idea of how your energetic matrix comprises these two forms of Qi.

Now, each and every field and energetic channel are connected together into one integrated unit. You could think of them as being like a series of cogs that are all influencing one another as they move. When the lower Dan Tian goes through this sudden recalibrating, it will begin to affect the movement of Qi elsewhere too. The result of this is something called Zi Fa Gong (自發功); this is commonly known as 'spontaneous and natural Qi flow'. Zi Fa Gong is a process of spontaneous movements that the body can go through of its own accord. They take place as a result of the Qi moving at a higher degree through your body. If we understand that the movement of Qi stretches the Huang, then we can understand how this may happen. The soft tissues of the body lengthen, stretch and vibrate as a result of the increased movement of energy running through their length, and the result of this is that your body can move involuntarily in a variety of interesting ways. Zi Fa Gong is very much misunderstood within the internal arts community, and so a large part of the next chapter is dedicated to explaining these bodily reactions. For now, it is enough to know that Zi Fa Gong is a normal reaction to the consolidation and movement of the lower Dan Tian.

When your body enters the Zi Fa Gong process and begins to tremble, shake or twist around the region of the lower abdomen, then there is no need to rotate the lower Dan Tian any more. Your work is done here, the key is in the ignition, from now on you simply need to sink the Qi whilst stood in Wuji so that it can begin to 'ground' your experiences. The process of sinking the Qi should be your next practice and your key priority in your development.

Sinking the Qi

Learning how to sink your Qi is a key skill within the internal arts and yet a skill that eludes many people. Without the ability to sink your Qi, it will not begin to move smoothly into the channel system, meaning that it will never mobilise in the right way. In the case of consolidating the lower Dan Tian, we now have a field built within the lower abdomen. We wish for this field to start distributing Qi around our channel system, and so we must sink our body's Qi towards this point. No doubt, the increased energetic flow resulting from your work with the lower Dan Tian has generated a certain degree of Zi Fa Gong; this is normal. But we wish to move beyond this process, and so we need to learn how to sink our Qi down. To do this, we move through the following process:

1. Relaxing the contractive muscles
2. Sinking the mass actively through the body
3. Filling the lower abdomen
4. Expanding the lower abdominal region
5. Stretching the connective tissues of the body
6. Connecting the soft tissues into one unit
7. Stressing the soft tissues through increased release of mass
8. Generating expansive 'space' within the body

This process was mentioned in Chapter 1 and you have actually already started to move through it. Because of your practice of regulating the breath and body, you have already begun to relax the contractive muscles, sink the mass actively through the body, and fill the lower abdomen under the influence of your centre of gravity. Now it is time to progress past this stage. Let us visit each part of the process one step at a time; as with the previous exercise of moving through the five keywords of breathing, they are essentially a type of causation chain with each stage leading to the next stage when your skill level hits a certain level.

Relaxing the Contractive Muscles

Through the use of Wuji as a standing practice, you should have aligned the body in such a way that the large active muscles can 'hang from the bones'. The stabilising muscles have disentangled themselves from the active muscles, and so the efficiency of your muscular system should have improved greatly. As the large contractive muscles begin to relax and lengthen, they will no longer serve to 'catch' your mass as you relax. The result of this is that your mass should be able to travel down to the floor via the Huang.

Sinking the Mass Actively Through the Body

It is here, in the second stage of sinking your Qi, that many practitioners fall foul of becoming stuck. They are often held back by one simple error: they are not distinguishing between sinking 'passively' and 'actively'. It is the active sink that we need to move our mass in the correct manner through our body. To understand the difference, think of it like this – active sinking influences every part of our body as our mass moves *through* our body to the floor; passive sinking is different from this, as our mass is simply dropped to the floor, without it affecting our body at all. It is as if we have sunk our mass and missed our body on the way down!

Sadly, passive sinking is the default mode for our body, and so if we do not consciously work towards actively sinking, then we shall not stumble across it in our training.

To actively sink, allow your mind to absorb into the awareness and then into the body. The interaction between your mind and the body will cause the Qi to influence the Huang; though you may not yet feel it at this stage, the Huang will stretch as a result of your Qi. They then become like a series of elastic slings that are stretched out within your body, especially within the torso. Then, gradually begin to relax and sink your mass down to the ground. Go slowly and take your time. If you have managed to actively sink, then you will feel how your body mass is affecting each and every internal sling inside of you on its way down to the ground. If you manage it, then well done, you have realised that the dropping of your mass correctly enables it to serve as a catalyst for change within the body. If we passively sink, then we lose this catalyst.

I would like to reiterate here that this is an error many people make in their practice; I would advise looking at what you are doing and really checking that you understand active sinking. If in doubt, go and find an experienced teacher to help you with this. It can sometimes be helpful to put your hands on the teacher's body and feel how their body functions when they actively sink; in my experience, many students are surprised at the sensations and what this process feels like.

Filling the Lower Abdomen

When you actively sink to the floor, you will find that the lower abdomen starts to 'fill'. This will not happen beyond a very tiny amount if you passively sink; it requires the correct dropping of mass through your body. The 'filling' that starts to take place is a direct by-product of the correct sinking method and will begin to manifest of its own accord as a result of the previous stage of practice.

What is actually happening is that the sinking of your mass is starting to stretch the Huang in a very specific manner. It will lead to the feeling of the inside of your torso becoming shaped as shown in Figure 8.17. Note that this is an 'internal' shaping and not an external structure that can necessarily be seen on the outside of your body.

This can be quite deceptive, body awareness is a strange thing; it can feel as though you are becoming avocado-shaped in your body, but when you look in a mirror you look just like you did before. If anything, the only slight change may be a relaxation to the lower abdominal muscles that can cause the belly to round ever so slightly. But this is not an excuse for developing a large gut; that is primarily due to your lifestyle!

As your mass begins to shape the inside of your body in this fashion, there is a downwards movement of Qi inside you; the mass leads the Qi. The Qi will then begin to fill the space of your abdomen. When this is combined with the awakening of the lower Dan Tian, then you are building a very good foundation indeed.

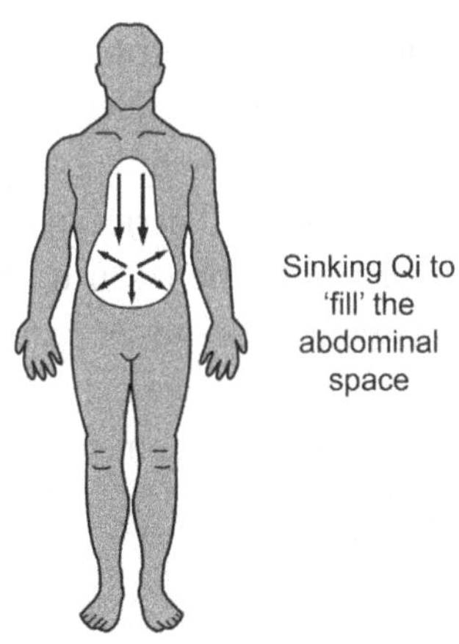

Figure 8.17: Filling the Lower Abdomen

Expanding the Lower Abdominal Region

As a result of the sinking, when your lower abdomen is starting to fill in the right way, it will begin to feel as though it expands. Note that this expansion is internal; it is a feeling, not a swelling of your gut. It will feel like there is a slight pushing outwards of your Qi from within the abdominal cavity, from the base of your perineum all the way up to the diaphragm. This pressure feels very strong, and some have likened this feeling to being 'packed' inside of the abdomen. When this is combined with the inwards-pulling of the lower Dan Tian as a result of the Yin Qi field upon the Huang and abdominal wall, you are starting to develop a high level of skill in Dan Tian building.

Stretching the Connective Tissues of the Body

The active sinking within your body will stretch the Huang; the filling of the abdomen with Qi will stretch the sinew channels. It is as if the filling of the abdomen is starting to lengthen the sinew channels, the connective tissues that run near to the surface of the body. They will pull and tighten in a very specific manner. It will feel as though the more you sink, the more your outer body starts to stretch. It is a very distinct and strong feeling. As the sinew channels lengthen, they become more conductive. In this way, the more you sink, the more you help to open the channels.

Connecting the Soft Tissues into One Unit

When a certain degree of sinking has taken place, then the Huang and sinew channels will start to influence one another. They will join together in a very specific way. This will mean that you are now one integrated physical whole. Some have mistakenly thought that 'connection' within the internal arts means that your joints and muscles move as one unit; this is not true. Internal connection is when your whole body, from the inside to the outside, is merged as one large elasticated series of soft-tissue connections. You will know when this happens, as when you move one part of your body, even something as small as your little finger, you will feel a series of connected movements and stretches all the way through various parts of your body. This kind of connection can only come through correctly sinking the Qi.

Stressing the Soft Tissues through Increased Release of Mass

Once the body is connected together into one unit, we continue to stretch the body under the release of more mass. The active sinking must continue so that our mass is used as a stressor for the connective tissues. This will help them to continue growing and developing. Essentially, it is a cycle. The more we sink, the more we stress the Huang and they grow, and this enables us to sink and stress them more. In this way, we keep building and developing our structure through consistent practice of sinking. The more we build these connective tissues, the more the channels open and the more our Qi flows.

Generating Expansive 'Space' Within the Body

The final result of all this sinking will begin to manifest when you have managed to sink to a high enough degree. Do not be surprised if this takes some time; it can be a lengthy process. Nothing within these arts can be hurried.

If we look at Figure 8.18, we can see what happens when we have sunk to the right level.

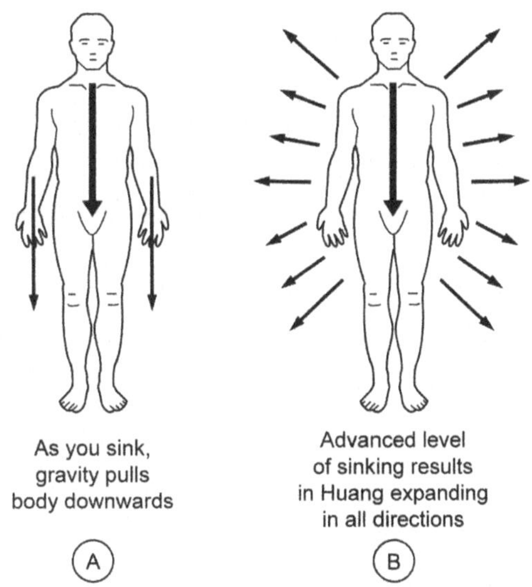

Figure 8.18: The Result of Sinking to a High Enough Degree

Image A shows the direction that your body will move when you sink as a beginner or when you are passively sinking. In this way, the more we relax, the more gravity gets a hold of us and pulls us down towards the ground. In B, we have sunk correctly over a long period of time. Now, the honeycomb nature of the Huang means that, when I sink, my mass is distributed out through the Huang and sinew channels in all directions. The sinking establishes a kind of spherical stretch and so my body will expand. All I do is sink and my body opens up as in B. It is as if the sinking of the mass initiates an expansion of the Huang that inflates you from the inside. This will then, in turn, circulate the Qi out through to your entire body. This is a correct result of sinking in the right way.

Why Sink?

The reason I have outlined the sinking process here, in this chapter, is because it should become of great importance to you once you have managed to awaken the lower Dan Tian. The Dan Tian will mobilise the Qi, and we now wish it to move in the right direction – down towards the lower abdomen. It is here, in the lower Dan Tian area, that the Qi is then directed into the channel system, and here that we need to aim for. Few people naturally have Qi that sinks in the right way; it generally goes up and outwards for most people. This is another reaction to the lower abdomen no longer being our physical centre and 'grounding point'. If we can sink the Qi down at this stage in our practice, then it will greatly help us to use the lower Dan Tian in the best way for our Nei Gong training.

On another level, the awakening of the lower Dan Tian will generally send most people into the Zi Fa Gong process (we explore this in greater detail in the next chapter). Whilst the Zi Fa Gong process is normal and extremely helpful, it will actually only evolve in the right direction if we sink our Qi properly. So, the sinking of our Qi, after the awakening of the lower Dan Tian, is the key to utilising Zi Fa Gong to the maximum benefit in our practice. To summarise: wake up that energy system, and then sink the Qi! This will take you a fair while, I should think.

The Microcosmic Orbit

Whilst there are numerous cycles and circulations of Qi that we wish to establish within the body, the most famous of these is, no doubt, the Xiao Zhou Tian (小周天), or microcosmic orbit. It is the key circulation of Qi that takes place up the back of the body, via the Governing channel, and then down through the front of the body within the Conception channel. It forms a loop of rotating Qi that is shown in Figure 8.19. I was actually taught it as the 'small water wheel' of Qi, and in previous books I have used this name for it. I have since learnt that most people know it as the 'microcosmic orbit' and there was much confusion as people have asked me the difference between the two. They are the same thing, it is just that different traditions and teachers use different names. In order to save confusion, from now on I shall refer to it in my writings by its more commonly known name.

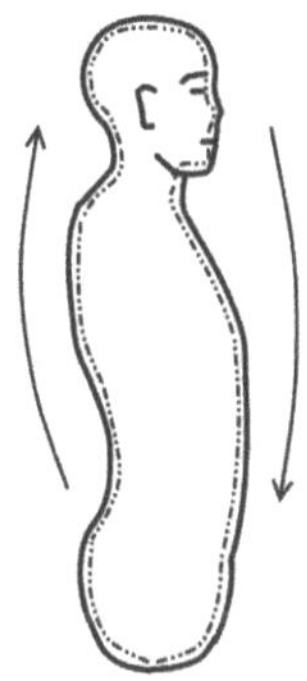

Figure 8.19: The Microcosmic Orbit

The reason this particular circulation of Qi should be introduced here, in this chapter, is because of its extremely close connection to the consolidation and turning of the lower Dan Tian.

The microcosmic orbit is one of the most fundamental skills that we need to attain within our practice. We establish its earliest functions via the use of the lower Dan Tian, and then later we return to it, as there are many stages involved in its evolution. Many people are unaware of this; though we have the possibility of working with some aspects of the microcosmic orbit early on in our training, there are many more advanced stages of practice with this circulation that come much further down the line. The development of the orbit is traditionally divided into five main stages, though I subdivide it further. These stages are as follows:

1. The physical establishing of the circuit
2. The rotation of Qi
    a. 'neutral' Qi
    b. Yang Qi
    c. Yin Qi

3. The rotation of congenital fluid
    a. Ding fluid
    b. marrow washing
4. The rotation of light
    a. refracted
    b. pure
5. The rotation of the alchemical pill

As you can see, I have subdivided three of the stages of circulation up into further levels of attainment. This is to help you understand progression within the circulations. We shall return to these stages and discuss them in detail below. First, let us look at the functions and mechanics of the microcosmic orbit.

Why Do We Need the Microcosmic Orbit?

Though there is a fair amount of writing on the microcosmic orbit in the English language, there is a surprising lack of information on why exactly we need this orbit. It is often presented purely as a way to move towards enlightenment, but there is a lot more to the orbit than this. It is important for many reasons, one of the key ones being safety.

We could list the following key functions of the microcosmic orbit:

- To regulate Yin and Yang
- To distribute Qi to the channels
- To recycle substances
- To protect us from excess
- To transform the body
- To transform the mind

Each of these is now explored below in greater detail.

To Regulate Yin and Yang

Throughout the various processes of Nei Gong, you are going to be playing around with Yin and Yang to a certain degree. Some aspects of Qi development will make you calmer, or Yin, and some parts of the process can be stimulating, and so make you more Yang. These temporary fluctuations are quite normal and to be expected for any practice that works on a deep internal level. The only time this becomes a problem is if the body becomes stuck in either one of these patterns. Many issues can develop in people with an incorrect practice who have made their mind and body too Yang.

By opening the length of the microcosmic orbit, we actually help to balance Yin and Yang within our system. The Governing channel along our back serves to regulate the Yang aspects of our body, whilst the Conception channel governs Yin. When we successfully circulate our Qi along these two channels, then the body is able to return itself to a state of balance much more effectively if we ever move towards one of these two extremes. This can be very important, as later on in our practice we will need to develop and move a lot of Qi, more than the body may be used to. In this case, it is normal for the body to temporarily become too Yang in nature. It is as if we are overstimulating our system. The role of the microcosmic orbit here is to stop this change of state from being an issue, as it helps our internal environment return to a central point of balance fairly quickly.

Though these regulations take place on an energetic level, there are, of course, physiological components to this process as well. The opening of the Governing channel serves to develop and strengthen the sympathetic aspect of the nervous system, whilst the Conception channel is closely connected to the function of the vagus nerve and parasympathetic nervous system. When we can regulate these two components of our body successfully, then we will have benefitted our physical body's functioning immensely as well as our stress levels.

To Distribute Qi to the Channels

The Governing and Conception channels are also known to serve as kinds of reservoirs for our Qi within Chinese medical teachings. The rest of the channel system works like small rivers and waterways that come off the reservoirs. When we circulate Qi to a higher degree within the microcosmic orbit, we actually help to deliver more Qi through the channel system; this helps with mind/body connection as well as aiding us in the process of opening the channels.

To Recycle Substances

The movement of energy along the line of the microcosmic orbit is likened to nature's water cycle. Water becomes clouds, which then become rain, and so the water is returned to its source. The inter-transformation of Jing, Qi and Shen are viewed in the same manner within Daoist teachings – or at least they should be. One of the key practices of Daoism is to convert Jing upwards into Qi and then, from here, into Shen. This can be done with or without the microcosmic orbit in place. In one of the earlier systems I practised in my youth, there was no microcosmic orbit, just strong energy work with a conversion of Jing to Qi. Without the orbit, there was no recycling, Jing was converted upwards, but there was no reverse of this process taking place; consequently, I became very drained by this practice. I have seen this error in others as well. We need the orbit in place so that anything we convert upwards can also recycle back down again in the same manner as water transforms within the cycles of nature.

To Protect Us from Excess

If we make an error in our practice, it is possible to send a sudden surge of Qi up into the head; the result of this is an instant headache, blurred vision and dizziness. If this is repeated over a long time, then we run the risk of developing more serious conditions, most likely psychological illness. Though we obviously don't plan on doing this, we have the microcosmic orbit there as a safety net. In case we make an error and too much Qi goes upwards, then we have the microcosmic orbit serving as a kind of earth wire in an electrical circuit.

To Transform the Body

Aside from its function as a safety net, the Qi moves through the orbit, then reaches the rest of our body. It is here, through this circulation of energetic information, that we can really begin to change the direction of our body's evolution. The better our orbit, the more efficient the practices are at developing our health and practice.

To Transform the Mind

One of the key ways that our brain and upper Dan Tian receive Qi and Jing is through the circulation of the microcosmic orbit. Many of the teachings of the Marrow-Washing Classic (see Chapter 7) concern the higher-stage substances that rotate within the microcosmic orbit.

The Lesser Microcosmic Orbit

Once the lower Dan Tian begins to make full rotations, it will generally start to awaken the 'lesser microcosmic orbit' of its own accord. This is a rotation of Qi along the pathway shown in Figure 8.20. This rotation moves through the lower back, along the underside of the diaphragm, and then down the front of the abdomen where it makes a full cycle.

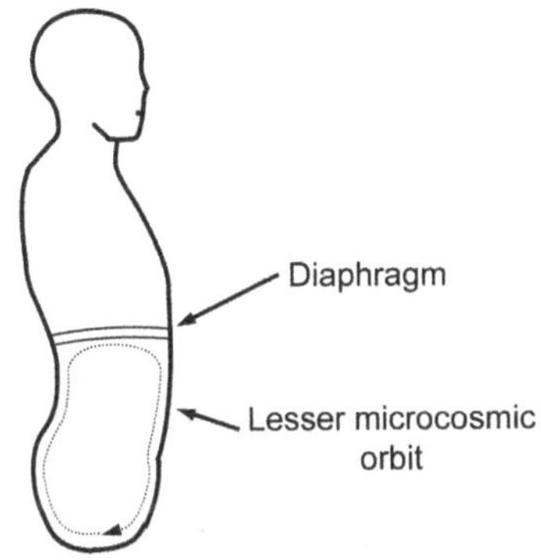

Figure 8.20: The Lesser Microcosmic Orbit

This small rotation of Qi is a direct result of the turning of the lower Dan Tian. It helps to establish the power for the remainder of the microcosmic orbit, as well as helping to create enough space in the lower back for Qi to easily pass through.

The opening of the lower back is an important part of the process, as it ensures that no blockages appear within the early stages of the circulation. It has long been recognised that Qi can stagnate anywhere along the line of the microcosmic orbit. These points of potential stagnation are classically named the 'clipping passes', and they are shown in Figure 8.21. To complete the full circulation of the microcosmic orbit, we need to get our Qi to move past these points.

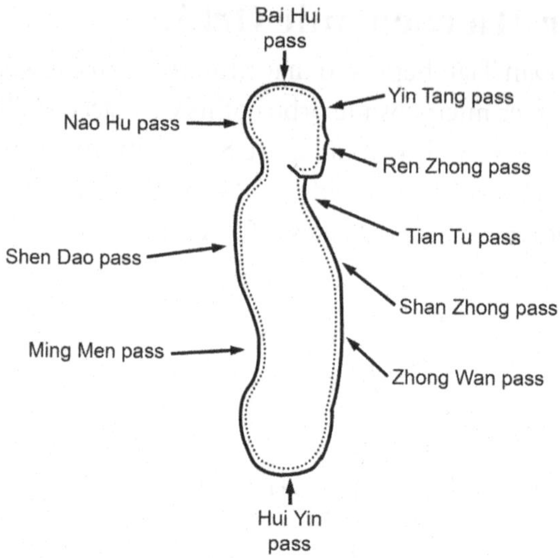

Figure 8.21: The Clipping Passes

We shall now look briefly at the kinds of problems that can arise from long-term blockages that occur at any of these points.

Hui Yin (會陰) Pass

If there is a chronic blockage of Qi within the Hui Yin pass, then it is possible for depletion of Jing and Qi to start happening. The practitioner's energy will drop into a chronically poor state. They can become pale in the face, dizzy and fuzzy-headed. This is because the Jing in this region of the body is blocked and so cannot move or function properly.

Ming Men (命門) Pass

If there is a major blockage in the Ming Men pass, then the back will be cold to the touch. As Qi moves into this region of the body, it can become stuck; this will result in sharp pains in the lower back that may radiate out into the legs causing sciatica-type symptoms.

Shen Dao (神道) Pass

If Qi is chronically blocked at this point, then there will be pain in the upper back that may radiate out into the arms. In extreme cases, there can be a sudden sharp pain in the heart; in this instance, stop practice and seek help immediately.

Nao Hu (腦戶) Pass

This is a very dangerous region for Qi to become stuck in. This can lead to headaches, usually followed by blinding lights in your eyes that cause pain; if this is allowed to continue, then it will, no doubt, lead to psychological illness.

Bai Hui (百會) Pass

As with the previous point, Qi blockages here will lead to headaches and the potential for psychological issues. Be very wary of pain in the crown of the head during microcosmic orbit practice; this is a sure sign you need some assistance.

Yin Tang (印堂) Pass

Blockages here will begin with eye and sinus pain; they will then move into hallucinations and psychic illness, including the potential for invasion of the body and mind by malevolent spirits. Obviously, we would definitely like to avoid problems with this point!

Ren Zhong (水溝) Pass

This is not such a dangerous blockage and is actually the most common for many people. When Qi tries to get past here, it can lead to itching sensations appearing all over the face. These itchy areas are quite random and pop up around your whole head. They are a result of the Qi hitting the Ren Zhong pass and 'firing off' in random directions as they meet the resistance of this point. This is actually the only blockage that you should just leave be; it will clear when it is ready. Try not to scratch these itches, as this will disturb the process of the point's opening.

Tian Tu (天突) Pass

This is another very dangerous point for Qi to become stuck within. Blockages are usually an issue here for those who have been depressed for a long time. When the Qi becomes stuck at this point, it will first manifest as a shortness of breath and then, if left unattended, it can lead to breathlessness and choking. Blockages here generally need assistance from an experienced Qi Gong teacher.

Shan Zhong (膻中) Pass

If Qi becomes blocked here, then it can lead to pain and stagnation of Qi in the chest. This will lead to palpitations, which can be problematic. You should immediately stop the practice and seek help if this happens. In women, stagnant Qi here can also lead to pain and stagnation in the breasts.

Zhong Wan (中脘) Pass

If Qi blocks here, then it is possible for your digestive system to become negatively impacted. It can become hard to digest food, and in extreme (but rare) cases it can lead to chronic muscle pain and wastage.

Problems Are Not Always Clearing Reactions!

The list of problems that can arise as a result of practising the microcosmic orbit has been included simply because of how many people I have now met who have come from schools that did not understand these issues. Now that I have taught around the world for a number of years, I have met people who have practised under teachers who simply told them that the symptoms were signs of the body 'clearing itself' and that the issue will pass. In fact, the body was not 'clearing', it was developing an issue due to a chronic blockage being present. Understanding the difference between a problem and a 'clearing reaction' is quite important if you are going to move into deep internal work; this is a part of the reason why people who teach in-depth Nei Gong really should be practitioners of Chinese medicine as well or, at least, have a good knowledge of Chinese medical theory.

That being said, the vast majority of people will not have the issues listed above. They will manage to practise the microcosmic orbit with little to no difficulty. If you are, however, one of those people who experience these issues developing when the microcosmic orbit begins, then you should seek out an experienced practitioner to help you move beyond this blockage.

The Logic of the Lesser Microcosmic Orbit

There are various ways of working with the lesser microcosmic orbit of Qi. Some schools favour externalised movements, others use guided intention, and with the method discussed here, the primary mechanism is the rotation of the lower Dan Tian. The logic behind using the lower Dan Tian as a driving force is that a practitioner never actually has to have any interaction between their own energetic movements and their mind. The general rule is that if the mind is involved, then there is more chance of a mistake being made. If a person is to use their intention to lead energy around the circulation of the Governing and Conception channels, then at some point they have to rest their awareness on each of the clipping passes in turn. If they mistakenly use an overly strong intention (which is quite likely if you have a direct goal of leading Qi somewhere), then there is the potential for energy blocking at one of the passes. It was a clear principle within traditional Daoist methods that one did not use the mind to lead Qi through the microcosmic orbit or, indeed, any of the channels; this is a teaching that is often not adhered to in many contemporary schools of Qi Gong.

As the lesser microcosmic orbit begins to awaken, there are a number of clear signs that it is taking place:

- The space between the bones of the lower back start to open up; your lumbar literally lengthens. This can feel like a forceful but pleasant stretch in your lower spine. As this happens, you can feel an increase of energy flow here. It makes the lower back very warm to the touch. Because of the back of your body becoming longer and the front of the body remaining the same, it can actually tip you forwards a little. Do not be surprised if you start to sway forwards onto your toes or even stumble forwards a little as if you are losing your balance; this is a normal result of the spine opening. As your body becomes used to it, this reaction will start to subside.

- The lumbar opening will enable Qi to move up towards the Ming Men point and the Ming Huo (命火) or 'Ming fire'. The Ming fire is an expansion of Qi within the lumbar region of the back; it is essentially another of those spherical fields of Qi that exist in various parts of the body. In many people, the Ming fire is weak, the ball of Qi in their lower back is not expansive enough; the result of this is that they have a weakness to the flow of Qi through this area of their body. When the lesser microcosmic orbit starts to open up the back, then this ball of Qi expands and strengthens. It generates a field of warmth around the lumbar which can actually be felt a few inches from the back. It is as if the heat that can be felt is radiating from the spine itself. The Ming fire opens and then serves as a further driving force for Qi along the length of the Governing channel. We need this Ming fire to open so that we can complete the full microcosmic orbit.

- As the rotation of Qi moves into the abdominal muscles, it can cause them to undulate and move like waves of their own accord. This only happens for a short while, but it is a clear and useful sign of progress. It is a completely natural occurrence that you have no control over; the pulling of the muscles is coming from inside, as the Qi of the orbit magnetically draws in the Huang in a wave-like fashion. When this happens, it is a surprise to see just how much power there is in the Qi of the microcosmic orbit.

When the lumbar spine has lengthened, the heat of the Ming fire has awakened and the spontaneous undulation of the abdominal muscles has manifested, then it is time to start turning the lesser microcosmic orbit into the full orbit. This should not be too difficult a development. If, however, you are stuck here and you cannot attain the results described above, then do not move on – instead, return to the previous stages outlined in this book and look to your foundations. The problem will always lie somewhere in the foundations, or else you just need more time. The microcosmic orbit can often take a few years of practice to attain for many people; this is a realistic timescale.

Developing into the Full Microcosmic Orbit

When you have managed to experience the lesser microcosmic orbit, and only when you have managed this, it is time to move on. To do this, we need to move our Qi along the full length of the Governing channel. This is fairly simple to do, providing we have done the previous practices to an efficient enough level.

First, make sure your Wuji posture is good, sink your breath and awareness as before, and then allow the lesser microcosmic orbit to begin. Stay here for some time, a few minutes or more, and then you begin to influence the lower Dan Tian in a different way by changing from 'passive' to 'active' breathing. To do this, stay relaxed, sink your Qi as best you can, and then change to reverse abdominal breathing as discussed in Chapter 5. Make this change of breathing methods subtle and make sure you manage to keep the correct qualities of your breathing as you change methods. Most importantly, your diaphragm should still be moving downwards as previously discussed. If the diaphragm moves upwards on inhalation, then the Qi of the lower abdomen will escape upwards and so the orbit cannot open. If the diaphragm sinks downwards on inhalation, then pressurisation of the Qi will begin to fully open the Governing channel. This process is shown in Figure 8.22.

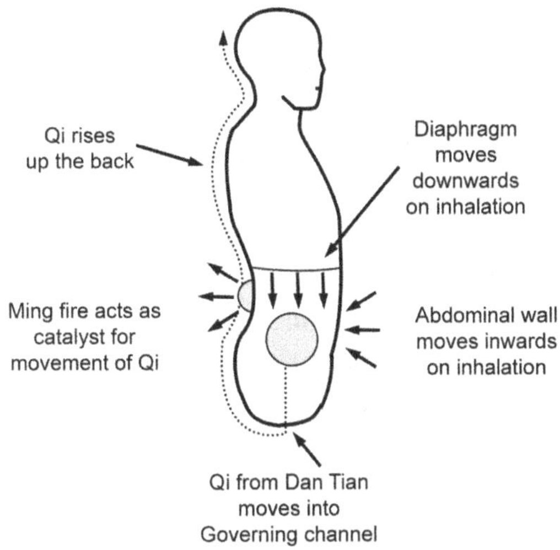

Figure 8.22: Opening the Governing Channel

Keep your inhalation and exhalation long and relaxed. As the Qi begins to react to this breathing method, it will rise into the lumbar region of the spine, meet the Ming fire, and then start to move its way along the length of your back. People seem to have different speeds with this process; some people's Qi moves with the inhalation up the length of the back, whilst others' moves more slowly, independent of their breathing rhythm.

As the Qi moves along the length of the back, it will feel like a high-frequency vibration moving up your spine. If there is a feeling of warmth, then this is muscular resistance; with time, it will fade and only the vibration will be left behind.

You should maintain the reverse abdominal breathing method, in Wuji, until the vibration along your back begins. When it has started, then you should switch back to passive breathing methods. In this way, you are just using the reverse abdominal breathing as an initiator of the process, a 'kick start', if you like; once it is going, then you can just allow it to happen and observe. If, after around half an hour of practice, the reverse abdominal breathing has not started to move this vibrating force, then it is too early for you. The lower Dan Tian is not ready to start this process, and so you should return to your foundation work.

As this vibration moves along your back, it can make your whole body lightly vibrate as a reaction to the Qi's influence. As it passes the vertebrae, they will open up and the spine will lengthen from inside of your body. In some people, they can make quiet 'cracking' noises as they open. As long as this does not come with pain, then you should not worry; it will pass as the Governing channel fully opens.

When it reaches the crown of the head, it will then travel down towards the sinuses and face. There is a distinct feeling of Qi vibrating around the inside of the head which is very pleasant; it is like a low humming inside the front part of your skull. From here, it will move down to the throat and into the length of the Conception channel. In women, this vibration will move through the chest and across the surface of the breasts before it continues down the front of the abdomen to the lower Dan Tian once more. In men, it can be harder to feel on the surface, as the vibration moves deeper into the torso, away from the surface of the body. Figure 8.23 shows these differences.

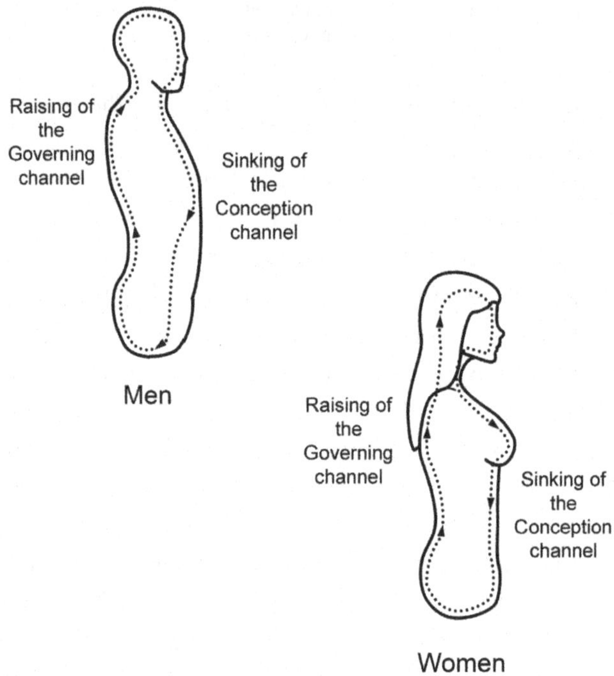

Figure 8.23: Male and Female Sinking of the Microcosmic Orbit

Once it reaches the lower abdomen, then the orbit is complete. It then tends to continue rotating within the body of its own accord. Sometimes, it will change back into the lesser microcosmic orbit for a while, and you will need to restart it with the reverse breathing method, and at other times, it will simply continue to cycle up your back and down your front.

When you have managed the orbit, then continue to practise in this way for as long as you like. Observe the unfolding process and, with time, it will become an inherent energetic cycle that is always there for you. It is likely that you will have to make the microcosmic orbit circulation a 'practice' for a few months, but after this time, you will find that it is always happening. Just drop your awareness into the body, and there it is.

It is important that you are aware that none of the problems caused by blockages in the clipping passes listed above are present. If they are, and issues are developing, then I would suggest finding an experienced practitioner or teacher to help you. You really don't want these kinds of issues to develop in your practice as, if they reach too chronic a stage, they can be difficult to rectify.

The Reverse Cycle of Women

For women, the energy flowing within the microcosmic orbit also has the ability to flow in the opposite direction. In this case, the Qi moving from the lower abdomen flows upwards along the line of the Conception channel, over the head, and then down the centre of the back. This flow is normally known either as the 'reversed orbit' or, sometimes, the 'wind path', though this second name tends to be more commonly applied to alchemy training rather than Nei Gong.

The reverse cycle of energy through this orbit is a very important aspect of training for female practitioners. Though men will also occasionally find that their own energy flows in this direction as well, it will only happen on rare occasions, and it will not assist them in their practice; it should just be ignored and left to change back when it is ready. They should never attempt to make this circulation happen through any kind of directed willpower.

Women will find that this orbit begins to take place of its own accord, and they should simply allow it to happen. It will be far more regular for women than it is for men, and will happen more and more, the deeper they go into their Nei Gong practice. Sometimes, it will even happen for women long before the regular direction of the first microcosmic orbit has opened, but generally, it will start to manifest a little later in their practice. Within the practice of alchemical meditation, women actually learn how to utilise this cycle in time with the phases of the moon, but within a practice such as Nei Gong, we do not worry. Nei Gong is not as advanced as alchemy, we are not working on such a deep level, and so there is no need for the connection of this cycle to the outer environment.

The key role of the reverse flow of energy in this orbit is to extract Jing from the Uterus. This Jing is then raised upwards, through the Conception channel, towards the chest where it is stored. This has the benefit of ensuring that women have a healthy amount of acquired Jing stored around the Heart centre. This is a natural place for women to store their Jing; it is quite unique to women, and male practitioners do not have Jing in their chest. Figure 8.24 shows the pathway of this flow of energy, as well as the movements of Jing which take place.

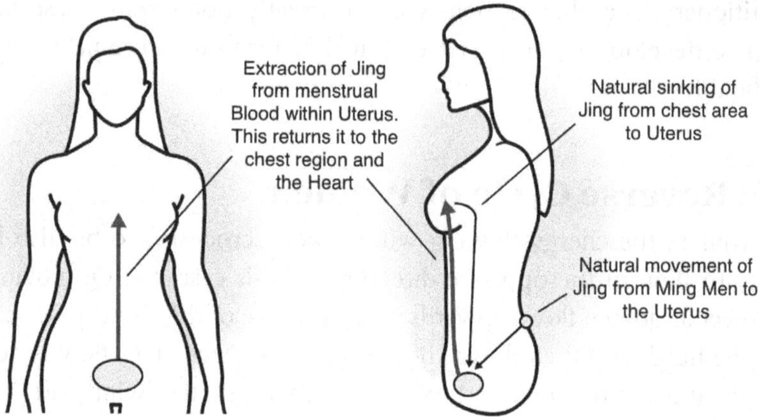

Figure 8.24: The Wind Path of Female Practice

As shown in Figure 8.24, the general direction of flow of Jing within a woman's body is from the region of the kidneys towards the Uterus where it becomes menstrual Blood. As well as this, there is a natural sinking motion which takes place as Jing from the region of the chest sinks downwards towards the Uterus. The reverse cycle of energy within the microcosmic orbit causes some of this Jing to be raised upwards, away from the Uterus and towards the chest, where it moves into the region of the breasts to be stored.

As this cycle begins to open up, there is a clear feeling of upwards movement which begins low down in the abdomen before rising into the chest region. Women will have the distinct sensation of their chest expanding outwards, and sometimes you will even find that your body physically begins to stretch around the ribcage and behind the breasts. As the Jing moves along this line, it is also normal to experience sensations of heat moving upwards towards the chest, and this can leave a woman with a feeling of warm energy expanding across the chest and breasts. If Jing moves into the nipples, then do not be surprised if they become somewhat swollen. This is a normal reaction to the energetic movement taking place within your body.

As the reverse flow begins to extract Jing from the menstrual Blood, it is normal for a woman's menstrual flow to lighten to a certain degree. Though there should never be a complete ending of a woman's period, it is fine for it to become a little lighter. This is simply because there is not as much Jing present to generate the material basis for the creation of Blood itself.

The key factor to keep in mind with regard to this direction of flow within the microcosmic orbit is that women will find that it happens of its own accord. You should find that sometimes it takes place for a small portion of your practice, and other times it will be for the whole practice session. On the other hand, there may be weeks on end where it does not manifest. Do not worry about any of this, and do not look for patterns; your body will know what is best. Continue with your training, and if the reverse flow starts to take place, then simply leave it to happen. Do not worry about any particular method at this time, simply observe what is taking place and give your Jing and Qi the space they need to move in the most efficient manner.

If you wish to know more about women's internal practice, then please refer to the book *Daoist Nei Gong for Women: The Art of the Lotus and the Moon* (Singing Dragon, 2016). This book was written by myself and my wife, Roni Edlund, and it covers a great deal of the female-specific aspects of Nei Gong practice. It is a helpful adjunct to this book for women and men who teach the internal arts to women.

The Stages of the Microcosmic Orbit

To conclude this rather lengthy chapter, it is wise to discuss the various stages of development that the microcosmic orbit goes through. Though many of these stages are very advanced (the final stages are hardly reached by any practitioner), it is helpful to see where the practice can go as it develops.

The Physical Establishing of the Circuit

All channels have a physical component to them. It is through the sinew channels or the Huang that Qi conducts. These physical lines of tissue serve as 'riverbeds' for the flow of Qi along their length. The microcosmic orbit is no exception to this rule; the physical aspect of the orbit has to be there for the energy work to take place. It is the combined raising of the head and sinking of the sternum that moves the tissues into the right place for the physical aspect of the orbit to develop. The biggest problems/risks develop when somebody has raised the head but not sunk the sternum. In this case, the chest is still 'full', and so the Conception channel is blocked. This means that Qi can rise up but not back down again. This can lead to excess Qi movement to the brain, a cause of certain Qi Gong sicknesses.

The Rotation of Qi

The methods and results discussed in this chapter are for the circulation of Qi along the length of the microcosmic orbit. Initially, this will be what I call 'neutral Qi'. This is the Qi of the body that is driven by the lower Dan Tian and the momentum of the lesser microcosmic orbit combined with the influence of the Ming fire. This is the Qi that feels like a vibrating wave moving along your back and down your front. This is the foundation of the orbit and the part of your practice that establishes the various safety mechanisms and Yin/Yang balancing properties of the microcosmic orbit. This is generally the furthest you will go into the microcosmic orbit's energetic circulations for a long time in your practice; the stages beyond this will begin to unfold of their own accord over a lengthy period of time.

The next stage of energetic circulation is the rotation of pure Yang Qi through the Conception and Governing channels. Not many practitioners reach this stage in their training, because it involves going very deep into Nei Gong and converting neutral Qi to a very specific form of Yang Qi. We will discuss these types of Qi in the next chapter.

When pure Yang Qi moves along the length of the back, it feels very uncomfortable. It moves quickly and feels like a powerful electric shock that rushes quickly up your spine, into the occiput, and then through into the middle of your brain, close to where the 'muddy pill' sits. The centre of your brain receives a powerful shock that causes a white flash to go off in your head, and your body to convulse. It is as if you have been plugged into a defibrillator and received its electrical zap into your head. When the Yang Qi rises into the microcosmic orbit, it will cause this reaction three times. These three times are not necessarily close together; the first for me was on a meditation retreat. It was so sudden and painful that I, rather embarrassingly, passed out. The teacher was happy with my progress, and I felt like an idiot! The second of the three shocks came several months later.

The reactions of the Yang Qi are known as the 'three thunder strikes' and they are a recognised aspect of alchemical training. They serve to flood the brain and upper Dan Tian with Yang Qi: a process which helps to open up several key spiritual centres within this region of the body. Once the three 'thunder strikes' have gone off, then the experience will not return.

Pure Yin Qi is equally unpleasant and equally rare. I have only known three or four of my students to contact this level of energy in their practice to date, and even then, only two of the circulations contained a lot of power. The Yin Qi circulation can come before, after or independent of the Yang Qi circulation; I have not yet spotted a pattern in this.

When pure Yin Qi moves through the microcosmic orbit, it feels as if you are trying to squeeze a marble through a drinking straw. It is uncomfortable and feels as if there is not enough room for Qi to move through the Governing channel's length. This rotation happens only once in your process and is very slow. Once it begins, it takes a few weeks to a couple of months for the single rotation to complete.

Because of the magnetic quality of Yin Qi, it pulls on the Huang as it passes by, meaning that your spine and back are strongly affected. The whole of your back can be realigned by this process and the muscular structure of the torso will change so that the Governing channel can fully open. This is where the pain comes from; though it is a beneficial process, the Qi does not always understand the idea of discomfort and so it can leave you with an aching back for the whole process. On top of this, there is a lot of emotional adjustment that takes place, as emotional debris trapped within the spaces between the vertebrae is squeezed out of you.

The Rotation of Congenital Fluid

The rotation of congenital fluid through your microcosmic orbit generally happens only within alchemical meditation practices, so I will not discuss it here in detail. Essentially, a cultivated form of Jing from the lower abdomen, Ding, and Lu travel like a warm, bubbling fluid through the orbit. This is the 'Ding fluid', and it has a strong rejuvenating effect upon the body. We generally need a specific breathing method known as the 'three animal carts' breathing method to help this circulation unfold. This is a breathing method specific to Daoist meditation systems and is not really relevant to Nei Gong practice.

The second type of congenital substance to move through the orbit is Jing that has been extracted from the sexual fluids. This is an aspect of the marrow washing that we looked at in Chapter 7. The pathway of Qi that you have built through microcosmic orbit training serves as a major pathway for the Jing, Qi, Shen conversion process. This helps to nourish the brain, bone and marrow of the body, as well as serving as the connection between microcosmic orbit training and spiritual cultivation.

The Rotation of Light

Once again, this is primarily an alchemical stage of development, but I shall include it here for completeness. I also want to make clear that the microcosmic orbit is a series of developmental stages that evolve, through your practice, over time. It is not something that is simply completed when the Qi has made a cycle through your body.

The circulation of Shen along the microcosmic orbit is important for various spiritual components of alchemical training. As your Shen moves along the Governing and Conception channels, it passes its influence into the rest of the channel system, and so the mind/body connection is changed to a 'spirit/body' connection. It is through this highly advanced method that a practitioner of alchemy can adjust their entire body's functioning and even convert the body into pure light at extremely high levels.

There are two types of Shen rotated through the orbit. The first is 'refracted' light. This is an expression of the five spiritual energies discussed in detail in Chapter 11. These five lights are able to then build a stronger connection with the body's functioning. It is also with this practice that many of the debris of 'cause and effect' are cleared from the body's channels. As you can imagine, this is a very high-level endeavour and few manage to attain this level in their practice. Its methods are still held in strict secrecy within the Daoist lineages.

The second form of light is pure 'unrefracted' light that is a manifestation of pure spirit. When this substance moves through the microcosmic orbit, it lights it up like a silvery band that extends around the body. This was named the Fa Lun (法輪) or 'wheel of law', a name that linked its use to the 'cause and effect' quality of Heaven's influence.

The Rotation of the Alchemical Pill

The final stage for alchemical Daoists is the combining of Jing, Qi, Shen, Yin and Yang into one single unit. This then forms the ingredients of the 'alchemical pill'. It is an oversimplified explanation, but basically the 'pill' is then decreased in density until it reaches the level of Qi; almost tangible in alchemical terms. It is then circulated through the microcosmic orbit nine times (though this may well be a metaphorical number; it is beyond my capabilities or full understanding), and this process of circulation is the equivalent of 'swallowing' the pill.

These are steps towards attainment of spiritual immortality. Once again, these are alchemical processes and very advanced. Many of you reading this may well not even believe in these stages being real; this is okay, it is not my job to convince you. I am simply outlining the classically understood stages of development for the microcosmic orbit.

Though some of the stages outlined above are very advanced in nature, it is always interesting to have an overview of an entire process. Within Nei Gong, and at this stage, it is the circulation of neutral Qi that we are concerned with. Keep working on the above practices until you have attained Gong at this stage. In the next chapter, we shall start to look at the nature of the channels, opening them, and the two main divisions of Qi.

Chapter 9

MOVEMENT OF THE YANG QI

The awakening of the lower Dan Tian and the beginning of the microcosmic orbit are important stages in Nei Gong development. In addition to the functions focused upon in the previous chapter, they also begin the movement of Qi through the channel system. The large energetic pathways that run up the length of your back and then down the front of your body serve as a kind of 'mobile reservoir' for the body's Qi. From here, Qi moves into the subsidiary branches of the rest of the channel system, including the organ channels that run near to the surface of the body. This is the vitally important stage known simply as 'opening the channels'. It is the basis for making your energetic system run in an efficient manner. Whether you seek Qi Gong practice for health, martial arts or spiritual development, opening the channels is an integral part of your journey.

Revisiting Qi

So far, we have looked at Qi in various ways. Initially, we discussed in Chapter 1 how the definition of Qi varies from art to art, then we looked at the experiences of Qi within the body and, from here, moved into discussions of the nature of Yin and Yang Qi. It is now, at the stage of opening the channels of the body, that we really need to look at the nature of Qi in greater detail. What are Yin Qi and Yang Qi? Where do they come from? How do we convert and use them in our practice? These are the kinds of issues we need to clarify once we enter energy work of this kind.

The first thing to understand is that the Qi of the channel system primarily falls under the heading of Yang Qi. It moves in a somewhat linear fashion along the length of the channels. It conducts its way through the material of the Huang or sinew channels, depending upon which part of the body it is moving through, and carries with it vital energy as well as conscious information. It tends to be experienced as a vibratory force that is moving through the 'riverbed' of the body's soft tissues for the majority of people. At various stages in your development it can also be felt as an electrical-type current that is moving through the body, but that is unusual in the earlier stages of your practice.

Generally, most people will not be able to feel their Qi very easily; some people can, but they are certainly in the minority. Instead, what people generally feel is one of the Ba Chu or 'eight experiences' of Qi that we discussed in Chapter 1. These are not your Qi per se but rather the way that Qi is interacting with your body.

The eight experiences are as follows:

- *Diao (shaking):* Feeling like you are shaking inside is due to the movement of Qi, primarily Yang Qi, reacting with your body's tissues. As the tissues begin to unbind as a reaction to the movement of Qi, they shake.
- *Yi (excitement):* This indicates a hyperactivity of the inside of the body and sometimes the mind; it can leave you 'buzzing' for some time afterwards. This is a sign of the Qi moving at an increased rate. You are feeling the body's sensation to increased Qi flow and the energy that is produced by this process.
- *Leng (feeling cold):* Feelings of cold are usually how the body processes a region of the body with a chronic deficiency of Qi, or else, if the cold feels as if it is moving along a channel, it is usually how you experience an energetic pathogen leaving the system. In this case, it is the reaction of the movement of Qi that you are feeling.
- *Re (feeling hot):* Though there are types of heat associated with Jing and circulation of essence, there is also the general heat that can be felt throughout the body during Qi Gong practice. This heat is down to an increased flow of blood, or else resistance in the channel system as Qi is trying to conduct along its length.
- *Fu (feeling light):* As Qi moves upwards in the body, it can be a little 'unrooting', which makes you feel light and as if you could float. Many of these kinds of somatic experiences where the whole body's feeling is changed are because of the movement of Yin Qi.
- *Chen (feeling as if sinking):* As the more Yin types of Qi, including Water Qi, are experienced, they can feel as if you are becoming heavier or being drawn down towards the ground.

- *Jian (feeling tight):* If Qi conducts strongly through a channel, then it can actually tighten the channel temporarily. This is because the connective tissues of the channel are reacting to the increased information of the Qi passing along their length.
- *Ruan (feeling soft):* As channels open and release tension from their length, it is normal for the body to suddenly feel as if it is softening or slackening to a certain degree. This is the by-product of Qi helping the channel system to free itself up.

As you can see from the list above, it is the reaction to your Qi that you are feeling rather than Qi itself. This becomes important because there are actually a couple of experiences of Qi that we shall discuss soon that are literally Qi itself. In the beginning, you are generally feeling how the body is reacting to the energy you are producing and moving. You could think of it like this: you can't actually feel the wind; all you can feel is how the wind reacts with your body when it makes contact with it. What we think of as the feeling of wind is actually how our body processes the experience of having wind stimulate the nervous system and all of the effects that come from this. For a long time in our practice, the experience of Qi is the same.

Tuning into Qi

Though it really is not very important, my experience is that most students are keen to feel their own Qi as soon as possible. What is more important is the way that the movement of Qi is transforming your body as a result of your practice. That being said, if you have never felt your Qi, then it can be an exciting prospect to tangibly connect with its flow.

Essentially, your brain is like a radio and the realms of physicality, Qi and spirit are like different radio stations. Since most people are tuned into the 'station' of the physical body, they cannot easily feel their Qi. To adjust the channel, we can adjust our awareness. There are various ways to do this, but the simplest is to use the lower Dan Tian as a kind of converter for your awareness.

By settling your awareness into the lower Dan Tian and going through the various stages of regulating the breath and mind that were discussed in Chapters 5 and 6, you should have managed to calm your mind and anchor it into the lower Dan Tian. This is the preparation helping to 'adjust the frequency of your awareness' so that it can begin to connect with your Qi.

To practise 'adjusting the frequency', simply sit in a meditative position and make yourself as comfortable as possible. Make sure that your spine is upright and that you are sat with your eyes closed.

After a few minutes of sitting in this way and establishing the correct qualities in your body, you should begin to 'listen' to your lower Dan Tian. The word 'listening' is chosen on purpose because there are only a few senses we can use to interact with the world. Wherever we place our awareness, we are going to engage one of the sense faculties. If you 'look' at the lower Dan Tian, you will start to see colours and other visual phenomena; this will actually prevent you from adjusting the awareness to the frequency of Qi. This is because the mind, more than anything, really likes visual stimuli. If we give our awareness the instruction to 'look' – no matter how relaxed – then this gives permission for the start of visual stimulation. The acquired mind is then engaged, the imagination kicks in, and then our practice is halted.

If you try to 'feel' the lower Dan Tian, then you will interact with the physical body. The nervous system will activate and you will suddenly become aware of a whole range of tactile experiences; none of these will be Qi; at best they will be one of the 'eight experiences' of how Qi is interacting with you. These interactions are still not Qi itself.

'Smelling' or 'tasting' the lower Dan Tian does not make a lot of sense. 'Smelling' would involve trying to sniff the Dan Tian! Sniffing involves using the nose and this is a very mechanical process that will bring you into the body. 'Tasting' as a sense is always focused into the mouth, it is a sense that cannot be projected out from the locale of the mouth and head.

That leaves us with the sense of 'listening'. Listening is perfect for this kind of interaction. It engages a sense faculty that can be projected to various locations; in this case we are 'listening' to the lower Dan Tian region. It will not engage any visual reactions and it passively moves you away from entering into the realm of tactile feelings. Instead, we can sink the awareness to the lower Dan Tian and then simply 'listen': relax as much as you can, as if you are casually listening to something in the distance; you are not intently trying to hear something with focus, it is a casual 'half-interested' form of listening.

If you can absorb your awareness into the lower Dan Tian region of the body and casually 'listen' for a length of time, then you will start to find that your awareness begins to 'tune into' the frequency of Qi. This principle is shown in Figure 9.1.

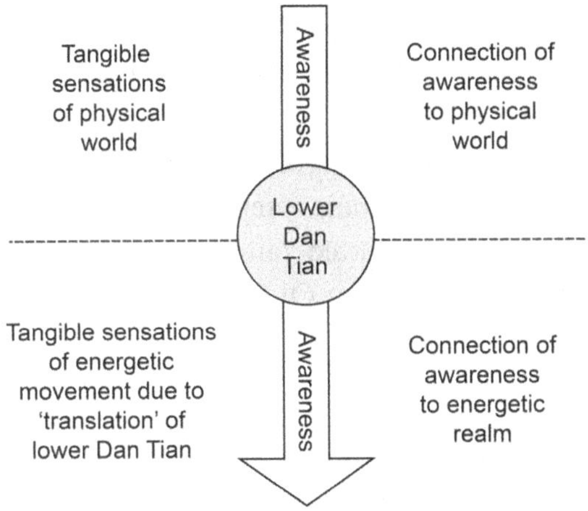

Figure 9.1: Tuning into Qi

The reason that this happens is because the lower Dan Tian is a kind of translator between the physical and the energetic frequencies. In the case of 'substances', it converts Jing (the densest of the San Bao) upwards into Qi (less dense than Jing). It does this by adjusting the energetic frequency of the substance so that it changes form. Remember, Jing and Qi are the same 'thing', they are just in different states: two different points on a spectrum of conversion. It is one role of the lower Dan Tian to be involved in this change; in this way, it acts like a step-up transformer in an electrical circuit.

When our awareness is placed into the lower Dan Tian and allowed to passively 'listen', then it also goes through this kind of conversion. It steps up the frequency away from physicality into the energetic level. When this happens, you will find that the sensation of Qi starts to open up for you and you can experience Yin and Yang forms of Qi as tactile experiences. It is quite common for the channels to become clear for you to feel, as well as the various fields of energetic information that surround the body. It just takes time and following these steps.

I should remind you here, though, to remember that this kind of sensation or awareness is not really that important right now. The change of the Nei Gong process will still occur, whether you can or cannot feel your own Qi. There are enough signs and experiences to be had within the body that show you how your process is unfolding. So, if you are a very insensitive person when it comes to perceiving these kinds of things, then do not worry. I personally was as sensitive as a brick for many years and had no idea what was going on inside of my energetic system. I simply ignored this issue, carried on with my practice and progressed along the path of the Nei Gong process regardless of my lack of sensitivity.

Fire, Water, Yin and Yang Qi

Within this book so far, 'Yin Qi' and 'Yang Qi' have been used as terms to describe the two main categories of Qi that move within the body. This has been a slight oversimplification of the terminology as, in fact, there are further subdivisions of each of these categories. Essentially, what we have are pure Yang Qi, pure Yin Qi, distorted Yang Qi and then, finally, distorted Yin Qi. The distorted versions of Yang Qi and Yin Qi are called Fire and Water respectively, as shown in Figure 9.2.

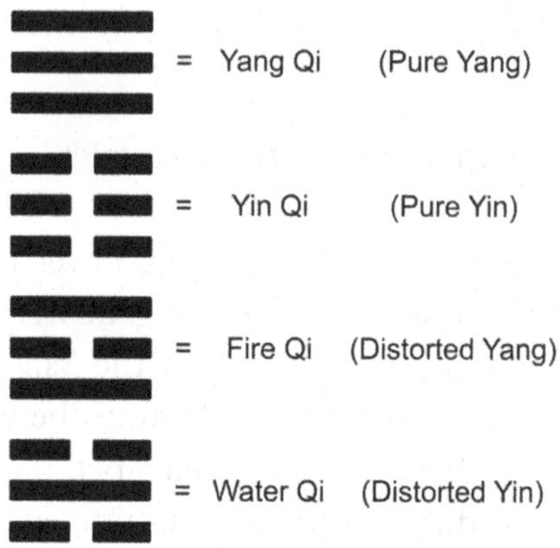

Figure 9.2: Yang, Yin, Fire and Water

As you can see, these types of Qi are represented by four trigrammatic symbols derived from the Yi Jing or Classic of Changes. This text is often known by its alternative spelling, the I Ching. Within the Yi Jing, various forms of Qi and how they transform into one another are represented by a series of symbols known as the Gua (卦) or 'trigrams'. The four symbols of Yang, Yin, Fire and Water shown in Figure 9.2 are half of the eight key symbols from which all forms of Qi are derived. The Yi Jing is a study of how the various forms of Qi are combined with one another and inter-transform. A skilled scholar of the Yi Jing can use the text to understand the nature of Qi as it transforms in the background to an event or situation that is unfolding at that time. If you are interested in this subject, I have written an introduction to the Yi Jing and its usage as a part of my previous book, *White Moon on the Mountain Peak: The Alchemical Firing Process of Nei Dan* (Singing Dragon, 2016).

We do not need to understand the Yi Jing fully for the practice of Nei Gong; we should just become familiar with a few of the basic symbols and concepts. Essentially, a solid line is a representation of Yang, whilst a broken line is Yin. Pure Yang is thus shown as three solid lines, whilst pure Yin is represented with three broken lines. Fire is Yang that has been 'distorted' by its interaction with Yin and so it is two solid lines with a broken line in its centre. Likewise, Water is pure Yin that has become distorted by its interactions with Yang. This is why it is depicted as two broken lines with a solid line between them. This is a diagrammatic representation of how pure Yin and pure Yang become transformed when they enter into the realm of manifestation. This is shown in Figure 9.3.

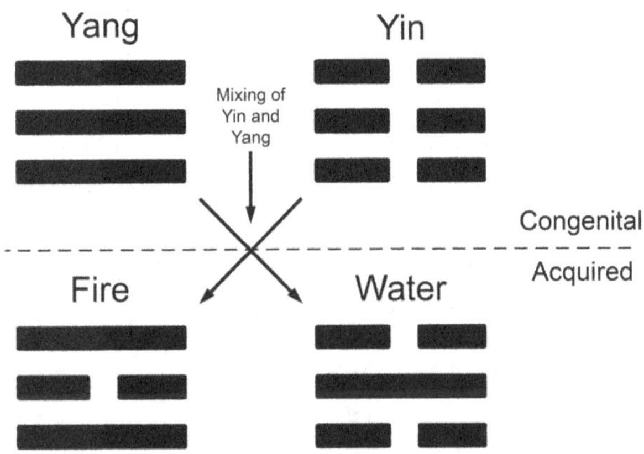

Figure 9.3: Yang and Yin Convert to Fire and Water

Within the process of creation, it is stated that Yang and Yin are Heaven and Earth respectively; everything exists in the middle, between these two poles, and is a mixture of these two; nothing, apart from Heaven and Earth, is pure Yin or pure Yang. These distorted forms of Yin and Yang are known as the Wan Wu (萬物), 'ten thousand things' or 'myriad things'. Within Daoist creation, the Wan Wu are the infinite manifestations of life that exist upon the earthly realm. They are generated within the space between Heaven and Earth as a manifestation of the multitude of ways in which Yin and Yang can interact as creative forces.

This process is reflected within the microcosm of human creation. Here, pure Yang (Heaven) is consciousness or spirit. It enters into pure Yin (Earth) which is our body. In this way, spirit and form come together as one unit. As soon as pure Yang enters into pure Yin, then a process of 'mixing' takes place. This begins in utero and represents the way that spirit causes the creation of human life even from its founding moments.

This process of spirit or consciousness merging with the body then continues and it is through the body that consciousness experiences life and the outside world. The Wan Wu that are created at this stage are the infinite streams of thoughts and mental 'movements' that are a result of the experience of life. The nature of mind, then, as discussed previously, governs much of the quality of Qi within our body and so in this way Yin and Yang have generated the potential for our inner energetic matrix. The continued formation of the Wan Wu governs which direction our personal energetic evolution then takes.

The state of pure Yin and Yang is the Xian Tian or 'congenital state', it is literally 'pre-Heaven' according to the Chinese characters, or 'before the distortion of becoming mind'. Once we are alive and functioning cognitively, then we are in the Hou Tian, 'acquired', 'post-Heaven' or 'after the distortion of becoming mind'. The Hou Tian state is dictated by the distorted versions of Yin and Yang Qi – Water and Fire respectively. We can see this from the two arrangements of the eight Gua which are shown in Figure 9.4. They are known as the 'congenital' and 'acquired' arrangements.

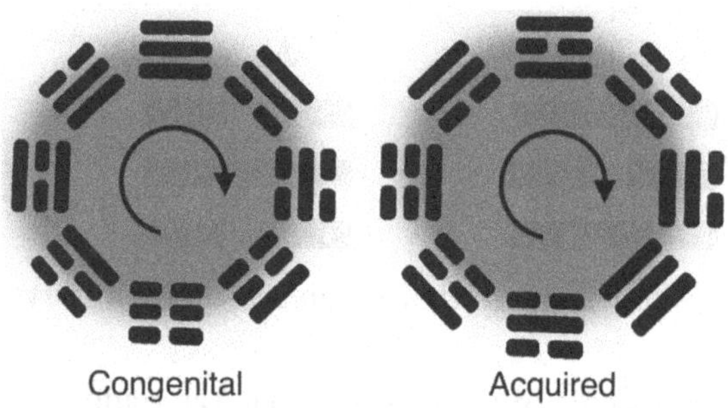

Figure 9.4: The Congenital and Acquired Gua Arrangements

What is shown is that in the congenital state, life is organised according to the two poles of pure Yin and Yang, Earth and Heaven. This is why they are sat in the key positions at the top and bottom of the arrangement. In the acquired state – life – the two key positions are held by distorted Yin and distorted Yang, Water and Fire.

If we look at this in another way, we can see that we actually have the potential for pure Yin and Yang within the body; they are there, they always have been. They were seeded into us at the point of our creation. It is just that locating the pure forms of Yin and Yang is very difficult.

Pure Yang exists at the very centre of our consciousness, it is the seed of spirit. Unfortunately, it is buried beneath a whole mire of distorted Qi – Fire Qi. This is essentially our 'true nature' and the 'acquired nature' that surrounds it.

Pure Yin sits within the centre of our Jing; it is the seed for the generation of our physical form. As Yang is the seed of our consciousness, Yin is the seed of our physical aspect. Once this pure Yin 'seed' moves into action, then it becomes distorted and thus it is known as Water. These ideas are shown in Figure 9.5, which shows how we understand life through Fire and Water but contain within us, somewhere, the potential for Yang and Yin.

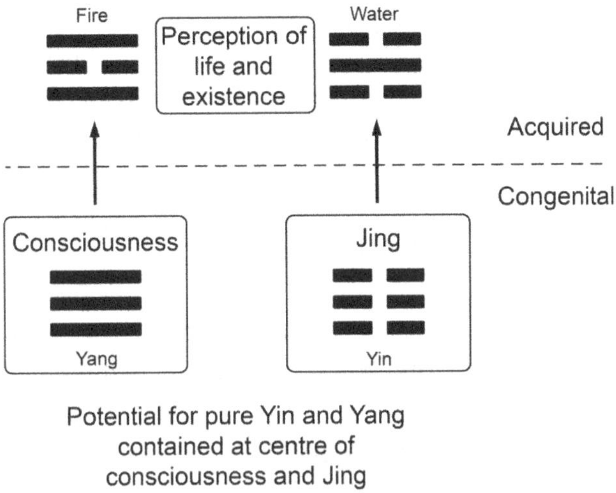

Figure 9.5: The Seeds of Yin and Yang

It is a key aim of Nei Gong, and indeed most Daoist practices, to locate Yin and Yang. It is stated classically that we need to 'convert Yin and Yang to Fire and Water'. This conversion enables us to work with the purest forms of Qi that exist within us; they are the very seeds of our existence. In the majority of cases, these two pure forms of Qi are then generated and merged, a stage known as 'merging Yin and Yang' or 'unification of the whole'. Needless to say, this is very difficult. Hardly anybody who enters into the Daoist arts ever manages to locate and build a large amount of pure Yin and Yang Qi. Fewer still manage to recombine them into one unit; this would be very high-level Nei Gong practice indeed.

Alchemical meditation practitioners will have their own method of locating and working with Yin and Yang. Though there are some shared principles, there are differences between the alchemical meditation and Nei Gong methodologies. They are complementary practices but both quite unique in their approach to the challenge of working with these two primal forces.

Within Nei Gong, one simple rule is recognised: it is almost impossible to locate true Yin. For this reason, practitioners look to generate pure Yang. When pure Yang is generated, pure Yin will be drawn to it naturally. In this way, however much Yang you build, you will attain the same amount of Yin. They are attracted to one another in a 'magnetic' manner. We shall return to this process in Chapter 11 when we look at the highest levels of Nei Gong practice.

Pure Yin and pure Yang are to be found at a state of 'pure' consciousness, as in experiencing the realm of consciousness without the veils of acquired mind being in the way. This can only be experienced through finding a balance between mental stability and relaxation. This will result in an entering into stillness, a state that brings you to 'emptiness' – the realm of pure Yang. Once again, we shall return to this at a later stage in the book when we look at the final stages of Nei Gong training.

A Slight Error in Terminology

When we talk of Yin Qi and Yang Qi within the body, what we are discussing is actually Water Qi and Fire Qi. Because of the highly advanced processes involved in locating pure Yin Qi and Yang Qi, we will not be utilising these in our practice for a very long time and many of us (maybe) never will. Instead, what we use in our training are the distorted versions of these two forms of Qi. They are the energetic expression of these two poles, and it is these expressions that move through our body giving us life. This means that rather than it being Yang Qi moving through our channel system, it is actually Fire Qi – distorted Yang Qi. Rather than it being Yin Qi moving in fields through the body, it is Water Qi – distorted Yin Qi.

Because the spirit is said to reside in the Heart centre, the source of Fire was located as being within the chest. This is the home of pure Yang and out of this place comes our Fire Qi. Water, on the other hand, was located within the region of the lower abdomen and kidneys. This is because the kidneys and Ming Men house pure Yin and from here comes distorted Yin – Water. The strongest influence of Water is felt in the fields of the lower abdomen, around the lower Dan Tian. The strongest influence of Fire is felt within the region of the heart, where the mind begins to extend its influence out into the channel system. Figure 9.6 shows the sources of Fire and Water within the body.

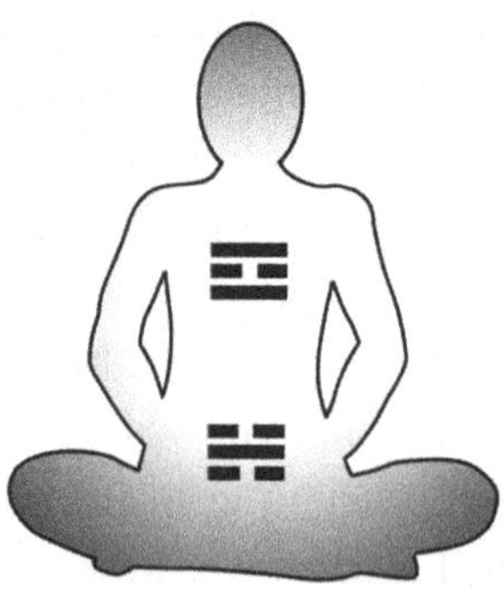

Figure 9.6: The Body's Fire and Water Centres

Because of the sheer amount of different aspects of the training that are named Fire and Water, we avoid as much confusion as we can by simply referring to our Qi as Yin and Yang. It is for this reason that I use the terms Yin Qi and Yang Qi when I actually mean distorted Yin and distorted Yang, or Hou Tian Yin and Hou Tian Yang. It is distorted Yang that moves through your channels; this is Qi that has been adjusted by the layers of acquired mind. It is distorted Yin that builds the fields around the lower Dan Tian; it is distorted by the nature of your Ming and how it is expressed through your Jing.

It is important at this stage to recognise what we are actually referring to in our practice. I shall continue to use the terms Yin and Yang within this chapter.

Opening the Channels

This brings us to a major aspect of the practice: opening the channels. This is very important in our training as it serves to facilitate and improve several key processes:

- First, the channels are each linked to major organs and associated systems within your body. As the channels open up to a higher degree, it helps to regulate the health and function of these organ systems. The regulation of these key organ systems, according to Chinese medical thought, is the basis of your internal health.
- The more the channels open, the greater the flow of Qi into your body. The more Qi flows through the body, the greater the level of connection that exists between your mind and your body.
- The channels are the key places where your body stores somatic memory of past traumas, emotional experiences and, basically, every event that has ever befallen you. These psychological experiences generate energy, a form of Qi, and this Qi is deposited around the body where it then 'sticks' within the channels' length. This is the basis for the development of blockages, energetic debris which compromises the flow of Qi along a channel's length.
- The channels have a kind of psychological feedback loop into the mind: blockages within the channel will impact the body's functioning, and the blocked channels will, in turn, send this information back to the mind. These blockages then cause further distortions of the acquired mind. In this way, a vicious cycle of increase in distortion within the

acquired mind and decrease in channel quality is established; it is these kinds of cycles that we are trying to impact through opening the channels.

The above functions are the key reasons why we want to increase the level of flow along the channels' length. As we can see, three of the points listed above (the first, third and fourth) are primarily concerned with improving various aspects of our mental and physical health. The second point is linked to increasing the mind/body connection. It is this function of opening the channels that we shall return to further down the line in our Nei Gong process. At this stage, it is the improvement of our level of well-being that we will be working on.

The Anatomy of a Channel

We have already looked in brief at the anatomy of a channel. We have discussed how they comprise two main aspects: a physical 'runner' or 'riverbed' as well as an energetic 'flow' along this physical pathway. The Qi essentially 'conducts' along the length of the channel. In this way, we could liken the channels to wires in an electric circuit. There are two required parts: the physical copper wires and the electricity that moves through the wires.

In classical terminology, it is stated that Qi should move through the channels like sound moves through a drum-skin. Traditional instructions involved 'turning your Huang and sinew channels into a drum-skin', pointing out the importance of pulling the Huang taut and elastically connecting it together. If we then 'bang the drum-skin', sound will travel and 'conduct' along its length. No doubt, the metaphor of sound was used as it moves through the drum-skin as a form of vibration, similar to how Qi is generally experienced when it moves along a channel pathway.

The Qi that travels along a channel's length can feel electrical in nature sometimes, but it also carries with it a kind of information. This 'information' is an expression of the quality of your mind. This means that your Qi has an emotional quality to it as well as the ability to carry memories and thought patterns along the channel's length into the body. Remember that this is Yang Qi (albeit distorted Yang Qi) and as such it is linked to both the Heart and the mind; your mental state directly governs the nature of the Qi that moves along the channel's length.

As the Qi travels along the physical aspect of the channel, it can either tighten or slacken it. This is largely to do with the emotional intent of the Qi moving along the channel's length. Chinese medicine even acknowledges the manner in which seven of your key emotional states would affect the Qi within your body:

- Anger 'raises' the Qi
- Joy 'slows' the Qi
- Sadness 'dissolves' the Qi
- Fear 'descends' the Qi
- Shock 'scatters' the Qi
- Worry 'knots' the Qi
- Guilt 'stagnates' the Qi

We can see from the above examples just how the mind governs our Qi's quality. It is easy enough to see from this how it would influence the nature of Qi within a channel. As the Qi 'conducts' its way along the channel, it begins to engage the Huang or the sinew channels. This action is in accordance with the teachings of the Sinew-Changing Classic. This will then mean that the energetic movement will cause a direct change in the quality and level of binding within the Huang and sinews. Where the physical strands of these connective tissues become bound, there sits an emotional pathogenic residue which we need to clear from the channel in order to improve its functioning. The collective name for these types of energetic debris was Xie Qi (邪氣) or literally 'demonic Qi'. Note that the use of the term 'demonic' came from previous belief systems of all illnesses being afflictions from negative spirits. As Chinese medical theory developed and began to see most illnesses as coming from the mind, Xie Qi was translated as 'sick Qi', though the original characters were kept.

As the connective tissues start to become unbound, there is a great level of conduction along the channel's length and so the channel is said to be more open. As with everything, this opening happens in degrees, and as you develop within your practice, there are clear signs of when the channels have fully opened up. We shall discuss these towards the end of the chapter.

Channels of Light

It is interesting to note that the earliest-known name for the channel system was the 'hall of lights'. This was a reference to the body (the 'hall') being filled with channels of light. We generally associate the experience of visual light with Shen rather than Qi or Jing. This would indicate that there is a

Shen aspect to the channels as well. This is, of course, true: we have discussed already, several times, that the channels are a route whereby the mind interacts with the body. Whilst beginners learn that the channels are composed solely of Qi, more advanced students should be aware of the presence of Shen within the channels' length as well. It is a rule of Daoism that everything exists on three main levels: the physical, the energetic, and the spiritual or 'plane of consciousness'. The channel system is no exception to this.

In the earliest stages of our training, we are most aware of the physical aspect of the channels. We can see, work with, stretch and even touch some of the channel pathways on a physical level; these would be the sinew channel aspects of the channel system. As we go deeper, we can adjust the frequency of our awareness and so access the Qi aspect of the channel system. At this stage, we can feel and directly experience the energy of the channel system. This means going beyond the 'eight experiences' which are essentially halfway between physicality and energy; we are feeling the way in which the Qi interacts with our body. Beyond this level, within the realm of energetics, is where we experience Yang as a somewhat 'fluid' electrical current and Yin as a series of fields and spherical forms with a 'magnetic' quality to them. Deeper still, and we reach the stage of Shen, the consciousness aspect of the channel system. This can only be achieved through the development of 'inner vision', a skill that manifests out of Nei Gong training.

'Inner vision' is exactly what it sounds like: you are able to 'see' inside your body. It means that the brain is able to interpret energetic information and then translate it into a visual form that you can understand. When you look at the channel system through the use of 'inner vision', you will see that the channels are like a huge mass of glittering, silvery white lights. They extend through the body in a chaos of glittering lines that look like a huge tangled ball of wool. Amongst these tangled channels are a series of slightly thicker lines that extend along the more conventional routes that we are used to looking at in acupuncture books. These more prominent channels are around 1–3 mm in thickness, whereas the more tangled and less ordered lines are much thinner. Deeper still into the body, and the congenital channels are around 3–5 mm in thickness. At later stages, you will be able to perceive these channels in other people and you will see that, on average, they are about the same thickness in most people. Figure 9.7 shows a comparison of the channels' makeup with regard to the three levels of their manifestation.

As you can see, the physical aspect of the channel is the widest, the Qi aspect is slightly thinner, and the Shen lies at the channel's centre. It is here, through this thinner region of the channel, that emotional information travels to become Xie Qi once it is distributed outwards into the thicker 'tissue' aspects of the channel's pathway. This is the basis for the development of blockages according to psychological roots. Of course, blockages can work the other way too and be the result of physical trauma or sickness.

In extreme cases of sickness, whole channels can become stagnant and sick; these then take on a dark greyish hue. This darker area slows the Qi down within the channel's length. Clearing the channel and improving the person's health returns the channel to its former brightness.

It is interesting to note that quite a number of Qi Gong doctors have shared their experience of channel visuals through the use of the same skill and the accounts are generally very similar in nature.

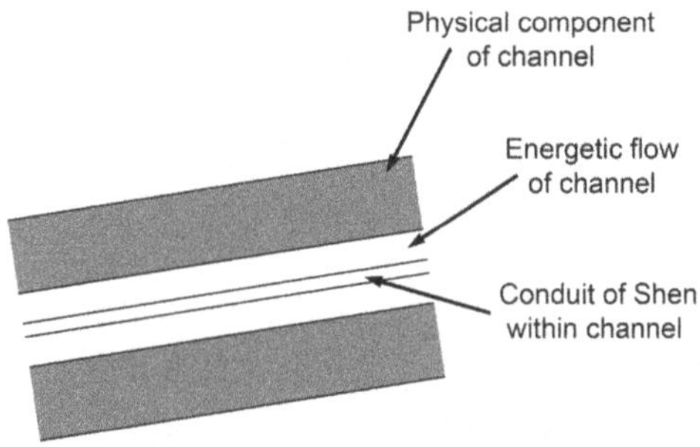

Figure 9.7: The Jing, Qi and Shen of the Channel

Zi Fa Gong

As we begin to work with the lower Dan Tian and open the microcosmic orbit of Qi through the Governing and Conception channels, we will start to send more energetic information through the entire channel system. In the earliest stages of practice, this will take place in the channels near to the surface of the body; it will take quite some time before this process moves deeper, into the congenital channel system.

As the channels open, it is likely (but not guaranteed) that you will experience the process known as Zi Fa Gong, first discussed in Chapter 8. The literal translation of the term is 'self-expression quality'. If we look at what this means, it is indicating that the process is causing the nature of your 'self' to be expressed externally through your body, in particular through a series of spontaneous and uncontrolled movements. For this reason, Zi Fa Gong is usually known as 'spontaneous Qi movement' in the West. When this phenomenon begins, it is normal for the body to go through a series of dynamic phases that include shaking, folding at the waist, spinning, running and even producing expressive dance-like movements. Figure 9.8 shows a student going through the Zi Fa Gong process.

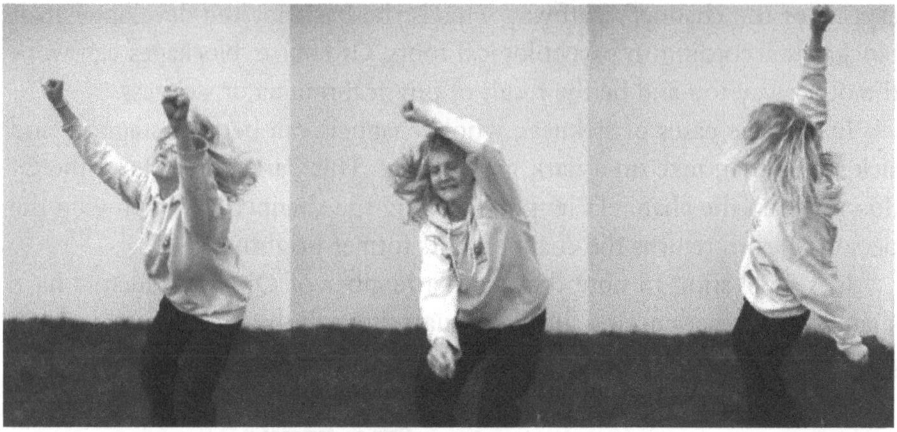

Figure 9.8: Zi Fa Gong

These movements are similar in nature to the spontaneous Kriya of Yogic traditions and serve to take you through a series of developmental stages:

- Initially, the process of Zi Fa Gong helps to clear out pathogenic debris from the channels of the body. This helps them to open and improve your health by shedding many of the energetic 'roots' of disease.
- After this, it helps to establish many of the trickier circulations and energetic cycles within the body. It would be difficult to use any kind of method or intention to open certain energetic branches and so we use the body's inherent abilities to build these connections for us.
- Later stages involve the development of Shou Yin (手印) – 'hand shape' or 'mudra', which, in Daoism, are a form of energetic and spiritual attunement. When the Zi Fa Gong process reaches this stage, then the body is essentially starting to refine very intricate and subtle levels of vibration using the mudra as a tool.
- Deep psychological switches can take place as the movement of the Zi Fa Gong process hits and reacts with the Heart centre and your nature. The quality of your Xing is a kind of antenna for contacting the spirit, and the Zi Fa Gong process can help to develop the Xing in a very efficient manner.
- The later stages of Zi Fa Gong take a person into a very deep and meditative state as the body's functioning switches from the acquired to the congenital channel system. It is here that obvious Zi Fa Gong processes begin to end and the process is ready to evolve onto more advanced stages.

Though the above stages of development are not necessarily 100 per cent linear, they are the stages that the vast majority of students will go through in their practice. Zi Fa Gong is a very powerful tool that comes out of the Nei Gong training; it can be used to create a very efficient energetic system in a relatively short time. Generally, people will move into Zi Fa Gong and out of it within a few years. During this time, many of the channels will have opened and the Nei Gong process will have unfolded within them to a fairly high level.

It should be noted, though, that Zi Fa Gong is started through the practice, but it should also end. If a person is still stuck within the Zi Fa Gong process after a few years of practice, then something has gone wrong. The movements that the body goes through should grow still again, apart from the occasional subtle adjustment that comes into your practice from time to time. I have encountered schools that deliberately kept students in this process for years on end and, essentially, these students were caught in a kind of trap. As with every aspect of our practice, we move into it, it unfolds, and then we progress onto something else; this is the natural evolution of the internal arts. If you are ever caught in one particular stage of development, then you have an error in your practice.

Personal Experience of Zi Fa Gong

I have encountered Zi Fa Gong processes within several schools of Nei Gong, Qi Gong and Yoga. I have seen this process being utilised in the West, in China, Taiwan, various parts of South-East Asia and in India. It is a process common to many systems in different parts of the world. I have seen it used for medicinal purposes, spiritual development and martial arts, and even as a way to deliberately possess yourself with spiritual entities. I should say, though, that I don't really endorse the last reason for the practice; self-inflicted possession always seemed like an odd thing to do to yourself! In each case, though the methods and uses are different, there are commonalities throughout the practice.

I have personally been taught Zi Fa Gong uses and methods by a number of teachers; below I give the key points I would like to make clear about Zi Fa Gong.

Out of the various teachers I encountered who used the process, many of them stated that they were the only ones doing so and theirs was the only method that induced such a reaction. Some teachers claimed that they stumbled across these reactions themselves and had actually created the system that induced the reactions; it is my personal experience that this is not the case and that Zi Fa Gong is an aspect of many practices and traditions.

Zi Fa Gong has always been there as a part of internal work. There are references to these reactions in several old texts on Dao Yin and Qi Gong practice. It is a recognised part of the training and should not be feared in any way. I have encountered many students who were frightened of this aspect of the training, as they had been told that it was a sign of becoming sick through Qi Gong training. This is not true; Zi Fa Gong and Chu Pian (出偏), or 'deviation', are different things.

It is, however, possible to do yourself harm with the process if you do not follow several key guidelines which I shall make clear in this chapter. Zi Fa Gong is a very strong tool and, as such, should be used with respect. I would suggest that you seek out a qualified and experienced teacher to help guide you properly through this process if you begin to manifest Zi Fa Gong in your training.

There is a great deal of secrecy around Zi Fa Gong. Powerful methods within Qi Gong were often kept secret. Perhaps this was wise in the past when people had to seek out masters for training, but in modern times things have changed. We have access to so much information, correct and incorrect, on the internet. There are so many methods that I have encountered, and many self-taught Qi Gong practitioners who entered into the Zi Fa Gong process. Since they are not armed with all of the information, they are at risk of harm and not able to move through it effectively; for this reason, I outline below the nature of Zi Fa Gong and how to use it properly.

Zi Fa Gong is frowned upon and, in some parts of China, hated as a practice. The repercussions of the cultural revolution and the political upheaval as a reaction to the Fa Lun Gong (法輪功) movement are still felt within the internal arts of China. This means that any esoteric or 'superstitious' aspects of their arts are still treated with mistrust. Even many Chinese-born teachers who are now in the West do not like Zi Fa Gong and will generally make wild claims about it being the result of mental illness or demonic influence.

As mentioned earlier, Zi Fa Gong should start, but it also should end. This is very important. There must be a developmental process involved in the practice. I have encountered a couple of groups that kept people in the process for a long time, sometimes many years or even decades. This is a complete nonsense and indicates that the method is not being utilised properly. As a tool, it should work through your body in a period of time that equates to a few years; in some people, it is much quicker. If you are still having these reactions after a lengthy period of time and they are not changing in nature, then you are doing something wrong.

Zi Fa Gong is not something 'high level'. It is a natural process that unfolds from within the body. In Taiwan and Indonesia I saw examples of it being sold to students as the result of either deities/immortals entering one's body (which it is not) or the Kundalini energy arising (which it isn't either). Zi Fa Gong is a natural process of change that the body can enter of its own accord when the circumstances are correct. It is as natural as flatulence and should be viewed as such! If it is seen in this down-to-earth manner, then it can be recognised for what it is: a natural part of the body's functioning. This stops people getting carried away and creating a cult-like mentality around it.

Whatever people need to clear will have an impact upon the nature, quality and duration of the Zi Fa Gong process. My own personal Zi Fa Gong process was over within a period of a few years. My first teacher in the process knew how to initiate it but didn't really know how to guide me through it, so, consequently, I spent a number of years not really developing in any way. I entered into Zi Fa Gong and stayed there, having the same bodily reactions for a long time. Whilst it improved my health to a certain degree, it did not progress.

The second teacher I met who used this process managed to take me through the process in six months. He understood exactly what the process was, why I was stuck and how I moved on in it. This is how the 'tool' of Zi Fa Gong should be used. It is a temporary 'clearing out' and 'realigning' process. In my personal case, I had two main conditions that needed adjusting: the first was a digestive condition and the second was accumulated energetic damage from recreational drug use. These two 'outer layers' were moved through, and then there was a process of change for my psychological state that had to take place. In most people that I have taught, I see a similar process: from sickness and imbalance of the body, through to the energetic system and then on to the mind.

Mechanics of Zi Fa Gong

Zi Fa Gong happens as a reaction to an increase in the movement of Yang Qi along the lines of the channel system. As this Qi moves through the channels, it carries with it functional information which generates action within several parts of the body. These are the energetic pathways of the channel system, the Huang and sinews, the nervous system and the mind.

The Energetic Pathways of the Channel System

When the Yang Qi increases flow along the energetic aspect of the channel system, it stimulates the channel to begin shedding Xie Qi that is caught in its length. The Xie Qi is a form of vibrational information that is related to the storage of a memory or event. It generally has an emotional quality to it and sits there in the channel causing a change to the overall Qi quality in that region of the body. When the flow of Qi increases along the channel's length, the Xie Qi can begin to move out of the channel. This process is called Xiao Dao (消導) or 'to guide out and dispel' the Xie Qi.

As well as removing stored energetic debris from the channel's length, there is also an overall change to the channel's quality. Every aspect of Xie Qi has an influence upon a channel's nature as well as causing a blockage. You could think of each channel having a whole spectrum of energetic resonances, and when we shed some of the Xie Qi, then the resonance changes. The quality of a channel is then also reflected back into the mind and our emotional state. This is why students who have been through Zi Fa Gong will often feel psychologically 'lighter' and happier.

A final aspect of changing the nature of the channel through Zi Fa Gong is that it is said to Tiao Ying Wei (调营卫), or 'adjust the way the channel nourishes and protects' the body. This means that a clearing of the energetic pathway of the channel should lead to an increase in vitality as well as strengthen your immune system.

The Huang and Sinews

It is a clear aspect of the Sinew-Changing Classic teachings that when Qi moves into the Huang, then they stretch. If the Huang stretch, then so do the sinew channels. Essentially, there is a reaction that takes place as Qi conducts along the length of the soft tissues of the Huang system. As these two elements interact with one another, the soft tissues begin to lengthen of their own accord. It is this facet of the body's internal functioning that we use to build many of the internal connections needed for Qi Gong training. The only reason that people don't generally experience this within their daily lives is because (1) not enough Qi is moving into the Huang, and (2) the contractive muscles on the 'outside' of the body are preventing the Huang from stretching. It is only when the contractive muscles (the activators) have been 'hung from the bones' that their influence is reduced. Then the Qi can move into the Huang and they will begin to lengthen of their own accord.

Many practitioners of Qi Gong will have stumbled across this, even if they are not aware of the mechanism involved. In this case it feels as if the arms are floating upwards. You are practising a simple Qi Gong exercise and, all of a sudden, it is as if the arms are being lifted upwards on a cushion of air; if you relax then the arms float higher instead of dropping to your sides. I have heard teachers saying that it is like being floated aloft on a 'cushion of Qi', but in actual fact the mechanism involved is that the muscles are not restricting the Huang. As there is an increase of Qi into the Huang, they begin to lengthen of their own accord. The result of the 'lengthening' of the Huang is that your arms move upwards with no apparent action involved; it feels as if they are floating.

This kind of 'effortless' lengthening of the Huang will take place all over your body during Zi Fa Gong, and this is the main reason why you will fold at the waist, bend over, turn around, walk forwards and make all manner of strange movements. The Huang are moving into action. Since there is little in the way of resistance from the muscles of the body, it can feel as if these movements are coming from nowhere. Often, your nervous system is not attuned to these types of movements either and so there can be a complete lack of body awareness when these movements arise. It can feel as if 'something else' other than you is moving you. This is the reason why some have incorrectly believed that spirits are entering the body and making the movements; it is not that, it is the Huang activating under the influence of the Yang Qi.

The Huang and sinew channels will have various adhesions and bindings in their length, and these will need to come out. As the soft tissues go through their spontaneous movements, they will begin to correct these issues. The result is that the physical aspects of the channels will open up and Qi flow will increase. It is also here, in these adhesions, that much of the Xie Qi becomes stuck. As the adhesions unbind, more of the Xie Qi will leave through the energetic aspect of the channel.

If an area of the Huang or sinew channels is particularly bound up, then it will interfere with the channels' lengthening; the result will be that the movements you go through can have a somewhat erratic quality to them. It is as if the Zi Fa Gong is 'sputtering' and taking on a jerky quality. This is quite normal. Traditionally, it would be said that you are 'hitting blockages' in the channels. Whilst this is true, essentially it is the unbinding of the Huang that will cause these 'sputtering' movements to soften out and become smoother in quality.

The Nervous System

The nervous system is clearly involved in the Zi Fa Gong process. I have met some practitioners who state that it is a purely energetic process and the body has nothing to do with it. I disagree with this – the body is moving, and so the body is involved.

The nervous system has a major part to play in the process. The Yang Qi moves through the channels and the Huang, but it is also related to the function of the nervous system. Zi Fa Gong is a very stimulating process, and the nervous system can become very 'activated' as a result of the process. This can result in all manner of unusual sensations along the length of the channels as the Zi Fa Gong process unfolds. The movement of Yang Qi brings with it all manner of unusual experiences as the sensory information contained within the Qi is 'read' by the nervous system.

There is also a very particular process involving the nervous system and how it deals with old injuries during the Zi Fa Gong process. The movement of Yang Qi activates nerve clusters around the site of old, stored injuries. The first experience of this is often a deep bruised sensation. This is the beginning of the process of tissue and chemical release that needs to take place in order to rid the body of the issue. From here, the nervous system sends bursts of electrical impulses that work on the site of the injury. This helps to adjust the Huang, clear the information contained within localised Xie Qi and bring both blood and nervous-system stimulation to the root of the problem. Since the nervous system is temporarily fired up and moving into action, it can add to the spontaneous movements that the practitioner is having. The consequence of this is generally a series of shakes and twists that are focused on the area where there are stored physical issues. As these issues clear, more adhesions leave the body, and there are often major changes to the posture and level of physical well-being of the practitioner.

The Mind

The sympathetic nervous system and the hypothalamus are connected to our emotional responses, and so naturally any process which affects the nervous system will likely have an emotional content to it. As well as this, the movement of Yang Qi is derived from the Heart centre in traditional Chinese thought, the seat of our emotional makeup. This means that during Zi Fa Gong, there are a whole host of emotional reactions that can come out of the process. Students will laugh, cry, shout and make a number of odd noises spontaneously. This is all a part of the process and should not be worried about. Within Chinese medical thought, you experience the nature of Qi when it is on the surface of your system. This means that when stuck Xie Qi related to an emotional event moves out of the body, there is a point when it is re-experienced. The information contained within the Qi is 'read' by the body and processed as an emotional reaction. This is a natural sign of the body shedding the pathogenic root of an issue. Within the 'alternative scene', these are known as emotional releases and they are common to many internal practices. Understanding how to work with these reactions is so important that we will return to them below when we look at how to move through the Zi Fa Gong process effectively.

As the mind goes through the releasing process of Zi Fa Gong, it can move back towards a central state. It is one of the major components of Zi Fa Gong that students will naturally let go of a whole host of emotional baggage. I have seen many students say goodbye to deeply depressed and anger-driven psychological states as a by-product of the Zi Fa Gong process. This is all a part of the body's own innate self-regulatory system whereby it wishes to make the functioning of our mind as efficient as it possibly can.

The Sequence of Reactions

It is quite amazing just how much variation there is in the Zi Fa Gong process from person to person. I have taught many hundreds of students over the years and seen many of them move into and through the Zi Fa Gong process. I have seen almost as many variations on just how the body and energy system can react to the increased flow of Yang Qi through the channel system. Many of these movements are very comical to watch, whilst others are just baffling as to the possible root cause of the phenomena.

That being said, there are a few key stages that many people seem to go through. These are generally experienced in the following order:

- First, the body shakes. It generally begins in the legs, moves into the abdominal cavity, and then spreads to the arms. It can range from an erratic shaking to a subtle vibration that can only just be seen. The Yang Qi is moving through the Huang, and the process is just beginning.

- From here, people usually begin to bend at the waist or fall forwards. They often need to take a step forwards to catch themselves. Some fall down onto the ground. This is the start of the Huang lengthening (often the back of the body is opening as a result of the Governing channel's awakening) as well as the forward rotation of the lower Dan Tian affecting the centre of gravity.

- After the 'folding' phase, students tend to enter into a process whereby their limbs start to move in unexpected ways. The arms can rise or shake or the hands can clap together. The legs will move and shake and the torso can twist or arch forwards. This is all a part of the channels opening around the body.
- Students can then begin to exhibit some of the more extreme movements, including running (watch out for objects!), spinning, and even crawling around on the floor. This can all look rather odd, but it is just another aspect of the body's self-regulatory process.
- As subconscious patterns begin to release from within the nervous system, people will start to generate dance-like, Yogic asana or 'martial-type' movements. Often, these are related to habitual movements that have been repeated enough times that they are programmed into the student's nervous system and soft tissues. For example, many Aikido practitioners who enter into this process will go through a phase of spontaneously break-falling.
- This then all begins to die down, and students enter a smoother and more gradual process of release. The movements become smooth and undulating in quality; they manifest as subtle waves that move through the Huang and the joints of the body. The erraticness of the early stages of Zi Fa Gong is no more, and the Qi begins to flow smoothly around the body.
- Generally, this is where the Shou Yin hand shapes begin to appear, and the process moves into a deeper stage of development. We shall look at the Shou Yin below.
- When the majority of the Zi Fa Gong process is done with, students will either begin to stand very still in their practice, or else they will naturally find that they are drawn down to sit on the floor in a meditative posture. This is a sign that it is generally time to move on. There has been enough clearing and opening for the body to be effectively ready for the next parts of the Nei Gong process. The practice now needs to change in accordance with the student's level of readiness.

Throughout all of the above processes, there will be a whole host of emotional releases and sounds being produced. These are all a part of Zi Fa Gong and the Nei Gong process. It means that classes with a lot of beginners in them can be quite noisy affairs. It is far from the quiet, meditative atmosphere that many associate with Qi Gong.

Emotional Releases

Emotional releases are a natural and common reaction to internal practice. This is the process of expressing stuck emotional trauma that is being held by the body, mind, channels or nervous system. Generally, as trauma is released, the emotional suppression of the energy is countered, and the person starts to cry, laugh or even scream out loud. I grew up around all kinds of alternative arts, and I remember seeing a class of twenty people having very extreme emotional releases in a Kriya Yoga class when I was around ten years old. I was very confused by all the crying and wailing and really did not understand the process at all. It was not what I pictured when I thought of Yoga!

Fast-forward many years, and now I am teaching a form of Qi Gong where these kinds of releases are commonplace. They are a very important part of the internal development process, as they help us to shed Xie Qi related to emotional issues. In some cases, this is just 'surface' emotional stuff and, as such, has very little impact upon our mental state; in other cases, these releases can come from deep inside, and the root of a very traumatic experience can be let go of.

Now, this may all sound good and, yes, it can be, but it can also be the most destructive part of the internal arts. Emotional releases are a powerful form of energetic movement. Anything that is powerful needs treating with respect, and so the following guidelines should be understood when looking at the nature of emotional releases within a practice such as Nei Gong.

Understanding Suppression Versus Indulgence

Emotional suppression can be a very damaging thing for our psychological health. Within modern society, it is often deemed negative to express your emotions, and so many people suppress them and squeeze them down into their being. Feelings of frustration, anger and worry are held in the body. In this way, they turn into a type of Xie Qi that can have negative impacts upon our health; often, these issues develop many years down the line, after a long time of festering away inside of the energetic matrix. We need to shed this Xie Qi and end the emotional suppression that has led to the root of this issue.

On the opposite end of the scale is overindulgence in our emotional imbalances. This is a problem too, especially in the case of emotional releases that develop out of Zi Fa Gong and other internal arts practice. If you indulge in an emotion, then you overidentify with it; the result of this is that you never actually let go of the energetic root of the problem. Though it may look as if you are releasing an emotional trauma, you are actually reinforcing it back into the body.

These two extremes – emotional suppression and emotional indulgence – are shown as a graph in Figure 9.9. Between these extremes, we have a point of 'balance'.

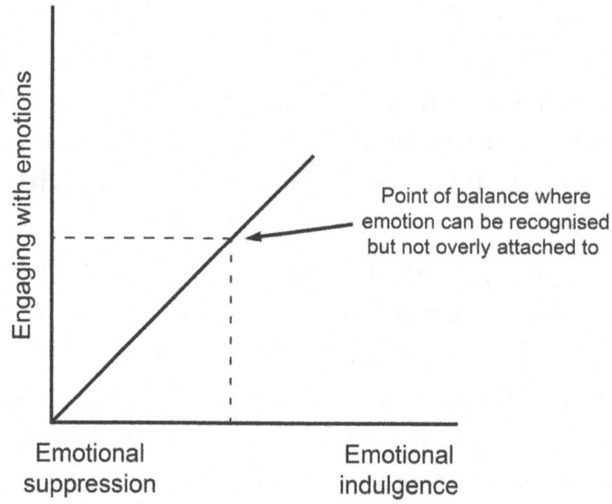

Figure 9.9: The Emotional Release Graph

The process of Zi Fa Gong will bring our emotions out to the surface and allow us to let go of them, but in order to do this effectively, we have to find this perfect point of mental balance that is the 'sweet spot' for letting go of trauma-related emotional energy. I have a simple way of doing this. I make sure that the student understands one thing: they do not need to experience the psychological aspect of an emotion to let go of the energetic root of it. This is extremely important for our development. Understanding this principle will make the difference between shedding emotional trauma and becoming stuck in it for a long time.

So, what do I mean by this? Well, an emotional release is a form of energy. Energy comes with expression. It is the expression of energy that is important, not the emotion itself. So, if I have a student who is crying, I will ask them, 'How do you feel right now?' If they answer that they feel very sad, then I stop them from practising. I send them off for a hot drink, a walk around the room, and to basically chill out and calm down for a few minutes. Only when they no longer feel sad do I let them return to practise. In the majority of cases, though, when I ask a crying student how they feel, they answer that they feel fine. They often cannot understand why they are crying. They are not sad, so why the tears? This is the perfect state to be in for releasing energetic roots to emotional trauma. The energy is leaving, we can see this. The student is having the energetic expression of sadness – tears; they are crying. But they do not 'feel' sad. There is no emotional connection to the expression of the Xie Qi. This means that they will not identify with the release; it is, instead, just a bodily reaction.

If, however, they actually 'feel' sad, then this is a trap. Whilst it may be better than suppression of the emotion, the student is now identifying with the process of release. Essentially, an emotional reaction is a form of stimulation for the acquired mind; it is an aspect of the five poisons, remember. As the emotional stimulation manifests within our mind, a further layer of the acquired mind is built and emotion is anchored into our sense of self.

Herein lies the nature of the trap; emotional releases can feel great, they are a form of catharsis. This is especially true if you have previously been suppressing your emotions. This has led to many internal arts practitioners entering into these kinds of releases and essentially indulging in them. Even though they have not meant to, they have been subconsciously anchoring these emotions back into the acquired mind. It is a sense of 'emotional neutrality' combined with energetic release that is needed to effectively move through the release of emotions. I have used the example of sadness above, but it is equally true for other emotions. Laughter can come without any obvious reason, and shouting can be present without any feelings of anger.

In practice, you can apply this by ensuring that you do not 'feel' emotional during your practice. If strong emotions arise, then stop, go and do something else; return to your training when you feel more centred in yourself.

If a student cannot find this point of balance and emotional neutrality, then they can become stuck in a loop of emotional release for many years. I have known of people in Yogic groups that use a lot of releasing processes; they have been stuck in the same cycle of crying and wailing for years on end. In contrast to this, an effective use of Zi Fa Gong according to the guidelines here can take you through the emotional release process in a matter of weeks.

Emotional Releases Are Yang in Nature

All emotional releases involve a strong movement of Yang Qi. The result of this is that the body and nervous system move into a more Yang state of being. Whilst this is fine in short bursts, we don't wish to cause the body to move into this state for too long or to a high degree. On top of this, the release of emotional energy is tiring for the heart and the emotional centre within this area of the chest. Do not fry yourself! If the emotional release makes your body shake violently, your face turn red or your heart rate speed up, then stop immediately and relax. This is another situation where you should take it easy, calm down and return to your practice at some other time. We wish to keep the process as smooth as possible; we don't need to stress the body to let go of stuck energies. Many mistakenly think that 'intense' is better when this is really not the case.

Light-Hearted Is Better

To be 'light-hearted' means that the Qi of the heart is 'light', it is not heavy and sinking. It does not anchor in to experienced emotional states and is not holding on to trauma. I have seen this time and time again in the practice: those who take a light-hearted approach to their practice move quickly and pleasantly through it, those who are overly serious in their approach to the practice find it much harder work. There is often an air of being overly serious within these arts, and this can be a real curse. If I have a room full of people going through Zi Fa Gong and the Nei Gong process, then I can spot the ones who will find it difficult to progress; they are the ones with a deadpan expression on their face and an almost militaristic approach to what they are doing. The ones who are laughing and smiling at what is going on will find the process much smoother and move through it a lot faster. For this reason, I would say that the teacher of Nei Gong has a very important role here: they should make sure that students in the classes are happy, smiling and generally having a good time; there really is no need to flagellate yourself with the training – life is hard enough already!

I have had students come to me from other schools who have been very surprised at my manner when I teach. I laugh, tell jokes, and generally try to ensure that the courses are fun as well as focused on what we are doing. I hear from so many students who tell me horror stories of classes they have been to where they have been shouted at, ordered around and essentially made to feel like their class is a form of Qi Gong boot camp. This really is not healthy. The more fun and enjoyment in the class, the easier it is for the body to release Xie Qi, and the more easily the Qi will flow. If the heart is light, then it will move the Yang Qi in a healthier fashion.

I should also point out that Qi Gong is not meditation. Silence is not required; it is okay for there to be laughter in the class when you are training together. It is also important to note that it is possible to have enjoyment and focus at the same time; these two are not in conflict with one another.

If these above guidelines are adhered to in the practice, then you will find that the emotional releases will unfold and evolve in the correct fashion. You will move through them, and the mind will naturally begin to become more centred as a result of your Nei Gong process.

It is one of the greatest strengths of Zi Fa Gong and the Nei Gong process that there is a certain degree of 'not knowing' with regard to how the body sheds its emotional trauma. Emotionally charged Xie Qi can be released as tears, shouting or any number of physically expressed Zi Fa Gong reactions. What the root of many of these reactions may be is unknown to us; there are too many variables involved in the Zi Fa Gong process. This does not matter. The body should be allowed to process and release these issues as it sees fit. We do not need to become overly involved. We are like casual bystanders who are observing but not getting involved in what is taking place. In this way, I have had students change their entire outlook on life and then find, to their surprise, that when they try to recall the memory of a traumatic event, they cannot find an emotional connection to it. Though the memory of the event is there, it is as if the traumatic aspect of it is missing. This has happened for events ranging from post-traumatic reactions to being at war, through to sexual abuse during childhood. This is shown in Figure 9.10.

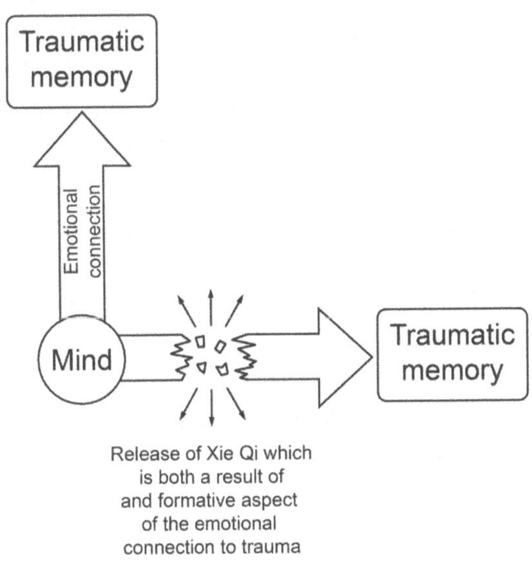

Figure 9.10: Shedding Emotional Connection to Trauma

The Six Healing Sounds

A note should be made on the Liu Zi Jue (六字訣), or 'six healing sounds', which are a famous form of medical Qi Gong. In these practices, students generally make a series of movements whilst expressing one of six sounds. This is in accordance with the classical phrase 'There is only one way to inhale, but six ways to exhale,' which was a key teaching of Daoist Tao Hong Jing (陶弘景). The idea is that each of the six sounds will help to purge Xie Qi from the key organs of the body. These six sounds are listed in Table 9.1.

Table 9.1: Six Healing Sounds

Sound	Pronunciation	Organ
嘘 Xu	Shu or Shh	Liver
呵 He	Her or Har	Heart
呼 Hu	Who	Spleen
呬 Si	Sir or Sss	Lung
吹 Chui	Chwey	Kidneys
嘻 Xi	She	Triple Warmer

In my experience, the actual body movements that go with each sound are not really that important. If you stand neutrally and make the sounds in a low, even tone on your exhalation, then they will do their job. Sound is vibration, and certain vibrations connect with different organs and forms of Qi; this is the basis of how making the sound can help to heal the related organ system.

The above description of the sounds is an externalised version of their functions, though. Whilst it can be helpful to practise them, it is nowhere near as effective as allowing them to happen of their own accord. This is what happens through the Zi Fa Gong process. For some, but not all, students, these sounds will be produced spontaneously as the related organ systems begin to clear of Xie Qi. As they exhale, they produce these sounds as well as the sounds in Table 9.2. Either or both of these reactions may be experienced.

Table 9.2: Six Sound Reactions

Sound reaction	Organ system
Shouting or growling	Liver
Laughing	Heart

Singing or yawning	Spleen
Sighing	Lung
Sexual-type groans	Kidneys
Humming	Triple Warmer

I should reiterate that these sounds are produced automatically and completely spontaneously. They are not generated in any deliberate way and are a reaction to the movement of Qi coming from the related organ system. Qi is a vibration, it will express itself in a variety of formats; one of these is through sound. The sounds can vary from quiet to very loud; they can be quite surprising sometimes. As with all reactions, they should be acknowledged but not overly identified with, or else you will not progress past them very quickly.

Prostrations

Another common reaction to Zi Fa Gong are prostrations. These can be in the form of kneeling-type prostrations, or else they can be fully stretched-out prostrations. Both of these variants are shown in Figure 9.11.

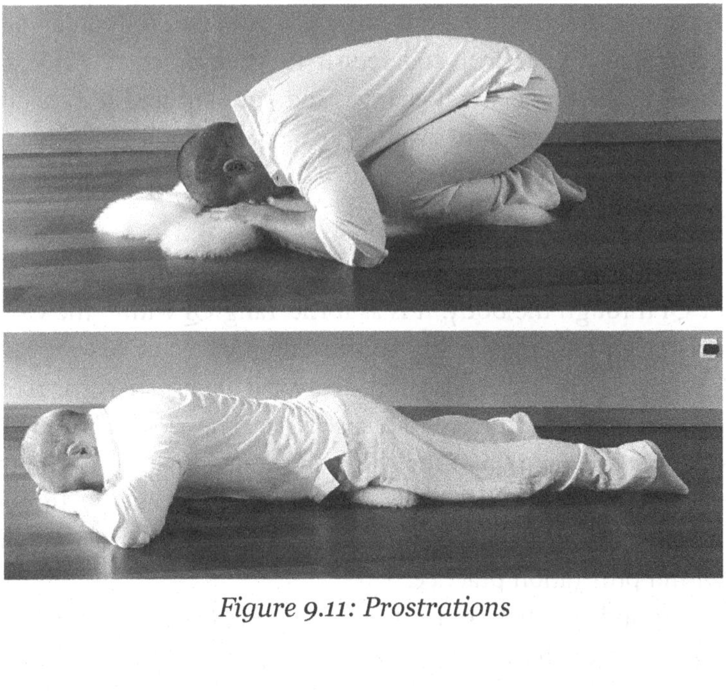

Figure 9.11: Prostrations

Prostrations have long been an important part of many spiritual traditions. Christianity, Islam, Buddhism and indeed Daoism all have their own forms of prostration. In religious contexts, the explanation of prostrations and their function is often linked to the idea of moving closer to God, or to show reverence and humility before a higher power. Whilst these ideas may be true, it is not the major function of prostrations within the art of Nei Gong. Within Nei Gong, prostrations are used as a way of bringing Yin and Yang close together. This is referring to the two forms of Qi: the Yang Qi of the practitioner's mind and channel system, combined with the Yin Qi of the planet. Initially, prostrations occur as a result of Zi Fa Gong during standing practice, but after a while, prostrations will go through the following developmental stages:

- Initially, your body will want to move closer to the ground during your Nei Gong practice. This will be experienced as a feeling of being pulled down to the floor during your practice sessions. It can happen slowly at first but then, after a while, do not be surprised if it takes a hold of you and pulls you quite quickly towards the floor. If this happens, please be aware of sharp objects and furniture around you that may be a risk.
- When you are taken to the floor, at first, you can get up immediately. It is as if the 'magnetic' pull of the ground does not have a hold of you any more, the 'circuit' is broken, if you like. You can immediately get back to your feet and return to your practice. After a while, though, the process will change, and you will find it difficult to get up off the floor straight away. The 'magnetic' pull of the planet does not relinquish its connection to you for some time; in some cases, this can be for several minutes.
- Once stuck on the floor, you can become aware of a strong movement of Qi through the body. It is as if the Yang Qi within the Governing channel is moving quickly and forming an arc across the length of your back. This is because of the classical Daoist energetic rule of Yin and Yang being attracted to one another. The Yin field of the Earth is drawing the Yang Qi of the channel system into a big circuit through your body, which will help you to move the energy through the microcosmic orbit more effectively. This is really the first milestone within prostration practice.

  As odd as it may sound, the Qi within the palms of the hands and the centre of the forehead can also feel as if they are being drawn into the ground when you are in a prostration position. This is the development of literal 'grounding' of the body's Qi – a movement of Yang Qi that connects you into the Yin Qi field of the Earth.

- After a while of experiencing prostrations in this manner, you will find that the process ends. It tends to end very suddenly, and the body is no longer inclined to be drawn down towards the floor. The process has already completed all of the work it needs to; it has established all of the changes and energetic adjustments that are required for efficient prostration usage.

  It is at this stage in your development that you can use prostrations as an 'external tool'.

This process of entering into prostrations in this manner can take quite some time. It is, in part, slowed down by the fact that it is rarely a continuous process. The above stages can come and go over a lengthy period of time when you are practising your art. Once again, do not add to this process; allow it to unfold naturally for you and let the body lead you through it naturally.

External Prostration Usage

Once the above process has concluded for you, then you may effectively start to use prostrations as a practice. This means that you do not need them to appear within Zi Fa Gong; they are no longer required to be initiated from within the Zi Fa Gong process. You can now practise prostrations as an exercise in its own right. If you practise them prior to the above process unfolding for you, then you are unlikely to have the necessary internal conditions in place for them to have a great deal of benefit; they will essentially be quite empty in nature until you have 'built the engine' for them. This is because there has to be a certain type of energetic potential built into the action of a prostration. This energetic potential can be built in two key ways – through religious devotion or through Nei Gong development.

Religious devotion works, as the practitioner enters a state of divine humility before a higher power. Those who can touch upon this kind of profound humility will open up a kind of energetic vacuum within themselves, and this will activate the 'mechanics' of the act of prostration. Nei Gong development is a better way for those who lack a connection to a religious or devotional root. It leads to the same quality being built inside of the body but in a different manner.

It is said that prostrations are (within Daoism) for purification of the Xing, dissolving of feelings of conceit, and for strengthening Yin and Yang. Let us look at each of these in turn.

Purification of the Xing

Anybody who has experienced a full energetic prostration within their Nei Gong practice will attest to the fact that it can have a somewhat dumbfounding effect upon the mind. It is quite normal to sit up after prostration and feel unaware of where you are or what is going on around. This feeling generally lasts for a few minutes and is akin to waking up in the morning after a very deep sleep. The look on a student's face is always interesting to see after a prostration, as they generally look pretty vacant in the eyes but have a large sleepy grin across their face. It is definitely a very pleasant state to be in.

The nature of the Qi movement initiated by a full and proper prostration serves to temporarily wipe the veils of the acquired mind out of the way of your true Xing. Though only a fleeting glimpse, it is one of the earliest times that a person will see the world without the lens of emotions and 'mind' being in the way. As the head touches the floor, the nature of your energetic relationship with the Qi of the planet means that there is a kind of discharge of Yang Qi out of the body. This then serves to clear the acquired mind for a short period of time. As prostrations are practised, it helps the acquired mind to become less of a distortion on the Xing. This is why prostrations were such a major part of many spiritual systems that were concerned with the nature and functions of consciousness.

Dissolving Conceit

Conceit is defined as having an excessive level of pride in oneself or one's achievements. This is in direct conflict with the energetic vacuum of humility that is considered an important quality for the Xing to have. The Xing needs to be 'empty' of an overly strong sense of self. It can only be empty if there is the vacuum of humility present as an overriding virtue. Conceit will never result in an 'empty cup'.

As the acquired mind's energy is discharged into the floor through prostration practice, it is these kinds of character traits that are worked through.

Strengthening Yin and Yang

Due to the increased energetic movement during prostration practice, the cycles of Yin and Yang Qi are both developed. The channel system is opened to a great degree by the movement of Yang Qi, and the fields of Yin Qi are nourished by their close connection to the planet's field. This helps in the Nei Gong process in general as well as strengthening our level of health.

Ten Thousand Prostrations

The above functions of prostration are the most valuable ones with regard to our practice, but doubtless there are a whole spread of further benefits of the practice that will take place as well. It is for this reason, the sheer potency of prostration practice, that they have been a mainstay of spiritual practice around the world. It is said that for a person to achieve a high level in their prostrations, they should practise ten thousand of them! Ten thousand is actually a metaphorical number in the Chinese language which is often equated with infinity. Essentially, it is stating that, as a practice, you can just keep going; there will always be refinement of the process taking place for you.

As a young Western student of these arts, I initially found prostrations to be a very difficult practice. Though I had encountered them in my early years of Buddhist study and then further on within Daoism, I always found them a challenge to do. This was purely from a point of my own biases towards the practice. I had always naturally been distrustful of religions and associated prostrations with cult-like behaviour and giving up your power to somebody else. I guess many of my associations came from watching things like Indiana Jones where the 'bad guys' always seemed to be prostrating before idols. All of these preconceived ideas around prostrations were a real burden and it took me a long time get over them; such is the depth of our social conditioning. For me, now, they are a practice of energetic work, no different from other forms of Qi Gong, as well as a form of humbling myself before the greater power of creation – whatever that may be!

Nowadays, it feels very natural for me to practise prostrations, and I always do at some point during my personal practice, sometimes a lot and other days just a few. If a true prostration really starts to unfold within me, then I will find that I am often held in that place, close to the ground, for quite some time. It can take me a full ten minutes to complete just one prostration practice. In this way, the practice is initiated by me, but then I allow it to take over and lead me into whatever work it deems the most beneficial.

I cannot give any further guidance on prostration practice than this. Many people want instructions including how many they should do, what time of the day, and so on. Prostrations (in a Nei Gong context) will unfold out of the process; the body will want to perform them and then this will build the 'engine' of the exercise. From here, when your body has the Gong of them, you can practise them as and when you like; trust your feelings.

Shou Yin

Shou Yin, or 'mudras' as they are more commonly known, are an important part of Daoist practice. Despite their widespread usage within the tradition, little is known about them in many contemporary Qi Gong schools. The use of Shou Yin has existed for countless generations, with each generation of realised masters developing their own methods which were passed down through the generations to modern practitioners. Figure 9.12 shows some examples of Daoist Shou Yin.

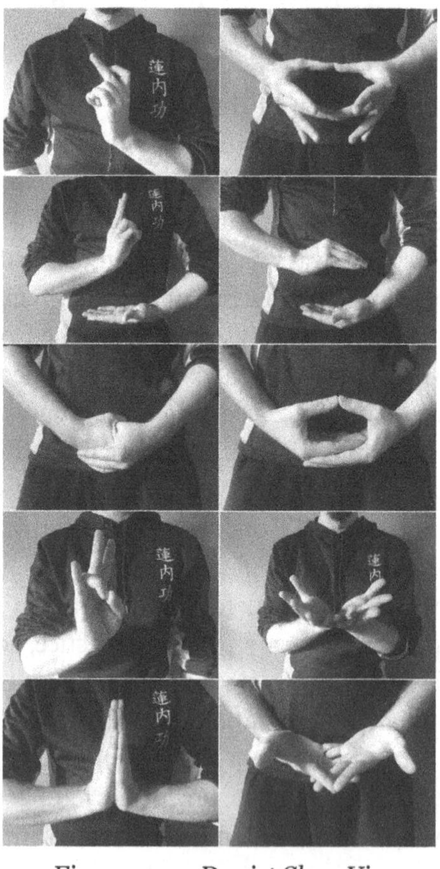

Figure 9.12: Daoist Shou Yin

Some of these hand positions are simple variations on open and closed fists, whilst some use complex shapes created by combining the fingers of both hands into a single shape. Whilst the workings of some of these positions are difficult to comprehend, the internal mechanisms of Shou Yin can be understood to fall into one or more of the following categories:

- The simplest level of Shou Yin works by extending or collapsing various lines of connective tissue within the body. The extensions of many internal lines of Huang and sinew channels culminate at the ends of the fingers. Through developing an understanding of these lines, ancient teachers worked out that by placing the hands into various positions, the physical lines of the body could be opened up in different ways. These lines then pull right through to the core of the body, meaning that each Shou Yin built in this way allows Qi to rush to various locations of the body.
- Some Shou Yin work by using placement of hands at different heights combined with archetypal shapes which your subconscious mind will automatically recognise as being associated with a specific energetic function. These basically work by drawing your awareness into a particular shape or state which then leads energy to shape itself in the same manner.
- A more complex level of Shou Yin works by connecting and disconnecting the energetic extremities of the channels running out to the fingers. By linking different fingers together into a ring shape, certain channels can be closed and looped together whilst others are extended and allowed to flow freely. The various combinations generated in this way then bring change to the overall energetic state of the body which a skilled practitioner of Nei Gong, meditation or martial arts can use at the correct time.
- Many more intricate Shou Yin are those which have been empowered by a realised master. Empowerment of Shou Yin involves taking the combined energetic resonance of all of the practitioners who have previously used the same symbol and then transferring it down into an individual student. This requires direct mind-to-mind transmission.
- The final category of Shou Yin is the most relevant to practitioners of Nei Gong as they enter into some of the more spiritually subtle levels of Zi Fa Gong reaction. These are hand shapes and finger connections that manifest spontaneously within the practice.

> A student entering into this level of the practice can produce the most delicate and often unusual Shou Yin that they either hold aloft or else connect with their body by placing their produced hand shape on various body regions. Sometimes these Shou Yin are held for a long time and other practitioners will move quickly through a series of complex hand shapes. It is these 'spontaneous Shou Yin' that create the deepest change within a practitioner of Nei Gong.

Spontaneous Shou Yin have a strong effect upon us as they are initially produced within the subconscious. They are an expression of what our inner self knows is needed at that current moment. If we do not hinder nor embellish this process, then it will enable the body to begin a whole series of very subtle attunements of Qi and Shen that we would not be capable of consciously making ourselves. At this stage, we should step back and adhere to the principle of Wu Wei: we allow the body to do what it needs to do whilst we simply observe as it takes place. Figure 9.13 shows a student producing Shou Yin out of their practice.

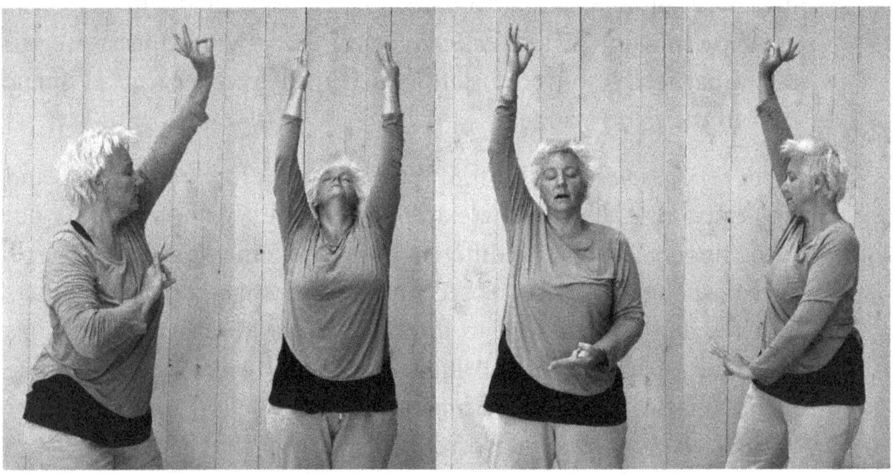

Figure 9.13: Spontaneous Shou Yin

Generally, this process of spontaneous Shou Yin production will come and then end after a few months of practice. It will then resurface on the odd occasion when the energetic matrix wishes to make a few self-changes.

Zi Fa Gong as a Tool

The above discussion of Zi Fa Gong should be enough to introduce you to the process and give you an understanding of what is taking place when the process begins to take a hold of you. The limitless amount of ways in which the body can move and Zi Fa Gong can manifest means that a full catalogue of the process would be almost impossible. You could fill volume after volume with only the expressions of Zi Fa Gong I have witnessed, and it would still only be scratching the surface. Moreover, it would not really serve much of a purpose. It is the practice of energetic 'self-expression' and, as such, to overly intellectualise the process may actually hinder its development.

Zi Fa Gong is a very striking process when people first see it, as it looks very crazy. It is an energetic expression of the nature of acquired mind. This means that it is rarely very 'ordered' in nature. The human mind is a very chaotic thing and so the energy that it expresses is a reflection of this chaos. Over time, though, as the process develops, changes to the practitioner's energetic system take place, and so the process becomes smoother. In this way, you are able to clearly observe an order developing out of the chaos as Xie Qi is cleared and harmonisation is moved towards.

Zi Fa Gong is a fundamental aspect of the internal arts but still only a very small part of it. We need to move into it and then out of it again. It will help us to clear certain blockages and build certain qualities into the energy body, but then we need to progress past it into deeper levels of development; this is the way to keep following the path of Daoism. In order to do this, we need to keep several key guidelines in mind when we practise:

- Do not add to or embellish the Zi Fa Gong process in any way. To become overly involved in the process in this way will lock you into a pattern that is difficult to move out of. I have seen many people try to generate a kind of 'fake Zi Fa Gong', and the result is not helpful in any way. Just stay back, get out of your own way and observe how the process naturally unfolds for you.

- At the same time, do not hinder it. It is a completely spontaneous process and, as such, we should not stop it. I have seen many students try to tense their body and fight against it, as they do not wish to lose control. Any sense of self-control is based in illusion anyway. Generally, these students eventually lose the battle; the movement of Qi is too strong and they end up sprawled rather unceremoniously on the floor, all sense of dignity gone!

- Keep a light-hearted approach to it. The happier you are, the more your Qi flows! Do not be overly serious in mindset, as this tightens the Qi. Don't judge, don't overfocus and don't overevaluate. Just enjoy the oddness of the Zi Fa Gong process. Laugh at the strange things your body wants to do.

- Zi Fa Gong is a very energetically stimulating process. Keep this in mind. Do not let the Qi rise up too strongly, as it can make the nervous system too Yang. Stay calm. If the body becomes overly Yang in nature, your heart rate goes up and things feel a little too excitable, then stop. Relax, calm down and restart when things feel more chilled. Powerful energetic tools should be used in a sensible manner. Almost all of the people I have met who have harmed themselves with arts like Nei Gong have often approached them with a lack of 'common sense'.
- To move through the process, do not attach. This is why I try to tell people that Zi Fa Gong is a very natural bodily process; it is no more special than any other process that takes place within the body, and we should accept it as that. In this way, you will progress past it into the deeper parts of Nei Gong development. It is over-attachment to the process that slows it down.
- Make sure that you approach your practice with a fair sense of balance. Though Zi Fa Gong will arise in your training, do not make this all that you do. Make sure you take time to work on your body development, breathing, and any exercises that are a part of your system too. Any practice is about balance, and only practising Zi Fa Gong would not really be a balanced way to approach your art.

Grounding Zi Fa Gong

Now that you have Zi Fa Gong manifesting within your practice and you understand how to work with it safely, we can look at how to progress through the process, how to move past it. We wish for the process to help us in our internal development, but then we wish to move on to further stages of training. To do this, we need to understand the idea of 'grounding'. Grounding is a commonly used term within the internal arts that essentially means to sink and drop the Qi.

The reason this is important is essentially because of the nature of Zi Fa Gong; it is a movement of energetic information that rises through the body. Though the Yang Qi may circulate in many different ways, it will have a tendency to rise upwards within the practice of Zi Fa Gong. This means that whilst allowing the process to unfold for you, there is also a second process that involves simply 'listening' to what is happening inside. Absorb the awareness through the body using absorption into breath as a way to 'interface' your awareness with the various processes taking place within your body. If you listen to the body, then you will gradually find that you become aware of the energetic root of many of the movements that are being generated by your body. Before there is a shaking or a movement of a limb, you will feel a rising of Qi somewhere within the body.

When you can feel these movements of Qi, then relax. Sink the Qi through letting it go. The result of this is that the movement will still be there, but it will start to transform. What were previously sharp and jerking movements will change into smooth, rippling undulations through the tissues that serve as the channel pathways. This is where we wish to lead the Zi Fa Gong process by grounding the root of these actions. Release the root of the reactions to the ground, and they will take you through the Zi Fa Gong process in a smooth and rapidly unfolding manner. Those who cannot ground will find that the process is more erratic and takes a lot longer to move through.

Keep It in Your Practice

As stated above, Zi Fa Gong brings with it a lot of energetic movement; it is a powerful technique. This means that it needs to be treated in the correct way. I have included information on the process within this chapter to help you understand exactly what is taking place, but really, you would be best to work with a teacher of these arts to help guide you efficiently through the process.

There are various guidelines in this chapter that will help you to understand the safe way to progress through this practice, but still, just in case there are issues, we need to draw the discussion to a close with one important fact: Zi Fa Gong should be kept to within your standing Qi Gong practice. It should not be carried over from your practice into the rest of your life. The Wuji posture essentially becomes a kind of trigger for your practice, and when you are no longer practising, then you do not wish for Zi Fa Gong to be there.

This means that, after practising, you should walk around and stretch the body out so that your mind moves from your breath and Qi back into your body. The higher your level of conscious connection to the physical body, the less you will be connected to your Qi flow and so the less your Yang Qi will start to generate the potential for movement. This process of ending your training by calming down your mind, walking briskly around the room and then stretching your body out in a purely physical manner is important for returning your body to 'normality' after your practice. I have always personally found that a cup of tea helps as well, but then, I am British, and that tends to be our answer to anything!

If in the very rare instance that your movements do not subside when you have finished practising, then jump up and down a few times, shaking your limbs. This will disrupt the flow of Qi in your channels temporarily; then, if there is a person on hand to help, get them to firmly (but not too painfully hard) slap you a few times on the lower back around the region of the Ming Men, as shown in Figure 9.14. This will disrupt the Qi moving through the Governing channel. When the Qi flow through the Governing channel is temporarily disrupted, it will stop driving Yang Qi through the rest of the channel system, and this will end the Zi Fa Gong process.

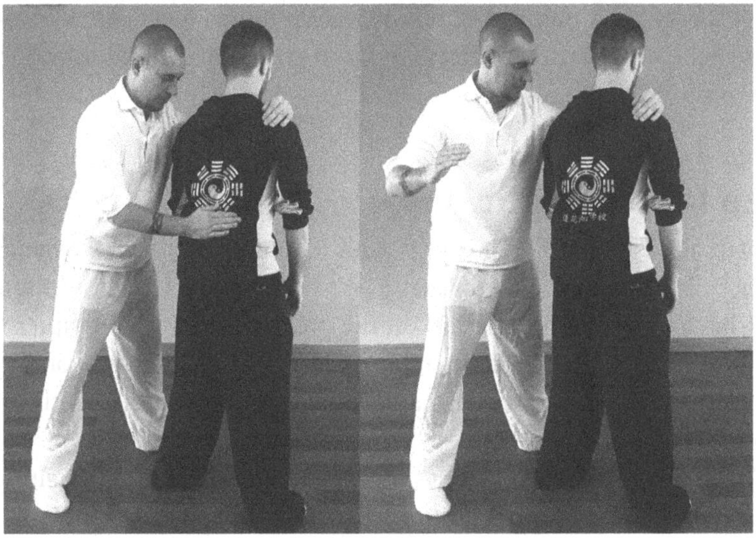

Figure 9.14: Slapping Ming Men

If you find that this spilling over of Zi Fa Gong into life outside of your practice is a common occurrence, then stop the practice. You should seek out an experienced teacher to help guide you through the process. In general, though, you should be fine. It is, after all, your Qi that is moving, and it is your mind that is involved in that Qi's generation. If you tell your Qi to stop and you really want it to, then it will. In my experience, those who have not been able to control the movements outside of practice are those who, to some degree, are overly attached to the uncontrollable nature of the process. Zi Fa Gong is a massively powerful and helpful tool, but it is just that – a tool. It should be understood and used as such.

Zi Fa Gong Ending

The process of Zi Fa Gong will continue and then begin to subside. You will know when much of the work has been done, as you will generally find that when your Yang Qi begins to move, it will cause you to slowly sit down on the floor and enter into a meditation-type posture. This transference through into sitting on the ground happens naturally and, once again, should not be added to, embellished or created deliberately. It is as if your body takes over for you and sits you down. As you sit down, there is a feeling of profound quiet that comes over your mind and energy system. This is the body's innate way of showing you that much of your energetic matrix is now actively circulating, and it is time to move on.

Generally, I find that students who reach this stage will either stand in Wuji quietly, with no Zi Fa Gong, sit down as discussed above, or enter into some of the more structured forms of Zi Fa Gong including Shou Yin and prostration. Generally, when your body is transferring between these different states, you have built a solid foundation; well done, you have managed to complete a lot of developmental work within the energy body!

Chapter 10

THE ART OF QI GONG

The previous chapter looked at one very specific series of reactions that can arise out of your internal practice. It is not a guaranteed reaction; most but not all students of Nei Gong go through it to some degree. What is important to realise, though, is that, more than anything else, we need to open the various channels of the body. Opening the channels should be our prime concern when we are looking at the movement of Yang Qi. The Zi Fa Gong process previously outlined is an early reaction to the opening of the channels under the force of Yang Qi. It comes and then it goes. Beyond this process, we have a period of learning how to balance the processes of purging, nourishing and regulating our energy body. This is primarily accomplished through the practice of various moving Qi Gong exercises combined with a series of important principles. Figure 10.1 shows the comparative length of time and focus that should be given to various aspects of the movement of Yang Qi.

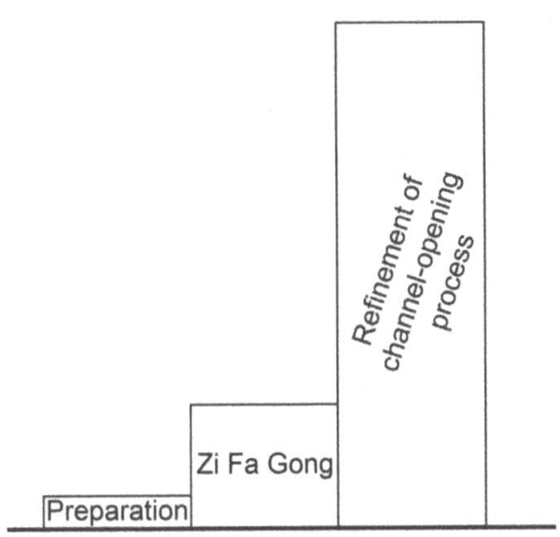

Figure 10.1: The Channel-Opening Process

As you can see, though the experience of Zi Fa Gong may be quite striking, it only forms a very small percentage of the time spent in opening the channels. Zi Fa Gong can help to open the length of the channels in a rather rudimentary fashion but then, beyond this, we need to learn how to balance the nature of the Qi flow within these channels' length. This will lead to the final stages of channel opening. To use my own practice as an example, I finished the Zi Fa Gong process in a relatively short space of time, and it then took me another five or six years of work to complete the processes outlined within this chapter. Some of the timescales I am giving in this book may sound very long but I am simply being realistic; these arts are a life study and not a quick 'weekend course to mastery' practice. Qi Gong for relaxation is a fairly easy practice; it can be a short-term goal to attain a level of calm in your art, but to really go deep – that takes time. Remember that in the past, Daoists would disappear into the mountains and dedicate their whole lives to these arts; this would suggest that we need to be patient and understand that development of these practices will take time.

Purging, Nourishing and Regulating Qi

Xie (泄) is 'to purge', Bu (補) is 'to nourish' and Li (理) is 'to regulate' or 'harmonise'. In order to further refine the quality of Qi within our channel system, it is these three principles that we need to understand and balance. It is a common error within the internal arts scene to not really understand how these three qualities need to be applied to your practice. Most Qi Gong practitioners that I meet have really only focused on one or two of these qualities, and even then, there is generally an overfocus on one of them. The result of this kind of imbalanced approach to practice is that your development is slowed or, in very rare cases, problems have developed. The three terms – Xi, Bu and Li – need to work together, as shown in Figure 10.2. It is here, in the central point of these three terms being balanced, that the body's Qi is harmonised.

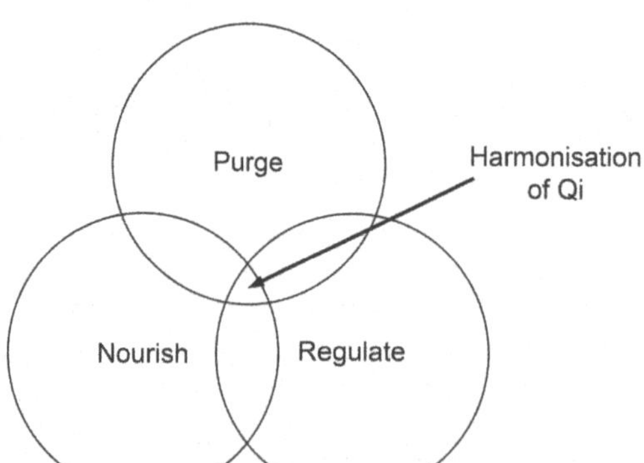

Figure 10.2: Purge, Nourish and Regulate

You could think of these three being as natural as exhaling (purge), inhaling (nourish), and having an even balance of these two (regulating). It is easy to understand how an uneven relationship between these three with regard to our breathing could be problematic, but these principles need to be applied to our Qi Gong training as well.

Purging

The mechanics behind purging pathogenic Qi from the body have already, to some extent, been discussed within this book. These are the processes of letting go and the Zi Fa Gong process. Letting go is essentially the process of Song that developed out of our evolution of the abdominal passive breathing methods we discussed in Chapter 5. The movement of Yang Qi then enables the channels to begin shedding stuck Xie Qi from within their length.

A third aspect of purging is the practice of Dao Yin exercises. Dao Yin can be translated as 'lead and guide' exercises. They are a very Yang, active form of internal practice whereby the joints of the body are opened up and pathogenic Qi is led out of the body through a combination of internal 'conduction' and focused intent. Dao Yin exercises are older than Qi Gong practices; their history stretches right back into the shamanic traditions of ancient China. Some teachers incorrectly state that Dao Yin is simply an older name for Qi Gong practice, but this is really not true: there are distinct qualitative differences between Dao Yin and Qi Gong; anybody who has practised both forms of exercises can attest to this.

Dao Yin exercises are an important part of Nei Gong practice, and you would be wise to study some to aid you in the purging part of your practice. This being said, they should only form a part of your practice and should not be the entirety of what you do; this will lead to imbalance developing – something we shall discuss below.

Nourishing

Nourishing the body is accomplished in two main ways: through the efficiency of our body's functioning and through advanced Sinew-Changing Classic principles. The first major aspect to understand is that our body produces Qi from two main sources – from the conversion of Jing to Qi and through a mixture of the air we breathe and the food we eat. The balance of these aspects of our life was known as the principles of Yang Sheng Fa (養生法) or 'life-nourishing principles' – more literally 'healthy living'. It is an often missed point that within Qi Gong training you will never build any real amount of Qi without looking at the nature of your lifestyle. No amount of trying to 'draw in Qi' from the environment or anything like this will ever be as effective as helping your body to function on a more efficient level. The vast majority of the Qi that we require for our health, practice and personal development is generated from within our body. This takes place on an energetic and cellular level. Whilst we may have an energetic resonance with our environment, we create the Qi we use up on a daily basis within our body. Figure 10.3 shows the main sources of Qi for beginner- and intermediate-level students of Nei Gong.

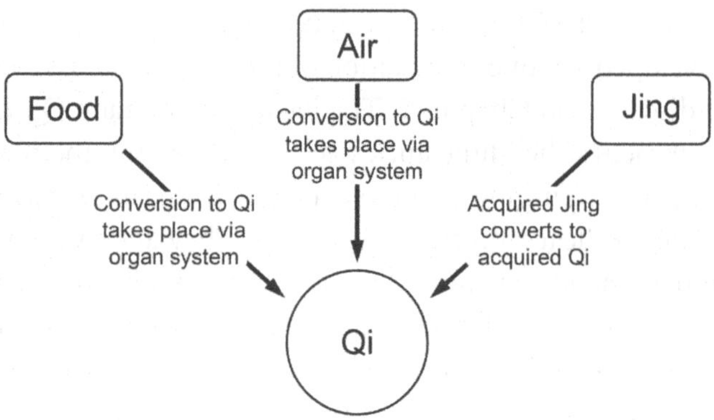

Figure 10.3: Sources of Qi

A full discussion of Yang Sheng Fa principles would be a very comprehensive task. It is the subject of many books from both Western and Eastern perspectives. Essentially, though, I generally tell my students to follow commonsense rules. Your Jing should be stilled, as explained previously in this book; do not overtax your body and mind. The more centred you can make yourself and the higher degree of balance you find in your life between healthy activity and rest, the more efficiently the Jing-to-Qi mechanic will take place.

There are disagreements within the internal arts world as to whether or not you can actually 'replenish' your Jing. Some say it is not possible, whilst others say there are hidden methods to achieve replenishment of Jing. The reason that people say it is not possible is that they are influenced by Chinese medical teachings; these teachings are aimed at 'regular' people, not those who study the internal arts. Jing can indeed be replenished, but it is not a basic-level practice. It comes under the heading of 'marrow washing' which we looked at briefly in Chapter 7. It is a practice that requires a high level of preparatory work and so, for a long time in your practice, you will instead be focusing on not 'burning up' your Jing and helping its cycles to run more efficiently.

The second main source of your Qi is the air that you breathe. The processes of regulating the breath discussed in Chapter 5 are concerned with making this process more efficient. Return to your breathing often and make its development a regular aspect of your life. The better connection we have to our breathing, the more balanced our mental state and the more efficient our Qi generation process. As well as this, look at where you live. The quality of the air you breathe is also important. I remember practising Qi Gong in the Tian Tan (天壇) park in central Beijing and finding the results very different from when I practised the same exercises in the Hua (华) mountain range a few days later. If you live in a city, then consider taking regular trips out into the countryside to breathe in some healthy 'Qi-building' air.

The third source of Qi is the food that you eat (as well as what you drink). Obviously, it is beyond the scope of this book to really go into different foods and their qualities in great detail. To keep it simple, avoid processed foods, refined sugars and, generally, junk food. Try to eat a healthy and balanced diet of green leafy vegetables and lean, organic meat; if you are vegetarian, then obviously adjust accordingly! There are plenty of books out there on Chinese food theory and therapy. I would advise looking into this instead of Western food theory if you are wishing to use your food as a way of building Qi. This is not because Western food theory is wrong in any way, not at all, it is just that it focuses on the nutritional quality of the food, whereas Chinese food therapy looks at the thermal and energetic properties of the food: an approach directly relatable to what we are seeking for our Qi Gong practice. Also, feel free to seek out qualified and experienced Chinese medical practitioners; make sure you get a full diagnosis (ensure that tongue observation and pulse diagnosis are included!) and then support your body's Qi-building mechanisms with herbal supplements.

I know this is an overly brief discussion of a very large topic, but you really need to explore this area of your practice. Qi Gong does not go well with a diet heavy in burgers, pizza and soft drinks!

The final way of building Qi is a little more advanced; it is related, once more, to that seminal text, the Sinew-Changing Classic. We shall return to this method later on in this chapter. You should recognise, though, that for a long time in your practice, Qi building will rely on the sources of Qi discussed here. Your food, your breathing and your Jing are where you should start.

Regulating

Regulation of the Qi is generally involved with two main factors – circulation and quality. Circulation of Qi relies on the opening of the channels as well as establishing the key orbits of the body, of which the microcosmic orbit is the first and most well known. We shall look at the various orbits of Qi that come after the microcosmic orbit later in this chapter.

The second factor involved in regulation of Qi is the quality. Though there are many factors involved in the quality of your Qi – such as pathogens present within the body, environmental energies of where you live and so on – the major factor is the state of your mind. The practice of regulating the mind as discussed in Chapter 6 is a good place to start with regard to helping to adjust the quality of your Qi. Think of the body as having an overall 'frequency' of Qi, and it is this that we wish to harmonise so that it is as healthy as possible. In general, it is meditative-type practices that help with development of the internal quality of Qi. The more stillness of mind that you can develop, the higher the quality of internal Qi.

Putting It Together

The reason why these ideas are important is that they will help you to establish the nature and content of your regular practice. We know that we need a flow of healthy Qi that is being generated within the body and moved through the channel system. We have looked at various tools and methods within this book and, no doubt, on top of this you will have your own practices as well. The way to now develop in the most efficient manner is to understand how to balance them and so build an effective practice. I have known many practitioners who did not build an effective practice as they did not understand how to balance their training sessions correctly. 'How' to practise is equally important as 'what' to practise.

So, in short, for *purging*, we need to start working towards developing the quality of 'Song' as a part of our breathing; this will then carry across into our mental state due to the interlinked nature of breath and mind. We should then look to have some kind of practice akin to Dao Yin training to help guide Qi out of the body; this works well when the Zi Fa Gong process begins to manifest within our training.

For *nourishing* the Qi of the body, we need to adopt a healthy lifestyle and look at the way we breathe. Our diet, level of activity and amount of rest are of prime concern to us. Look to understanding the Jing and how it is the foundation of everything that we do. Also remember that moving the body is an important part of our health; going for regular brisk walks or adopting a similar form of exercise is equally important for our Qi development as any complex internal practice.

For *regulation* of the Qi, we need to begin to understand the circulation of Qi through our body as well as making sure that we have an efficient Qi Gong exercise method which enables us to move and circulate Qi through the body. Movements should be soft and flowing and involve a high level of absorption of awareness into the body. These should be the Yin to the more 'expelling' practice of Yang Dao Yin.

Sitting behind all of this practice should be a regular practice of the Wuji standing posture, Dan Tian development and study of the fundamental principles of Qi Gong; without the principles, the art is lost.

Common Errors in Practice

I have seen people practise incorrectly as they have forgotten these three principles of purge, nourish and regulate. Below are some examples of ways in which people can make errors.

Always Purging (Too Yang)

I have encountered systems of practice almost entirely based on Dao Yin training. The systems were focused upon opening the joints, leading Qi through and out of the body and making the body too Yang. Generally, there was an overfocus on very active forms of breathing such as reverse breathing, and all of this was balanced with very little in the way of nourishment of the body. The result was that practitioners became too 'hyper' in their nature. Whilst they initially felt energised by the practice, they became unrooted and, in the end, drained by their practice. Always moving the Qi should be balanced with work to allow it to become soft and still.

Always Nourishing (Too Stagnant)

Other systems involve just 'bringing in' more Qi and building more energy all of the time. There is little in the way of clearing Xie Qi from the system and a lack of Yang in the practice. Xie Qi needs to be purged from the channels, or else the root of disease is not going to be cleared. Even if you have the most effective system of Qi building that there is, you will still just be burying the pathogenic quality of existing Qi underneath this gathered energy. If there is also a lack of circulation of Qi, no work on channels and orbits, then the Qi will become stagnant in quality; these people generally end up very 'sodden' in their quality and their bodies look swollen and stodgy. They need to purge the body of Xie Qi and move energy around their system to a higher degree.

Always Standing (Too Yin)

A very common error is within schools that overfocus on standing postures and static exercises; an example of this would be many Zhan Zhuang schools which solely do this type of static exercise. Whilst there is nothing inherently wrong with static Qi Gong postures – they are the place where most of the internal work is done – they should not be practised on their own. There should also be moving exercises that enable the Qi to flow and the body to relax whilst in a more dynamic state. Sadly, the vast majority of solely standing practitioners who I have met are very stiff, lack energetic movement within the body and are essentially making themselves too Yin.

Only Sitting (Denying the Body)

I am aware that by writing this, I am in the minority, but I do not feel that solely practising either meditation or seated forms of Qi Gong is healthy. There are exceptions, of course – those who can manage and develop a high-quality meditative practice will condition the quality of their mind to such an extent that it will take care of the body. These people, however, are rare. The vast majority of people who exclusively practise seated methods would benefit greatly from some movement. I call these people 'deniers of the body'. You have a body, you have Qi – move it. If you do not move your Qi, then it can become stagnant; on an even more basic level, if the body is not used, it will begin to lose function. As the old adage goes – 'Use it or lose it!'

Ignoring Yang Sheng Fa (Idiotic)

Even if we ignore the connection between Yang Sheng Fa and our practice of Nei Gong, there are countless studies showing that our quality of life and personal health are very closely connected. If we do not look after our body and energy system through a good diet, a healthy amount of exercise and positive health-related factors, then we will suffer the consequences. I have met Qi Gong practitioners who lived on junk food, drank copious amounts of alcohol and even smoked. The basis of regulation of quality of Qi is that we need to manage our health as best as we can. There is also the added factor of internal sensitivity. This means that if we practise an internal art to a high level, then we can actually make the impact of unhealthy food and drink worse. Your body will start to draw the energetic quality of your food out and you will become aware of just how damaging it is; consequently, the effects of this behaviour are heightened. You should look at these aspects of your personal well-being and consider them a part of your practice.

An Example System

A system of practice should include exercises of various types that work together in order to take a student through the internal process in a systematic and balanced manner. A system does not need to be huge with regard to how many exercises there are; in fact, often 'less is more', but there should be clear training in purging, nourishing and regulating. An example of this is the system I teach within my own school and practice. Though there are many practices not included here, these are the primary sets of exercises taught at a foundational level.

Ji Ben Qi Gong (基本氣功): Fundamental Qi Gong

The Ji Ben Qi Gong are eight simple moving exercises which are primarily designed to teach a person how to move their body in the correct way. They are designed to help a person restructure their form and sink their Qi through relaxation in order to refashion the body for more advanced internal practices. Each exercise is based around unification of the body, breath and awareness in order to circulate Qi through key internal pathways within the body.

Wu Xing Qi Gong (五行氣功): Five Elemental Movements Qi Gong

The five Wu Xing Qi Gong exercises are simple movements designed to help a person regulate the quality of Qi within their body. The exercises help to regulate the function of the five key organ systems of Chinese medical thought: the Kidneys, the Liver, the Heart, the Spleen and the Lungs. As the energetic strength of these organ systems is improved, it helps to regulate the quality of the body's Qi as well as assisting the body in production of Qi as its efficiency goes up.

Wu Dao Yin (五導引): Five Dao Yin Exercises

The five Wu Dao Yin exercises are moving forms of energetic purging. Each exercise is designed to target and open up key energetic centres within the body. As these centres are pulled open, they generate enough space within the energy body to help clear Xie Qi. The movements are then combined with focused awareness and specific breathing methods in order to lead the body towards a state of better health.

Long Dao Yin (龍導引): Dragon Dao Yin Exercises

The four Dragon Dao Yin exercises are a set of short sequences which specifically target the spine and associated channels. Through various stretching, twisting and undulating movements, the spinal column is squeezed and stretched in such a manner that it helps to purge Xie Qi from its length. This helps to generate space within the soft tissues of the body as well as opening up the core congenital networks which run through the torso. The more space is created, the higher the level of internal energy which the body may conduct along its length.

These four sets of exercises are practised alongside Wuji standing practice and development of mind, breath and Dan Tian. As you can see, some of the exercises are designed to move and circulate Qi in a softer manner, whilst the Dao Yin exercises are there to move and purge Xie Qi from the body. Together, these fundamental Qi Gong movements help to establish a healthy foundation for further internal development.

I have included these four sets as an example of practice. No doubt, you will have your own sets of exercises that you have been taught and practise. You do not need to know the exact sets described above; it is wise, however, to look at what you are doing and try to understand how the various exercises you have been taught fit into the purging, nourishing and regulating model. If you can understand these principles and adjust your regular practice in the right way, then you will develop in the most beneficial manner.

Stillness to Movement

The importance of the above discussion of how to apply and balance the nature of Qi Gong exercises as a part of your regular practice should not be underestimated. It is the same within any practice; I have seen this same error time and again in the martial arts as well. A misunderstanding of how to structure your training routines and how to organise your time can really hinder your development. This is another important role of the teacher: to help you understand exactly 'how' to practise what you have learnt.

This section should really be concluded with another key pointer: please keep in mind that the most change takes place during periods of stillness. This happens on a deep meditative level, but it also takes place within our exercises. The moving Qi Gong exercises that we practise are primarily designed to set up a series of 'causes', but the 'effects' are felt to a higher degree during our static practice. What I mean by this is that each moving exercise has a very clear function; the exercises are essentially 'goal orientated' in nature. So, you may have an exercise that is designed to send Qi to the organ of the Lungs, for example. When you carry out the exercise, with all of the correct principles in place, then the instruction is given to the body to direct your Qi in this specific manner. During the exercise, your Qi will begin to move, but the nature of any movement is that it will be likely to contain errors; these errors are a result of Wei or 'doing'. 'Doing' of the mind or 'doing' of the body are both more prone to involving mistakes than 'non-doing' or Wu Wei. That being said, the 'doing' is still required to initiate any event. This is the process of establishing the 'causes' within your body.

The next stage is to end the moving part of the exercise and transition into physical stillness. By doing this, you are entering into the Wu Wei phase of the exercise and so giving your body time to process the effects of the training. This process is summarised in Figure 10.4.

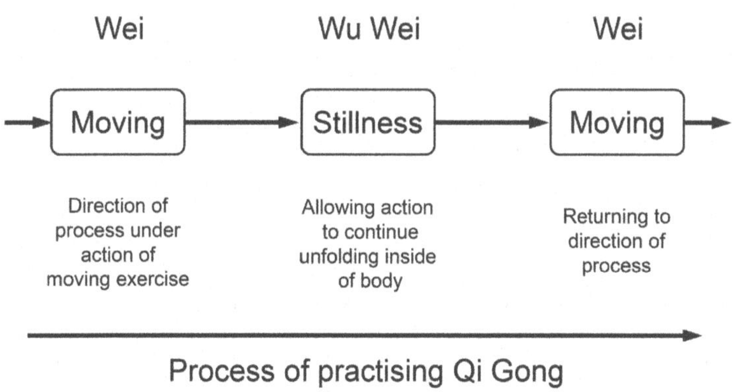

Figure 10.4: Moving and Stillness in Practice

When you are moving or actively performing an exercise, you are essentially directing a process. When you begin to stand still, then you give space for the body to unfold the fruits of your practice. This 'standing time' can vary from a few minutes to a full hour, there really is no rule. What is important, though, is that your body is given this time to change where there is very little involvement from yourself other than simply observing.

If I use an example of the Ji Ben Qi Gong, an exercise set from within my school of practice, it is based around eight simple movements. Each of these movements has a very simple function. The first exercise is called 'compressing the pearl' and it is aimed at helping the Qi within the lower abdomen to consolidate. This is its primary function, and it accomplishes this through a simple two-part movement that is repeated a number of times. It is very similar to many basic Qi Gong exercises from within other systems.

When practising 'compressing the pearl', it is repeated for a length of time. In the earlier stages of practice, students are given a number of repetitions or a length of time to practise the exercise. After some time, as internal awareness improves, it is repeated until it is starting to fulfil its function, to help consolidate the Qi within the lower abdomen. Once the Qi begins to move in the correct fashion, the students should stop the movement, transition into the Wuji standing posture and simply observe the body. This is the key: since the body has been given no further instructions, you have not carried out any other movements beyond 'compressing the pearl' and then standing in Wuji; it will continue to consolidate the Qi for a period of time of its own accord. This process is like an echo of the movement you performed, and it will continue for some time before the process begins to fade away and stop.

At this point in time, you should then return to the moving part of your practice, either back to 'compressing the pearl' or on to the next exercise. In this way, if you went through all eight of the simple Ji Ben Qi Gong exercises, you would stand for a period of time in Wuji after each exercise. Consequently, if people are really wanting to get the full benefit of the exercises, it can take an hour or longer to thoroughly perform all eight sections of the set.

The fact is that the most beneficial effects of the training are felt when you are standing still, as there is less room for error. There is always more power in the 'non-doing' than the 'doing'. It is important to make this clear as I have seen many Qi Gong practitioners miss out on the benefit of Wu Wei, because they do not stand between the exercises. They may have a set of ten movements which they move through, one after another. If they were to then stand still after practising all ten, a common practice, the full benefit of only the final Qi Gong movement would be felt. The power of each system is felt in that system's Wuji practice.

The Forty-Nine Major Hurdles of Liu Yi Ming

A very interesting set of guidelines for the practice of personal cultivation has been transmitted down through the generations within the Dragon Gate sect; these guidelines are from Liu Yi Ming (劉一明), an alchemical practitioner from within this particular tradition. Liu Yi Ming produced a number of writings, including the Tong Guan Wen (通關文), or Book of Surpassing Barriers, which focused upon those hurdles that may prevent a person from attaining Dao. Many of these hurdles are, at first glance, seemingly developed purely as ethical guidance, but on further examination are tools for mechanically changing a person's inner state. By realigning their behaviour through external governance, Master Liu was aiming to adjust the 'frequency' of their inner spirit and thus move them closer to the tradition of Daoism.

Listed below are the forty-nine major hurdles on the road to spiritual development. I have included the original Chinese since there is always room for interpretation when it comes down to translating Chinese to English; in this way, those who read Chinese can translate them for themselves.

- The hurdle of lust (色慾關)
- The hurdle of passionate love (恩愛關)
- The hurdle of fame (榮貴關)
- The hurdle of wealth (財利關)
- The hurdle of poverty (窮困關)
- The hurdle of vanity (色身關)
- The hurdle of arrogance (傲氣關)
- The hurdle of envy (嫉妒關)
- The hurdle of irritability (暴躁關)
- The hurdle of the untrue speech (口舌關)
- The hurdle of hatred (瞋恨關)
- The hurdle of perceived separation (人我關)
- The hurdle of poor climate (冷熱關)

- The hurdle of laziness (懶惰關)
- The hurdle of innate ability (才智關)
- The hurdle of being capricious (任性關)
- The hurdle of 'life factors' (患難關)
- The hurdle of scheming (詭詐關)
- The hurdle of second guessing (猜議關)
- The hurdle of empty esotericism (懸虛關)
- The hurdle of delusion (妄想關)
- The hurdle of fear of death (生死關)
- The hurdle of complacency (自滿關)
- The hurdle of fearing problems (畏难關)
- The hurdle of being slow (輕慢關)
- The hurdle of cowardice (懦弱關)
- The hurdle of stopping too soon (不久關)
- The hurdle of nihilism (暴棄關)
- The hurdle of accumulating debt (累債關)
- The hurdle of haughtiness (高大關)
- The hurdle of personal adornment (妝飾關)
- The hurdle of counterfeit knowledge (假知關)
- The hurdle of inner evil (陰惡關)
- The hurdle of too much alcohol (貪酒關)
- The hurdle of fearing the bitter (怕苦關)
- The hurdle of no faith (不信關)
- The hurdle of no master (無主關)
- The hurdle of short-cuts (速效關)
- The hurdle of carelessness (粗心關)
- The hurdle of procrastination (虛度關)

- The hurdle of lack of will (退志關)
- The hurdle of enjoying praise (誇揚關)
- The hurdle of hallucinations (幻景關)
- The hurdle of cause and effect (因果關)
- The hurdle of being over-enthralled with books (書魔關)
- The hurdle of reaching emptiness (着空關)
- The hurdle of becoming stuck in a phase (執相關)
- The hurdle of seeking the elixir in the bedroom (閨丹關)
- The hurdle of difficulty in lighting the furnace (爐火關)

Yi Dao Qi Dao

In the previous chapter, we looked at the use of the term 'listening', or Ting (聽), and why this term is used within the Chinese arts to refer to the more passive yet receptive state of our awareness that does not lead us into opening the floodgates of visual and tactile 'false positives' within our practice. It is this quality that we have been learning to apply in our practice. This began even in the earliest stages of learning how to relax and condition the mind; the use of our breathing as a vehicle for conscious absorption is also a major part of developing effective Ting.

Ting is a concept we shall return to in greater detail in the next few chapters as it essentially becomes one of the most important aspects of these arts: how to 'listen' correctly and then how to develop this skill further. For now, though, your 'absorption of awareness' practice that you have been developing is enough.

To begin to further your Qi Gong, you should allow the awareness to absorb its way into the entire body. At this stage, the lower Dan Tian is not so important and so you should allow your awareness to encompass the entire body, rather than just the lower abdominal region. To a certain extent, this should have started happening of its own accord anyway; the more you open the channels, the more the awareness is led through the channel system until it 'fills' the entirety of your body.

Especially for those who have experienced the benefits of the Zi Fa Gong process, as the channels are pushed open by the movements of the Yang Qi, the mind will begin to filter into all of the spaces of the body.

This is important as it brings us to a major Qi Gong maxim: Yi Dao Qi Dao (意到氣到). This is a very important phrase within the Qi Gong tradition, and it is often translated as 'Where the intention goes, energy follows' or something similar. The implications of this are often applied in a very 'Dao Yin manner' and so many practitioners are constantly using their intention or (worse) imagination to forcibly lead Qi through the channels of their body. Whilst it is true that you can forcibly lead Qi in this manner, it is not going to take you beyond the foundation stages of the art. Dao Yin exercises that lead Qi in this way are fine, but very foundation-level practices. The reason for this misunderstanding is due to a major misunderstanding of this classical phrase. As with many things within the Chinese arts, there are multiple ways to decipher the instructions; let us look at another way of understanding the concept of Yi Dao Qi Dao.

Yi Dao

Whilst it is true that 'Yi' in its simplest sense means our 'intention', it also has a more overarching implication. The Yi is an expression of the movement of our mind. Our intentions are one aspect of how our mind may move, but each and every thought that we have is also a movement. If we return to the concept of our consciousness being like a vast ocean and the movements of our mind generating waves on this ocean, then Yi is the movement that generates the waves, it is the wind. This means that whilst Yi is indeed our intention, our guided and conscious mental actions, it is also the subconscious movements of our mind that we have little control over. It also is everything from our emotional makeup through to our conditioned biases.

The term 'Dao' can be translated as 'to go' but it also, more correctly in this instance, can mean 'to arrive' at something, or the 'culmination of a journey'. In this way, when combined with the term 'Yi', we could understand it as meaning the 'culmination of the work you have done with your Qi to develop its quality'.

Qi Dao

'Qi' in this sense means the various forms of energy within our body as well as various transformative processes that take place within us according to our practice. This means that the term 'Qi' here is used in its widest and most inclusive sense.

'Dao' is the same as within 'Yi Dao': the 'arrival' or 'culmination of a journey'.

Looking Again at Yi Dao Qi Dao

If we now look again at this phrase, instead of 'Where the intention goes, energy follows,' we get 'The culmination of the work you have done to develop and regulate the conscious and subconscious movements of your mind will dictate the level of regulation and development of your internal energy as well as the processes of change that take place as a result of this.' Whilst this is a rather lengthy, and definitely not catchy, translation of the phrase Yi Dao Qi Dao, it does more accurately convey the teachings contained within this important Qi Gong phrase.

The implications of this are that it is the 'quality' of your Yi and not its actions that is important. It is also suggested that the results within the realm of Qi will unfold as a result of cause and effect according to the quality of your mind. This is very different from 'leading' Qi with your intention. In short, it is the difference between 'doing' and effective 'non-doing'. A mistranslation of the phrase, which results from not going deep enough, has transformed many people's practice from Wu Wei to Wei in focus.

Listening to Open the Channels

It is the quality of 'listening' that enables you to correctly apply Yi Dao Qi Dao to your practice. The absorption of your awareness into the body combined with the passive quality of Ting or 'listening' is what establishes the correct 'cause' within the body. Through the stages discussed up until this point in the text, you should have begun to move your Qi and consolidate the driving force of the lower Dan Tian. This will have started to open up the channels of the body and now, with your practice of static and moving Qi Gong, you can continue with this process. You are now at the stage of refinement of the channel-opening process. Your awareness will reach deeper into the body as a result of the work you have carried out so far and this means that your Yi will start to have an effect upon the Qi. This effect is that it begins to regulate itself and so the quality of the Qi within the channel system will develop further.

The higher the quality of the Qi within your channel system, the further you will go into the opening process. This is as a result of giving your body the correct level of 'attention' through the act of Ting. Give the body attention, and it will develop; always give it 'intention', and it will be subject to the various distortions contained within the acquired layers of your Yi.

All of this theory may sound a little complex, but it essentially comes down to practising your art of Qi Gong with the application of 'listening' to your body. The result of this is that the channels will open and develop further. You should continue with this practice until the major orbits of the body have been set in motion and the key congenital channels are opened according to the clear signs discussed in the section 'Signs of Channels Opening' below.

Key Orbit Openings

Most practitioners of Qi Gong will, no doubt, be familiar with the concept of the microcosmic orbit: the circulation of Qi that takes place along the length of the back and down the front of the body. What is less well known is that there are several other key rotations of Qi that we are trying to build through our practice as well. These include:

- the Girdling channel orbit
- the side branches orbit
- the circulation of Qi into the limbs.

These are all further circulations of Qi that will unfold as a result of your practice. There is little to 'do' in the way of helping these along. Though there are exercises that purport to focus on these specific circulations, it is my experience that they will open up in students when they are ready. It is simply a case of time, correct development of the principles of your practice and application of the teachings of Yi Dao Qi Dao.

The Girdling Channel Orbit

The Girdling channel is said to be the only channel within the body that travels in a horizontal fashion. It encompasses the waist and runs in the pathway shown in Figure 10.5. It has a slight dip down on the front of the lower abdomen as depicted.

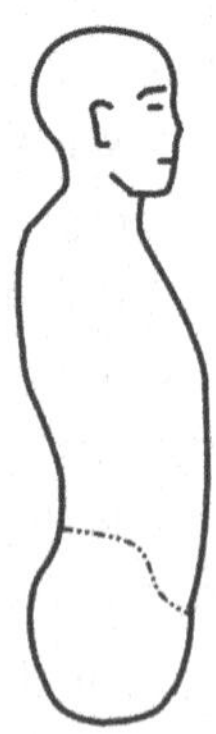

Figure 10.5: The Girdling Channel

The key functions of the Girdling channel are to regulate the Qi of the torso, to balance the Qi of the Liver, to support the Kidneys' functioning, to assist in the lower Dan Tian's formation and rotation, and to bind together all of the channels of the body. As the Girdling channel circulation begins to open up, there is a feeling of the Yin Qi being gathered around the torso; it is a gentle gathering, and in this way, you could think of the Girdling channel functioning like a kind of 'energetic corset'. Many people have a quality of Qi within the body that is too 'slack' and we want this to be changed.

Qi will circulate in both directions around the Girdling channel. The movement of Qi here has a very free and 'sluicing' quality to it when the channel begins to awaken.

Within Chinese medicine, it is said that the channel sits only in the region of the waist and 'binds' the rest of the channels, as depicted in Figure 10.6.

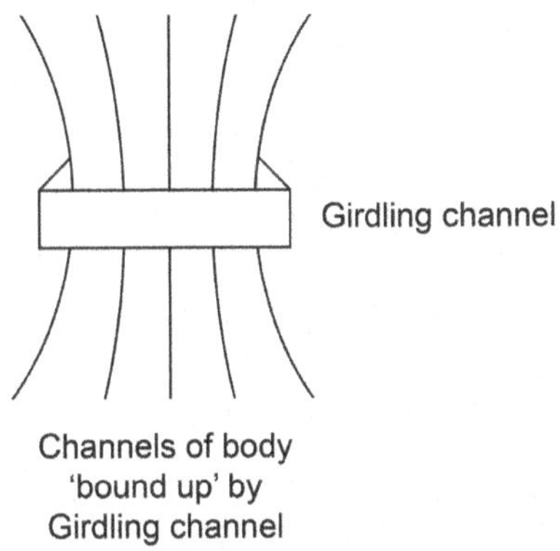

Figure 10.6: Binding the Channels

Problems with the binding function are made apparent through such symptoms as:

- swelling of the abdomen
- a feeling as if sitting in cold water from the waist down
- pain in the umbilical region and lower abdomen
- aching lumbar region
- irregular menstrual patterns
- infertility and impotence
- a lack of 'direction' in life.

It is these kinds of symptoms, as well as certain energetic conditions with the Kidneys and Liver that it can help with, that are treated within Chinese medicine using the Girdling channel. Treatment of the Girdling channel helps by 'binding up' the slackness in this area of the body. Understanding some Chinese medicine theory like this can help us to understand the nature of our energy body more clearly.

Nei Gong and alchemical schools take the location and function of the Girdling channel further by stating that, when fully activated, it runs as shown in Figure 10.7. In my experience, this is certainly the case: it can clearly be felt.

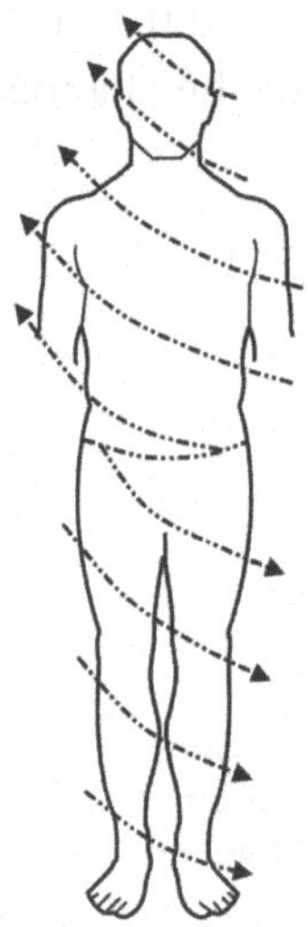

Figure 10.7: Nei Gong Girdling Channel

As the Girdling channel begins to expand outwards from the waist, it spirals around the channels of the body and 'binds' them all the way from head to toe. This helps them to develop in strength and efficiency. In this way, the Girdling channel is like an energetic coil that develops just beyond the surface of your skin. You can feel this taking place in your practice, and it comes with several clear signs that are discussed in the section 'Signs of Channels Opening' below.

The Side Branches Orbit

Within the torso are two branches of the congenital system that run along either side of your Central channel. They extend from the mid-point of the clavicle through to the pelvic cavity before they connect in to the rest of the congenital channel system as shown in Figure 10.8.

The side branches are deep within the torso and as such have very little connection to the surface of your body. They pass entirely through the Huang level of the body and have no relationship to the sinew channels; as such, they are very difficult to open and it takes a long time for Yang Qi to fully move along their length. We can assist their opening with lots of flexing of the torso and there are certain exercises that are designed to shift Qi through these channels, but ultimately it will, once again, come down to time and correct application of Qi Gong principles into our practice.

The natural flow for the side channels should be as depicted in Figure 10.8. The Qi should rise up through the left-hand side of the body and sink down on the right. It is for this reason that, according to Qi Gong terminology, the left side of your body is Yang, whilst the right is Yin. Note that this is in the opposite direction from the ascending and descending of the colon, something that often confuses people.

The rising of Qi on the left-hand side of the body serves to raise Qi through the Spleen system. Within Chinese medicine, the Spleen's Qi is said to be 'unhappy' when it chronically descends; this can lead to many symptoms, including:

- a 'bearing-down' sensation in the abdomen
- prolapse of internal organs
- urgency of defecation and urination
- a 'sagging' quality to the muscles of the abdomen
- haemorrhoids.

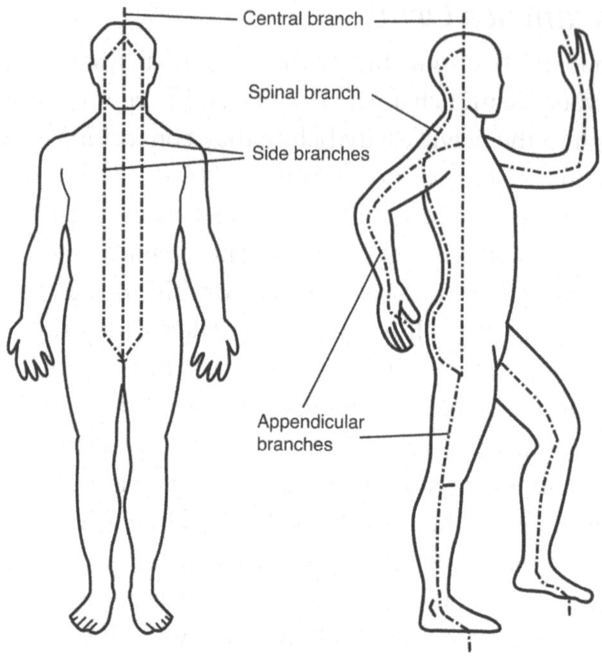

Figure 10.8: The Side Branches

It is the 'raising' of the Qi on the left-hand side of the body that is involved in preventing these issues from occurring. Chinese medical practitioners may work to support the functioning of the Spleen itself if these symptoms manifest or else, in the case of more Nei Gong-related systems, they may adjust the rotation of Qi through the two side branches.

The gradual descending of Qi on the right side of your torso ensures that the Liver is not too stimulated and that it remains functioning correctly. It is understood that if the Liver becomes imbalanced, then it may often start to raise the Qi on the right-hand side of the body, which results in a reversal of the side branches' circulation. This will manifest as symptoms such as:

- migraine-type headaches
- dizziness or acute bursts of tinnitus
- chronically dry mouth and throat
- insomnia
- irritability and stress-related symptoms.

Once again, this may be treated directly through the organ itself, the Liver, or some practitioners of Chinese medicine may work to balance the circulation of Qi through the side branches of the channel system.

These above symptoms are generally a sign of the organs related to the circulation of Qi within the side branches becoming negatively impacted by a reversal in the flow of Qi. On top of this, Qi may also stagnate within the circuit, which will result in symptoms such as:

- acid reflux
- swelling of the abdomen
- vomiting
- abdominal pain
- loose bowels
- undigested food in your stools.

These are symptoms that Chinese medical practitioners would know as being related to the Liver having a detrimental impact upon the Stomach's functioning; they can also occur as a result of stagnation of Qi flow within the side branches of the torso.

If the Governing and Conception channels can be said to regulate Yin and Yang within the channel system, the side branches can be said to regulate Yin and Yang within the space of the torso. This also means that they will impact upon the level of Yin and Yang within most organ systems too.

When Yang Qi begins to move into these channels, there is a feeling of warm fluid moving along their length, and many internal imbalances will start to fade away; for myself, this stage of channel opening was one of the greatest boons to my overall health. I was actually fortunate enough to have a teacher open this circulation for me directly using an empowered transmission; at that moment, a very severe chronic digestive condition I had suffered with for a long time was cleared up. I now only have slight recurrences of symptoms related to this condition if I am extremely tired and so have low Qi levels.

The Circulation of Qi into the Limbs

A further circulation of Qi needs to take place from the body out into the limbs. The Qi will then flow as shown in Figure 10.9. Note that this directional flow loops into and back from the limbs in a distinctly different manner from the directional Qi flow within the twelve organ channels that Chinese medical practitioners will be familiar with.

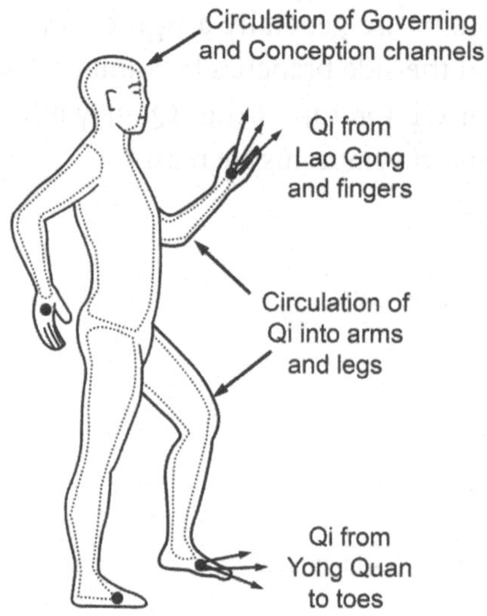

Figure 10.9: Circulation of Qi into Limbs

There is always Qi within your arms and legs; this Qi travels through the organ channels, the Huang and the sinew channels; but the circulation of increased Yang Qi has to take place. This is through the pathways that are an extension of the Thrusting channel system. This circulation of Yang Qi is important, as it serves to connect our deeper congenital channel system into the extremities. It is also here that the deepest level of purging Xie Qi will take place. Yang Qi can carry with it information of our most chronic pathogenic factors. When it can reach our extremities, it can carry with it the source of these pathogenic imbalances. It can often be quite amazing just how clear these pathogenic releases are. Figure 10.10 shows a student's reactions to pathogenic release, carried on the platform of the Yang Qi, out of the body via the limbs.

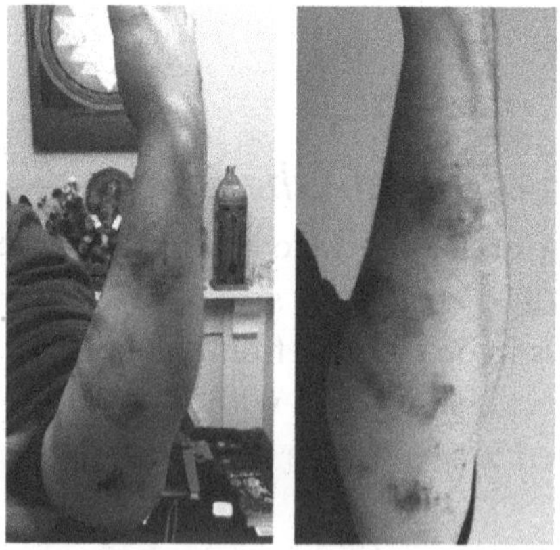

Figure 10.10: Pathogenic Release

What looks like black bruising on this gentleman's arm is actually a type of Xie Qi known as pathogenic Cold. It is shown here in a very extreme form. During purging-type practices in a class, this black discolouration began to appear within the channels of his arms. As the Yang Qi circulation increased through his body, it transported the black toxins along the channels towards his fingers. Over the course of the practice session, this black discolouration visibly moved out from his body, down his arms and out to his fingers where it dripped out onto the floor. The photos shown here were taken after the session where a few residues of the Xie Qi remained. Further sessions involved assisting these last remnants of the toxin to leave his body. To some, this may seem extreme: how is it possible that such a clear visual phenomenon can manifest? Well, from somebody who has practised and taught these arts for a long time, I can safely say that deep purging results really are this tangible. This kind of 'clearing out' can only take place when the Yang Qi reaches the extremities as there needs to be a strong energetic vehicle for the body to be able to get rid of this type of chronic imbalance. As a general guideline for your health – it is better to get these toxins out of the body rather than leave them there to fester and lead to chronic disease!

When the Yang Qi moves along the length of the extremities, it feels like an electrical pulse moving through the soft tissues. It increases circulation to the limbs, meaning that you will rarely have cold hands or feet: a rather unimportant but pleasant by-product of this stage being reached!

Signs of Channels Opening

All of the above circulations or orbits of Qi should open within the body after the main rotation of the microcosmic orbit has been attained. From here, the further the orbits develop, the more they serve to open up the organ channels and then smaller subsidiary branches of the energetic body. The Qi will 'overflow' from the deeper channels into the smaller surface channels as shown in Figure 10.11.

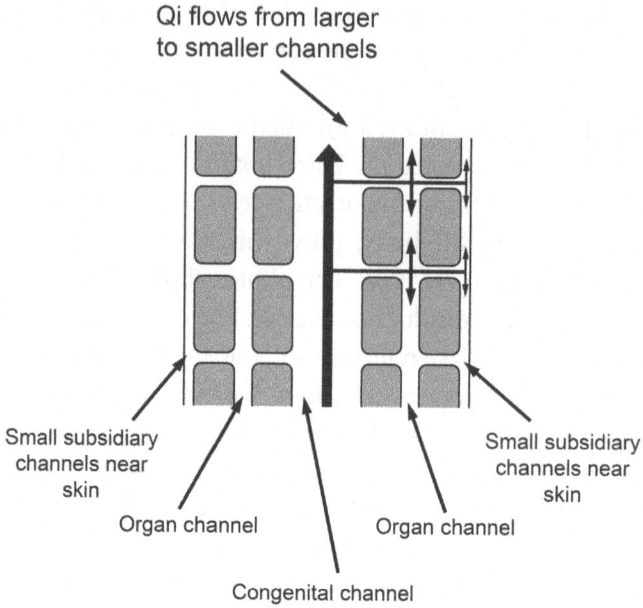

Figure 10.11: The Overflow of Qi into Channels

Now that we have looked at the various processes involved in opening the channels, we need to look at one of the most important parts of all this – how to know when they are open. Throughout all of the Daoist arts, there have always been clear signs of progress and indicators as to when you should move on in your practice. The greatest strength of a 'path' to follow is that there are markers along the way. It is rare that these markers are known by students of the internal arts, which is a real shame as knowing the right signs of progress is obviously a very useful tool when it comes to ascertaining just how you are doing!

Before I start looking at the signs of the channels being opened, it is important that we first return, once more, to the Sinew-Changing Classic and its teachings. Let us remind ourselves of three key points from within these teachings:

- The Qi must mobilise; the result of this is the engagement of the Huang. This will strengthen the Huang, which serves as a platform for the development of health.
- One should keep developing the Qi until the Huang fully stretches and the tendons are strong.
- The result of this is that the channels will open and the Qi will reach to every part of the body.

It is quite clearly outlined that once the Qi is mobilised and developed to a high enough degree, it will start to stretch and engage the Huang. In this way, the energetic will affect the physical. This is a very important aspect of our arts: any change we develop within the energetic realm must also be manifest upon the body. There is often a kind of 'divorce' between these two within the Qi Gong world; many believe that whatever we do with regard to our Qi and energetic system is irrelevant or somehow invisible in the body; this is really not the case. As stated previously in this book, when I visit my own teachers, they always test my progress by checking the quality of my Qi *and* how this is manifest within my physical body. If your Qi is not affecting the body, then you have not developed it far enough and so you should not seek to move on in your development.

Remember that the Sinew-Changing Classic could actually be called the 'Channel-Opening Classic' as this is its prime goal. So, how does moving and developing the Qi affect our channels? This is the first thing we need to understand.

Qi's Effects on the Huang

As we have already seen, the Huang is a kind of connective tissue. It is said to fill the spaces of the body and surround and uphold the viscera. It is everywhere within the body and serves as a conductor for the body's Qi. Each of the channels has a 'Huang component' to it, and then this transforms into the sinew channels and the tendons. To me, though, the Huang, the sinews and the tendons are one and the same; they are like a sliding gradient of density and strength. Deepest within the body lie the Huang, and as it reaches the surface, it becomes the sinew channels and then, at the end of the channels, lie the tendons. This is then repeated, so, if a channel was a tube, the Huang would be near to the tube's centre, whilst the sinew aspect of the channel would be near to the surface. These concepts are shown in Figure 10.12.

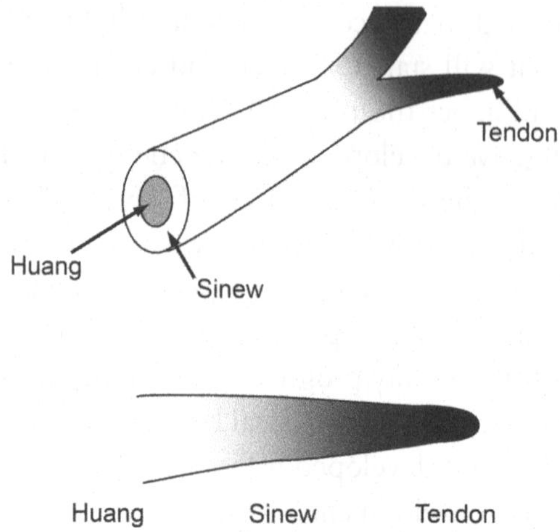

Figure 10.12: Huang, Sinew and Tendon

This means that with reference to the Sinew-Changing Classic and its teaching, we could say that the Huang, the sinews and even the tendons are affected in the same manner by our Qi; more specifically, the Yang Qi. This means that we could simplify all of this down to 'move the Qi to affect the physical aspect of the channel'.

The physical aspect of the channel is a kind of honeycomb structure that is both organic and malleable. It has a semi-plastic quality to it, meaning that even though it is soft and changeable, it can hold a structural shape. As discussed previously, this semi-plastic shape is then changed by our activities (or lack thereof) and also becomes blocked through the formation of adhesions. The Qi then passes through these structures via conduction, the flow of Qi along a channel's length. The more open the channel and the fewer adhesions or blockages, the more the Qi flows.

As the Qi moves into the honeycomb structure of the channel, it causes it to stretch. What was slack now becomes taut, as shown in Figure 10.13.

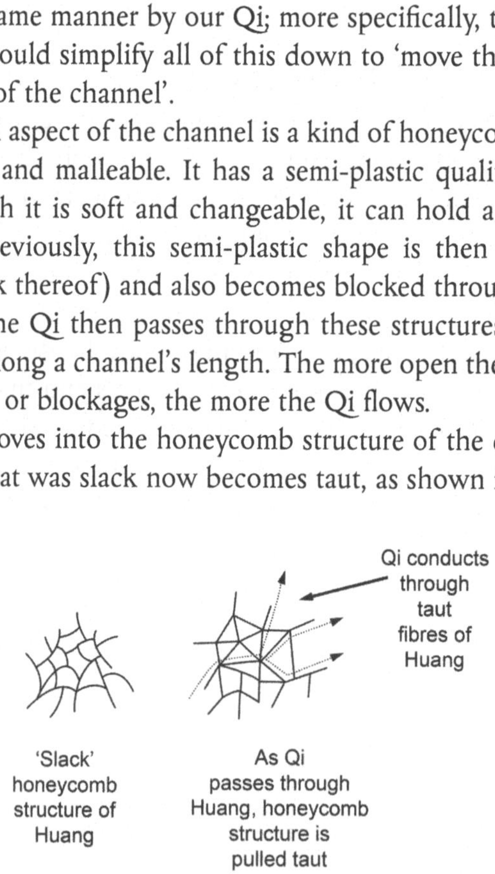

Figure 10.13: Opening of a Channel

The 'stretching' to tautness comes from the Qi moving into the channel's length. As the Qi conducts through the Huang, there is a reaction and the fibres of the Huang pull taut. This is what is alluded to within the Sinew-Changing Classic when it states that the Qi must mobilise; the result of this is the engagement of Huang. This happens to a very small degree in the early stages of practice, when the Qi is starting to move, but then continues to increase in power until the Huang is fully stretched out. The Sinew-Changing Classic advises that one should keep developing the Qi until the Huang stretches – the result of this is that the channels shall open and the Qi shall flow to every part of the body.

It is quite amazing, when you reach the level of the physical aspect of the channel fully engaging, just how powerful it is. On a physical level, it completely changes the feeling within your body. At first, in the early stages of Qi Gong, you relax and become softer. As you progress to this stage in your training, the body actually starts to feel 'hard' again, but this time the hardness is based upon expansion. It is like a hydraulic force moving through the channel's length; it expands outwards and feels inflated under the force of your Qi. Because of the honeycomb structure of the Huang, the influence of the Qi is felt in all directions and so the channel's length literally inflates outwards as shown in Figure 10.14.

This feeling of inflation spreads across the whole channel system but most clearly within the region where the congenital channels are said to have their influence. The thing to understand is that the feeling of inflation is not just a somatic experience that is yours alone to feel; it can also be clearly felt by others if they touch your body. I want to make this abundantly clear since I have met people who thought that they had reached the level of expansion when they had not. This is not to put anybody down in any way, not at all, this is not my aim – I just wish for people to understand what the individual signs of the channels opening are so that they know whether they have achieved it or not. The Qi Gong and Nei Gong world is rife with uncertainty and grey areas, so the clearer we can make signs of the progress, the better.

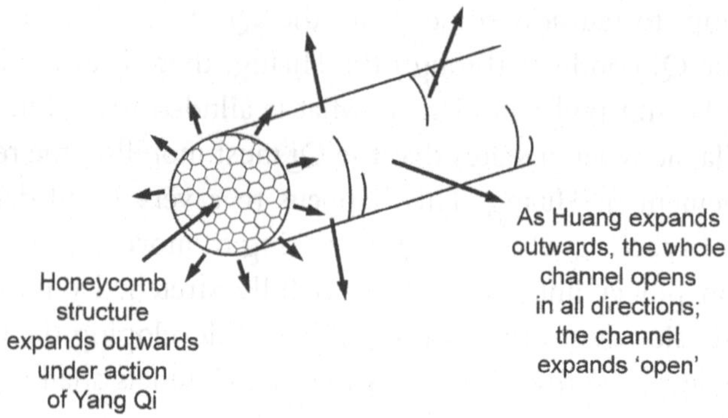

Figure 10.14: Inflation of the Channel Under the Influence of Yang Qi

Below are the signs of the main channels opening.

The Channels

Governing Channel

The Governing channel is the first channel to open; it stretches along the back of the body. When this channel opens, the soft tissues of the back will spread open from the Ming Men point which will be warm to the touch. This spreading of the soft tissues can be very clearly felt – it is as if there is a large sheet of elastic tissue which is opening up just beneath the surface of the skin. It opens up as shown in Figure 10.15.

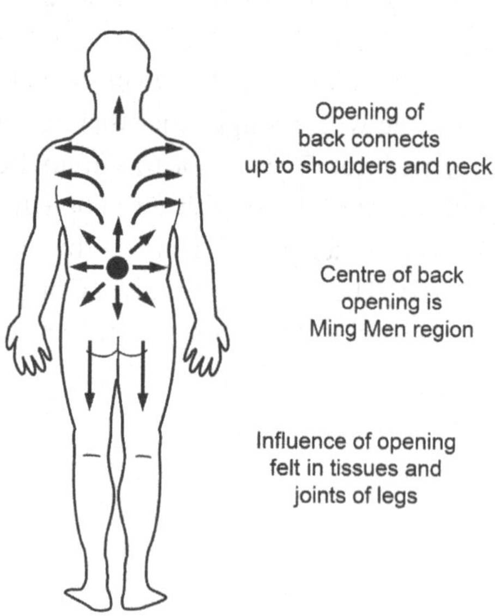

Figure 10.15: The Opening of the Back

The movement of this sheet of tissue can be felt by anybody who palpates your back as you drop into a Qi Gong position; it is as if the tissue just beneath the surface of your skin has come to life.

The opening of the Governing channel also serves to stimulate the nervous system in a very specific manner. This result is the Huang 'coming to life' all over the body. If you palpate a person who has their Governing channel open, it is as if the soft tissues of their body have a life all of their own, they can animate and move independently of the muscular system. If you have never felt it on somebody, it is a very strange feeling!

They say that the Governing channel controls all Yang of the body; Yang in this case is 'life' or activity. When the Governing channel has opened up to a high enough degree, then activity is there throughout the body. To the trained eye, you can also see it in a person when they move, especially when they perform Qi Gong exercises or a Taijiquan form. The animation of the Huang under the force of the Qi is the key.

Conception Channel

The Conception channel runs along the central line on the front of the body. It is closely linked to the vagus nerve and regulates the level of 'calm' we manifest within our mind. The first sign that we may become aware of is that we cannot 'panic' any more. That experience of the heart 'skipping a beat' or the mind entering into a state of anxiety simply does not happen. The opening of the Conception channel prevents us from getting into these kinds of states; if you still experience 'panic' in this way, then the Conception channel needs more work.

On a physical level, when the Conception channel opens, the depression in the region of the solar plexus is filled in. This is the depression shown in Figure 10.16.

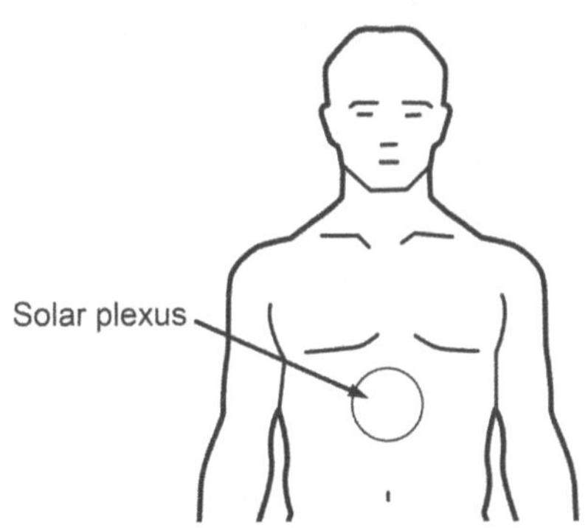

Figure 10.16: The Depression of the Solar Plexus

Unless a person carries a lot of body fat (in which case this sign can be difficult to palpate) each of us will have a natural depression in the muscular shape of the body just beneath the xiphoid process which sits on the bottom of the sternum. This shape changes when the Conception channel is fully opened. The expansion of the Huang under the action of the Qi is felt along the entire length of the Conception channel, but it can be felt most clearly within the region of the solar plexus. The depression is gone, and instead the solar plexus feels as if it is fully expanded outwards; you can hardly push it in on a person with a fully opened Conception channel as the force of the Qi is too high. Many people who have palpated this area on my torso have been surprised at how much power the Yang Qi can generate within a channel's length.

It should also be noted that men need the Governing channel to be open in order for the Conception channel to open; women, on the other hand, can open these channels either way around.

Girdling Channel

When the Girdling channel opens, aside from the health and psychological benefits, there is a strengthening of the Huang around the sides of the lower abdominal region. This is the area shown in Figure 10.17.

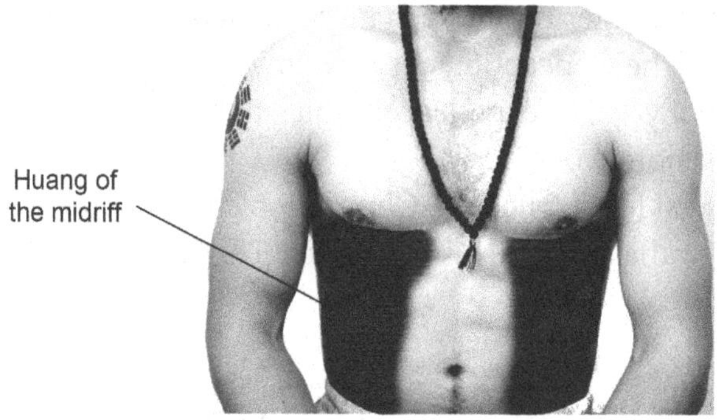

Figure 10.17: The Midriff

This is the region of the body where the oblique muscles run, but it is not the muscles themselves that are transformed; it is the Huang. The expansion of the Qi here means that the body has a very strong, elastic quality in this area. Once again, it is difficult to push your hands in to any great depth on a person's body if they have fully opened the Girdling channel. Even if they are relaxed, there is a large amount of hydraulic-feeling power expanding the Huang of their midriff outwards.

Side Branches

When the side branches open up within the body and there is a healthy flow of Qi within the torso, then the health of the Spleen and Liver are regulated. On a physical level, the Huang of the inside of the torso will also expand and open. This means that the joints of the whole body, including the spaces between the ribs, are expanded outwards by the Yang Qi's presence. This develops a very clear quality to the body that is difficult to describe in writing but can be clearly seen or felt by those who know what they are looking for.

Organ Channels

The result of the congenital channels opening to their full extent is that, with time, these effects will start to be felt within the smaller channels that are related to the organs. These are the channels generally depicted within acupuncture textbooks. The expansive quality can be felt, but to a lesser degree of strength, from within the congenital channels. If you palpate the body of somebody who has opened their channels, there will be a kind of 'pushing back' from the channels as they are pressed upon. It is the expansion of the channel that gives the feeling of being inflated, just beneath the skin. This feeling is subtler but, in my experience, is what most high-level Nei Gong teachers will test for as the organ channels will only fully open if the congenital channels are also opened to a high enough level.

Physical Signs

As with every aspect of these practices, there is change that takes place on a physical, energetic and consciousness level. These three 'bodies' of humanity are equally important in our expression of being and so we should expect to see transformation within all three of them. I have focused primarily on the 'physical' with regard to the signs of channels being opened, simply because they are the clearest and most tangible signs. It is important to recognise these signs, so you know where you are in these arts. With no signs of progress to understand, you are wandering along in the dark without a light. How else are you to know how your practice is developing and what you should be focusing on in your daily training?

Some of the stages I am going to outline in the final three chapters of the book can actually be dangerous to your health if the channels are not opened to a high enough degree. Many people underestimate the level of risk involved in high-level internal work, but they do so at their peril. The level of channel opening during these foundation stages of internal training really sets up the safety mechanisms for working at a more complex level. Understanding how open the channels are is vitally important in knowing if you should even think about moving on to more complex parts of the practice. Most of the more serious 'Qi deviation sickness' I have seen in people working with very intense Nei Gong practices resulted in moving to this stage before their channels were ready.

On a personal level, as a teacher, it can be helpful to know the signs of channel opening and other stages of attainment as it means I can directly tell, easily, where a person is in their practice. Inevitably, if you teach, you will have students ask you if they can progress on to more complex material than they really should be on. On top of this is the added complexity of new students telling you that they should skip the foundations of your system as they are already very advanced in their prior practices. Even if you don't want to get into the subtler levels of scanning a person's Qi to check their level, you can palpate and observe the quality of their channels on a physical level to see where they are in their practice. In this way, you can make sure that you drop new students into the correct part of your training system.

Chapter 11

ATTAINMENT OF INTERNAL VIBRATION/LIFE

Everything up until this point in the book has really been establishing the groundwork for entering into the more complex aspects of Nei Gong practice. It is really here, at this stage in your development, that progression without close tuition from a skilled teacher will be nigh on impossible. That being said, I shall discuss the process and explain the theory and experiences at this level, since having an overview of the whole process is always helpful. There is also the issue of the potential risk at this stage of your practice. Everything beyond here involves developing and utilising large amounts of Jing, Qi and Shen. If you think of your body like an electrical circuit, we are going to explore the process of adding more power into this circuit. If the circuit of the body has not been properly prepared, then it can start to short-circuit or 'burn up'. I have seen this happen to varying degrees in people who have tried to run before they can walk in these arts.

Please ensure that you read this chapter and look at it for information purposes, but check with a qualified teacher that you have carried out the groundwork to a high level before even attempting any of the work contained within these pages. The channels should be opened, the microcosmic orbit should be running, and the Qi should be well and truly established within the lower Dan Tian region before any of this work should begin. The channels ensure that excess energies can circulate through your system rather than getting stuck and building serious blockages, and the microcosmic orbit serves to 'earth' any excess energies that rise to the head as well as ensuring that anything that converts 'up' is converted back 'down'. Finally, the lower Dan Tian serves to 'ground' the Qi of the body; this is important as without your energetic base being 'bottom-heavy', you run the risk of the Shen becoming disturbed when you enter into direct work with the spirit.

It is here, at this stage in our development, that we wish to take our body beyond what is 'normal' with regard to levels of Qi. It is the real 'fuel-building' part of the practice. Our personal level of health and well-being will always have a set limit placed upon us by the inherent level of Jing and Qi we were gifted at birth. No matter how efficient we can make the running of our body, it will only take us to the limit of our own inherent capabilities. These limits are individual to us, and there is nothing in the way of justice or fairness involved in this; it just is what it is.

All of the channel opening, purging, nourishing, regulating and Dan Tian development will take our body to a state of efficient functioning. This is what the Daoists called 'returning to a youthful state'. They did not necessarily mean that we act like children, though that is not necessarily a bad thing, but rather that we can regain the abundant health and vitality we experienced in our youth. The assumption here is that you were healthy in your youth, of course!

Now, we wish to move beyond what is within our 'natural capability', to take our body and mind into states of functioning that are at very high levels indeed. This is where the risk comes in; we must have prepared our body for this in order to ensure that it can take the extra 'juice' we are going to work towards developing. This is all based on two things: the generation of extra Yang Qi and the filling of the lower Dan Tian with this Qi. No matter how often books will state that you 'fill' the Dan Tian right from the beginning in your practice, this is not true. Filling the Dan Tian with Qi is a difficult endeavour. There are various methods for doing so and all of them are complex. I am familiar with various systems' ways of doing this, and I will present to you here the safest of the methods that I am familiar with in the Daoist traditions. That being said, there is still risk involved, as adding Qi can lead to stagnation and sickness if the groundwork has not been set. It is for this reason that I always tell new students to forget about any kind of filling of the Dan Tian for a long time; just 'breathe' Qi in and out in your practice as if it were air.

Okay, enough with the discussion of risks! I apologise if I seem a little over-concerned in this introduction with the nature of this kind of work; I just want to ensure that everybody is aware of the risks and proceeds with the correct level of respect for these practices.

Shaping the Yi Through Theory

The mental quality of Ting, 'listening', has been explored within this book a few times already. We shall now look at it in a deeper fashion. This is always the way within Daoism and the internal arts: many of the skills and practices have already been looked at, but we often need to revisit our practices and take our understanding further. Many of the practices you start your training with will be constant exercises you return to over and over. We need to peel away the layers and go closer to the core of what even our most foundational concepts are and how they are applied. Our ability to 'listen' is most certainly one of these revisited concepts. It is within the quality of 'listening' that we can understand how to build more Yang Qi – the fuel we need to fill the lower Dan Tian.

To understand the nature of mental listening, we need to explore the theory behind its development as a skill. It is often this kind of theory that differentiates the knowledge-base of 'outer door' and 'inner door' students. For those who are not familiar with these terms, when you begin with a school or system, you are generally considered an 'outer door' student. This means that you are not a very close student, the teacher teaches you the 'public' aspect of the school's system. With time, if you show dedication, you are then taken as an 'inner door' student. Often, but not always, this is signified with a ceremonial event known as a Bai Shi (拜師). Once you are 'inner door', then many of the school's 'non-public' methods are shared with you. This has long been the way within the internal arts. I have personally been an 'outer door' and 'inner door' student of several teachers. In one case, I have even been Zhu Chu Shi Men (逐出師門) or literally 'thrown out of the door' after being accepted as 'inner door'. This was because I was not Asian and several senior members of the school took issue with this; challenges like this have, sadly, not been uncommon over the years.

The 'outer door' way of being taught is generally to simply be shown an exercise with little in the way of an explanation; certainly, this is generally the case within traditional Asian schools. The training usually goes something like 'This is what you do, this is how you do it, go away and do it lots of times!' An 'inner door' student might well be shown the same exercise, but they are given the 'why' and the 'how' of the practice as well, often in great amounts of detail. The reason for this goes back to your Yi and the afore-discussed principle of Yi Dao Qi Dao that we looked at in the previous chapter. With the mind being involved in the right way, there is a coming together of intention, energetic work and physical practice. This unification of mind, energy and body is where the most effective route into these arts is found.

So, if we look at this with regard to 'listening', then we can understand how this works. The skill of listening within these arts is essentially about conscious absorption of the awareness into the mechanisms of the mind and body so that you have the correct level of mind/body connection. It is here, at this perfect level of awareness, that your attention will serve as a catalyst for the development of personal evolution. Now, if I just tell you to 'listen' to your body, then this is not really an inaccurate instruction. It is true, that is what we are doing. But you are likely to need further instruction so that you actually manage to do this correctly. In this way, I 'shape the Yi' so that it can help you move towards the conscious development of the Gong of listening.

The Gong of Listening

The process of 'listening' is said to happen in three stages. These are 'listening' with your ears, then your mind, and finally 'listening' with your Qi. Each of these is now briefly discussed.

Er Ting (耳聽): Listening with the Ears

As mentioned before, if we begin to look at how we wish for our awareness to interact with our body, then we need to use the expression 'listen'. The other words teachers may use are 'observe/look' or 'feel'.

If we 'observe' or 'look' at what is taking place within the body, then we will start to give the mind permission to create visual feedback. If I look at my Dan Tian, for example, I will see colours, cloudy patterns or sometimes geometric shapes. Whilst these experiences are not 'wrong', they are not helpful either, as they are a form of stimulation for the mind. Giving the mind permission to have visual stimuli will often result in a whole stream of seemingly random thoughts popping into your head one after another; it can be like opening a floodgate of mental action.

As soon as you try to 'feel' what is going on, your body starts to produce reactions, and many of them. It is common to experience a feeling like ants walking on your skin. These somatic experiences can be very unhelpful, as they tend to draw your awareness towards these points. Anybody who has started their meditation only to find that they have an excruciatingly itchy nose will know what I mean by this.

If we 'listen', then we give our attention to whatever our subject is, and this engages our awareness in a more passive manner. The stiller we can allow our mind to grow, the better. It is like this: you cannot listen effectively if you are speaking at the same time; any conversation will show you the truth of this. Thinking is simply speaking without verbalising your thoughts. This means that it is difficult to listen whilst there is a lot of mental activity; you are essentially 'speaking to yourself' over the top of what you are trying to listen to. This is why we want the most mental stillness we can attain in these arts. The quieter your mind, the better you can listen. If we 'look' or 'feel', then we actually generate more movement of the mind and so this gets in the way of the listening process as well.

Initially, it is said, you will 'listen' with your ears. This is generally the first way that a new student will try to listen; obviously, this is because you are used to using your ears in this way. What the teachings are pointing at is that you use the most external and superficial method of trying to listen first (i.e. listening for actual sounds), but you should not be looking for an actual sound. Though auditory experiences may arise, they should be ignored, as they are not important and they will simply generate more mental activity; the acquired mind will enjoy the potential for stimulation!

Xin Ting (心聽): Listening with the Mind

After a while of 'listening with your ears', you will begin to be led towards the stage of 'listening with your mind'. This is another example of the method naturally unfolding for you if you stick with it – Wu Wei and continued practice is the key! The result of this development is that you will naturally begin to bypass the role of the ears and instead begin to 'listen' with your mind. Note that in the direct translation of the Chinese we can see that the character for 'heart' is used instead of 'intention' – 'Xin' instead of 'Yi'. 'Heart' is often used for mind to imply a certain degree of stillness rather than mental action: another reminder of the quality of mind required for effective listening.

When you 'listen with the mind', you actually use the energetic mechanic of listening without the physical aspect of the ears themselves. This begins to merge the awareness with the subject of the body without an external sense function being involved.

Now, a difficulty to be aware of is the engagement of the contemplation process. As soon as the mind starts to become our focus, contemplation starts to arise. This is especially the case if there is no external stimulation from the senses, as in the case of meditative practice. There is nothing for the mind to interact with, but it has faltered in its task of moving towards stillness and so, instead, it begins to 'contemplate'. This is a part of the reason why so many great realisations and insights have come out of meditation: it is the arrival of deep contemplative states. These are highly useful for many aspects of life but not what we are looking for in our practice of 'listening'. To move beyond this state, relax, let go, continue to allow the mind to absorb into what it is doing, and you will move beyond contemplation into deep listening – the final stage of 'listening with the Qi'.

Qi Ting (氣聽): Listening with the Qi

The final stage of Ting is something you have been preparing for with many of the earlier exercises outlined in this book. Up until now, you have been looking to regulate both the breath and mind so that your awareness can absorb into the breath and then, further, into the body. How well you have managed these prior stages will essentially dictate how well you will manage to begin to Qi Ting or 'listen with your Qi'.

When you reach the level of 'listening with your Qi', your awareness will begin to merge with the various flows and pulses of your energy system. It is at this stage that your mind will begin to fully merge and absorb itself into every little nook and cranny of the body. The more open the channels and the more active the Huang, the more 'space' your awareness can reach into. It is here, at this stage, that your mind will begin to melt with your body and flow like a fluid through your entire bodily system. The more you relax the mind, the more it is led through your body like fluid soaking into a sponge. It is here that the mind will begin to 'listen' at a very deep level and stabilise into the structure of your form. This is a profound level of absorption if you can attain it. Figure 11.1 shows the process of conscious absorption through the development of Ting.

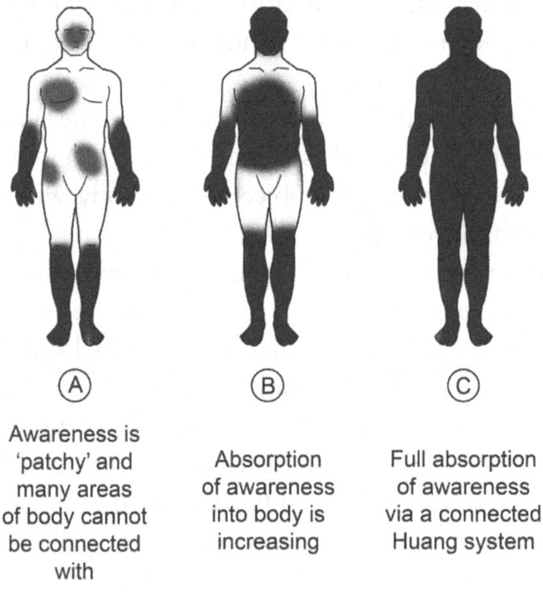

Figure 11.1: Development of Ting

You will know when you have managed to attain this stage of mental cultivation, as the feeling of being drawn into your body is very clear.

All you have to do is mentally 'let go' and your mind will be sucked into the soft tissues of your body as if it was a fluid being drawn into a porous object.

The attainment of this level of Ting is considered a milestone within your practice. It is known as the stage of Shen Qi Xiang He (神氣相合), or 'Shen and Qi harmonise with one another'. This phrase has often been misunderstood to mean that we need to place the mind into the lower Dan Tian and thus bring our attention to our Qi, but it is more complex than this. The process involved in attaining Shen Qi Xiang He is the absorption of the mind into the energetic processes of the body via the process of 'listening' outlined here. In this way, the 'mind' is quietened and the Shen can start to manifest. Shen develops from the stability of the mind within the 'structure' of the energetic matrix. As the two elements of Shen and Qi 'mix' with one another, they will give you access to the production of Yang Qi; we shall get to this very soon.

A Note on the 'Error' of Contemplation

We noted above that when we begin to shut off our sense faculties and absorb our mind into the body, we often find that we begin entering into deep contemplation. This is quite normal and a state that comes after you have silenced many of the thoughts that begin to enter into your mind. Generally, the way the process goes is this: thoughts, emotional movements, and then contemplation. The mind has stopped trying to distract you out of your practice and so now enters into a stiller state. When there is less mental resistance to the process of absorption, then there is a kind of 'bubbling over' of the mind. Though there is activity still, it is less distracted by the outside world and external stimuli. This where your mind works in a very efficient manner, and it can be a very useful tool. That being said, we wish to get past this state too; contemplation is not really going to help us to move towards full absorption of the awareness into the body, the Shen into the Qi, as it is still a form of activity, albeit a more helpful form of movement than the deluge of random thoughts you most likely passed through to get there!

The first thing to realise is that entering into a contemplative state is going to be almost impossible to avoid for a long time in your practice. This means you should not worry about it; resistance to contemplation will pull you back out towards the random thoughts that the acquired mind will generate to draw your attention. Figure 11.2 summarises this process.

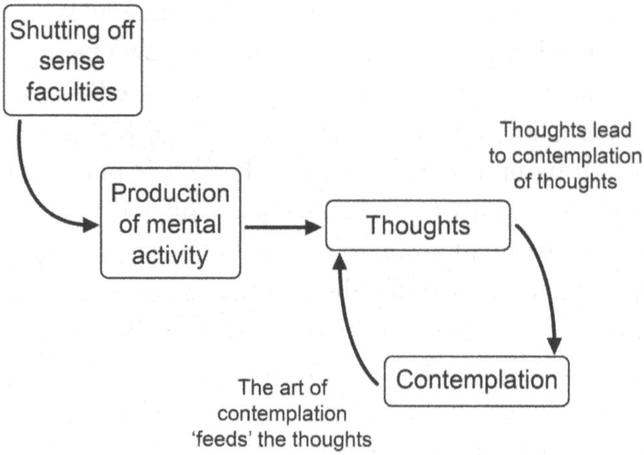

Figure 11.2: Contemplation and Thoughts

The first thing we need to understand when dealing with contemplation is that we will not move past it with any kind of mental force. Instead, we need to look for a form of 'satisfaction' for the mind. We don't add to the state by trying to use our conscious memory, active thought processes or anything like this, but we can give it a direction. We do this by 'planting the seed of theory'. Essentially, your mind is going to contemplate 'something', so why not just give it a nudge in the right direction? To do this, when you enter into a state of contemplation, simply bring the seed of gentle intention that your contemplation will be around the nature of your practice.

This may sound like an odd instruction, and certainly contrary to what many teachers would tell you, but I used to bring my contemplation to the classical scripture of Daoism. I would not 'think' of the scripture in an active sense, I would simply note that my mind was headed in that direction, it was stirring into a subtle form of action, so I would bring to mind, ever so briefly, the teachings of classics such as the Can Tong Qi (參同契) or the Wu Zhen Pian (悟真篇). As soon as my mind was seeded into contemplating these teachings, I would relax the mind and not become involved in the mind's processes. Though I don't really like to mix teachings from different traditions, some of the clearest guidance comes from the Buddhist Tantric teacher Tilopa who advised six mental approaches to developing the mind. These are:

- Don't try to recall
- Don't use your imagination

- Don't try to think
- Don't try to examine
- Don't attempt to govern
- Rest the mind

Though not from within the Daoist tradition, these six guidelines can be applied here very effectively. Allow the mind to continue with its contemplation without being involved and it will start to grow still. This will, in time, begin to lead you on to the stage of 'listening with the Qi'.

This was a tool I used extensively when spending time in monasteries on meditation retreat. Days consisted of teaching from scripture and then silent sitting. I quickly learnt to use the scripture to satisfy the mind. As I then ignored its machinations, I was able to develop beyond this stage into the kind of 'listening' I sought.

The Alchemical Nature of Listening to the Body

The reason why we wish to develop this quality of 'listening' is so that we can begin a very specific alchemical reaction within the body. This reaction is the generation of Yang Qi.

Generally, within Daoism, most of the processes involve three 'ingredients'. Three is a Yang number; in fact, it is the number of Heaven since it is the first uneven, or 'Yang', number aside from the number one which is instead linked to Dao and unification. For this reason, the number three is said to carry a particular type of resonance that can generate transformative power. This is why the number three is used extensively within practices such as Feng Shui and Chinese medicine (treatments involving three needles are said to have a strong effect upon the spirit).

In generating more Qi, we use three ingredients once more – the Shen, the Qi and the Huang. When these three come together, there is a type of reaction that takes place which we can use to generate more energy.

The Shen and the Qi are brought together through the principle of Shen Qi Xiang He discussed above. As we develop the quality of Ting, we enable the awareness to be absorbed into deeper processes until, with time, the mind and the 'energetic fluid' begin to merge with one another. These two then start to react with one another in a cyclical fashion. The more the mind is absorbed into the Qi, the stiller it grows. This stillness then starts to move the lens of acquired mind out of the way, and so the Shen begins to shine through. More Shen equals more stillness, and so the process continues. In this way, the processes of Ting and Shen Qi Xiang He are the alchemical gateway into meditative states of mind.

The Huang is the conductive vessel for the Qi and so, as the mind and energy begin to merge, the mind is drawn like a fluid through the entire body until it is essentially absorbed into the Huang. Once this has been achieved, then the three ingredients we require for increased energy production are in place.

Now, it would be easy to read the above description of the process and mistakenly think that it was very easy; you just put your mind into your body, right? No, I am afraid not; as with everything, it is not 'what' you do but 'how' you do it that is important. The above connection of mind, energy and body is a type of Gong that takes a long time to develop. There are clear signs of when it is starting to take place correctly, and these signs are related to the production of Yang Qi.

Full Absorption into the Body

To understand the process of absorption into the body, we first need to look at three terms that are used within the alternative arts scene. These terms are 'stillness', 'stability' and 'emptiness'. In Chinese, these are: Jing (靜) or 'stillness', Ding (定) or 'stabilise' and Xu (虛) or 'emptiness'. Often, these terms are used interchangeably when, in fact, they have very different meanings. Understanding a term's definition is a very important part of understanding what it is we are trying to achieve. To absorb the mind into the body and generate Yang Qi, we require stability of the mind; this quality is then further developed by how much mental stillness we can attain.

Stillness

The mind is 'still' when the 'waves' of the acquired mind are no longer present upon the 'ocean' of consciousness. We develop stillness within Daoism through the development of the quality of Ting combined with a growing awareness of letting go through Song. As with many things, stillness is a gradient rather than an absolute. This means that there are various levels of stillness depending upon your cultivation. If we place stillness onto a graph, as shown in Figure 11.3, we can see that we only need to attain a certain degree of stillness before we can attain the quality of 'mental stability'.

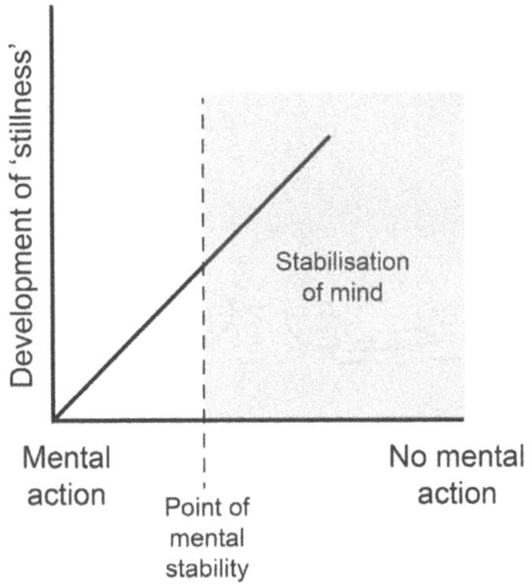

Figure 11.3: The Gradient of Stillness

The classical instruction is simply Jing Ding (靜定) or 'development of stillness leads to stability'.

Stability

When a certain degree of mental stillness has been achieved, then the mind will become 'stable'. It is this degree of stillness that we require for the production of extra energy within the body: more Yang Qi. Stability of the mind means that it is able to 'hold a shape'. To understand this, we need to see the 'fluid of the mind' as having a kind of form. When the mind is in motion, its form is always shifting. When we develop a high enough level of stillness, we can allow the shape of the mind to anchor into a structure, in this case our body. When the mind can anchor into our body, then it is given a place to stabilise and so the shifting of the mind's form grows still; we are now mentally stable.

Because of the associations we have with the term in the West, many have assumed that 'mentally stable' within the Daoist arts meant to be free from emotions. In part, this could be true – the emotions are forms of shifting energy, they cause the mind to move – but it is not how the term is being used. To 'Ding' the mind means for the Huang to be fully opened so that it can conduct the Qi, and so the mind can soak through into its structure and thus enable you to become fully absorbed into the body. When this happens, the shape of the mind is stable within your form. This process is summarised in Figure 11.4.

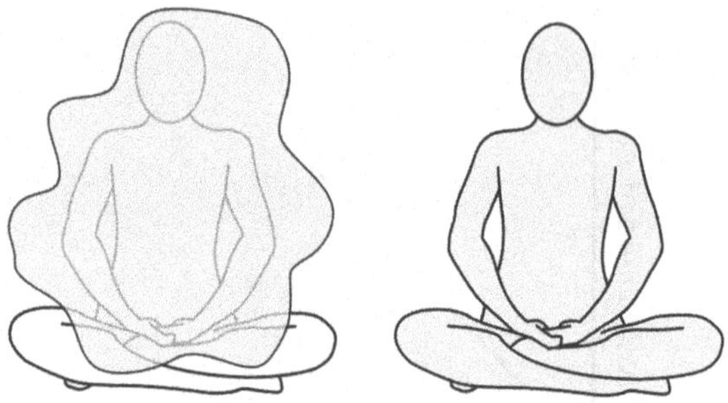

Figure 11.4: Stabilisation of the Mind

When the mind is stable, it helps a greater degree of stillness to develop, yet the terms 'stability' and 'stillness' refer to very different parts of the process of cultivating the mind.

Emptiness

The final term, 'emptiness', is often used interchangeably with 'stillness', but – at least within Daoism – they are not the same thing. We shall look at emptiness more in the next chapter, as it is very important when looking at understanding the mind and its evolution into Shen and Dao. For now, though, it is enough to understand that emptiness in Daoism essentially means 'empty of form'. This is an emptiness of 'thought forms' as well as a complete emptiness of 'form awareness'. This is reached by developing stillness to a high level.

Absorption Practice

To develop the Yang Qi, we need to go through the process described above and fully absorb the awareness into the body. When the correct level of Gong has been attained and the mind can 'listen' in the correct manner, then the Huang will actually start to produce more Yang Qi. It is one of the highest levels of development within the sinew-changing classical teachings that the 'sinews' will produce more Qi. In fact, even though the Sinew-Changing Classic says 'sinews', it is actually the Huang where this energy production takes place. Most likely this is on a cellular level, but since I am not a scientist in any way, I will keep things simple! The Daoists never discussed cells; they instead said that the 'sinews' (meaning Huang) produced more Qi when the unification of Shen, Qi and body could take place.

To practise this, it is easiest to sit in a meditative posture or in a chair, as shown in Figure 11.5.

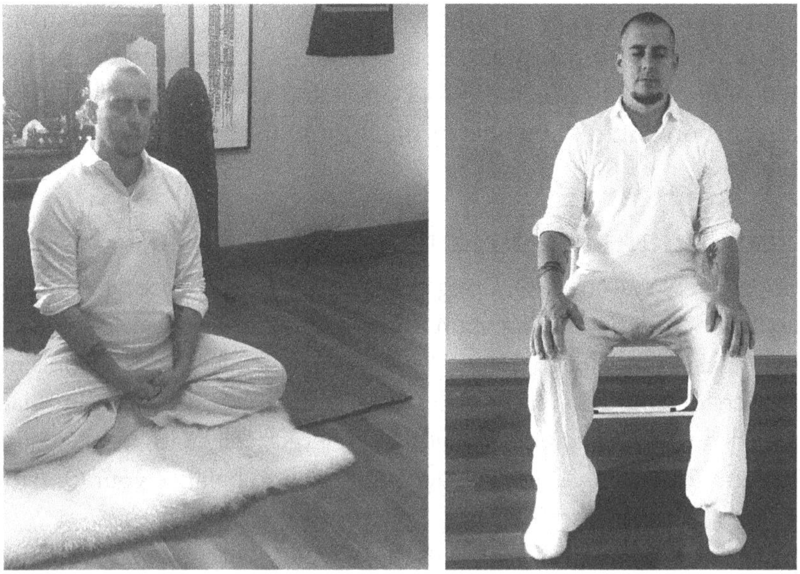

Figure 11.5: Absorption Postures

To be seated on the floor is preferred, as there are various energetic qualities to a seated meditation posture that are beneficial to the practice, but if you are injured or cannot be on the floor for whatever reason, then sit in a chair as shown. Just ensure that your back is upright, meaning that you should not use the backrest of the chair.

If the channel system is opened up, then the Qi will be conducting through the entirety of the body's Huang. This will enable the awareness to absorb all the way through the body, right to its core. You will have a stable awareness of your entire form.

When the mind is stabilised into the whole body, then keep 'stepping back' with the strength of your mind. It is said that the mind should be Gu (固), meaning 'firm' or 'unwavering' in quality, but at the same time Rou (柔), or 'soft'. You should keep relaxing the mind, or 'step back' with it, as I tell my students, until you find the right balance. The awareness will maintain the quality of listening through absorption into the body and yet be relaxed enough that there is as little mental focus as possible. It is all about that central point once more: too focused, and there will be mental action, so your ability to 'listen' is compromised; too much relaxation, and the mind will disperse out of the anchor of the Huang – this will result in daydreaming and thus mental activity once more. Firm but soft, this is the quality of mind we seek.

You should remain with this practice until the Yang Qi begins to appear within the body. When it begins to manifest, this means your mind is at the right point; use this as a marker. When the Yang Qi begins to manifest, then simply 'listen' to this process but try not to become too focused upon it. Focus will condense the mind to a point and so slow down the process. Remain anchored into the whole of the form as the process develops.

Tree-Balancing Practice

Almost every system of Qi Gong utilises working with trees, though to varying degrees depending upon the system. Such practice is generally known as Ping Heng Gong (平衡功) 'balancing and harmonising practice' or Shu Liao Fa (樹療法) 'tree therapy'. In general, Shu Liao Fa is the widespread name for working energetically with trees, whilst the term Ping Heng Gong can actually mean to balance your Qi with a variety of natural entities, not only trees.

The reason that trees were used so heavily within Daoist practice was that they were seen as great conduits of Qi that existed between the poles of Heaven and Earth. Generally, during the daytime, a tree 'breathes in' Qi, and so they can be used to help purge you of pathogenic energies. During the evening and night time, a tree 'breathes out', and so they can be used to help replenish deficiencies of your Qi. Remember, though, that these practices are adjunct practices to the wider arts of Nei Gong and, as such, are never going to be as strong as other parts of the system. They are simply used to assist you in regulating your own energy system in line with the Qi of the tree you are practising with.

There are various exercises and methods for working with trees, but these are not actually very important. If your energy system is awake, then it is not too difficult to connect with a tree's Qi; simply stand close to the tree, facing it, relax and begin your Qi Gong with a shared absorption of your awareness into your own body as well as into the trunk of the tree. Within a short while, there is a clear transference of Qi between yourself and the tree; once this starts to take place, simply relax and allow the process to work for you. Many of the Ba Chu can arise as well as a degree of Zi Fa Gong; all of these should be acknowledged and ignored, and then you can simply enjoy the experience of connecting with a tree's energetic field!

In general, a tall healthy tree is a good enough place to start your practice. This will ensure a healthy level of Qi within your 'practice partner', but then, there are also variations from tree to tree as they carry different vibrations that resonate with different internal organs. The list below is a starting point for your selection of trees to work with:

- Apple – Heart, Spleen and Lungs
- Ash – Spleen; also has a warming and moving action on the body's Qi
- Beech – Lungs; a very relaxing tree that can calm stress
- Birch – This is a detoxifying tree that purges pathogenic Qi strongly
- Cherry – Spleen; nourishes the Blood
- Cyprus – Kidneys; a strong nourishing tree for the body
- Elm – Intestines; a 'cleaning' tree for the guts
- Gingko – Kidneys, Liver; has a warming effect on the body's Qi
- Hawthorn – Spleen, Stomach and Liver; helps to move the Blood
- Hazel – Spleen, Stomach and Liver
- Holly – Clears pathogens, helps with arthritis
- Juniper – Kidneys and Liver
- Larch – Liver; a regulating tree for the body's Qi
- Maple – Heart; lifts the mood and helps clear depression
- Oak – Liver, Kidneys and Spine
- Pine – Liver, Spine; 'smooths' the Qi
- Rowan – Strengthens the immune system and helps prevent serious disease
- Spruce – Liver, Spine and tendons
- Sycamore – Spine, Liver and Kidneys

- Willow – Helps with all digestive disorders and calms the mind
- Yew – Spleen and pancreas

After you have finished your practice, you should sit down quietly with the tree, as close to its roots as possible, and simply breathe; many will find that this instruction is not really required, as there is a strong urge to do this anyway.

Attainment of Internal 'Life'

When the Yang Qi is starting to be produced within the Huang of the body, it will have a very clear quality to it. It is a form of internal vibration that is at a very high frequency. It can be felt all over the body and, for want of a better description, it feels like 'life' itself. Once you have felt this reaction, you will understand clearly why Qi has so often been translated into English as 'energy'. It is a warm, vibrating energy that manifests all over the body, from the level of the skin all the way through to your core. Basically, it will appear wherever you can apply Ting into the body. Some areas of the body produce more Qi than other areas, but still, the Huang of the entire body is a 'factory' for this process. Remember, though, that this is still 'distorted Yang Qi', as discussed in Chapter 9. It is still a form of Qi that is subject to the nature of our acquired mind; purifying the Yang Qi is a much later stage and really takes place through alchemical meditative training.

When the Qi begins to develop within your tissues, it will feel warm and 'activating'. It is a very clear vibration that shakes the whole of the inside of the body. It is very different from the vibration of Zi Fa Gong; it is a more subtle and faster energy that feels like it is energising the body.

Keep with this practice and, with time, it will begin to change into a stronger form. This will feel like a mild form of 'fluid electricity' that runs around inside of the body's channel system. It is not a painful sensation but definitely strong in quality. You are feeling the power within the 'circuitry' of your channel system at this stage.

It can take several weeks of working on this practice before the Yang Qi produced reaches this stage, so persevere. The less stability in your mind and the worse your ability to 'listen', the less efficient your production of Yang Qi will be.

Be careful with this practice, though: it is very Yang and stimulating in nature. Do not allow the body to become too 'hyper'. The absolute longest you should practise in this way is for an hour a session, and do not practise more than one session per day. If you go beyond this time, then you run the risk of causing yourself problems. The body needs time to normalise what is going on – if it leads to insomnia or headaches, then slow down and proceed more carefully; consider returning to the foundation work of opening the channels, as perhaps your body is not prepared enough for this kind of work.

Progressing into the Core

Keep with this practice on a regular basis until the Yang Qi is ready to move. You will know this is taking place as the feeling of vibration or electrical current will begin to shift into the central core of your body. It will move into your middle as if there is a column through the centre of your body, as shown in Figure 11.6.

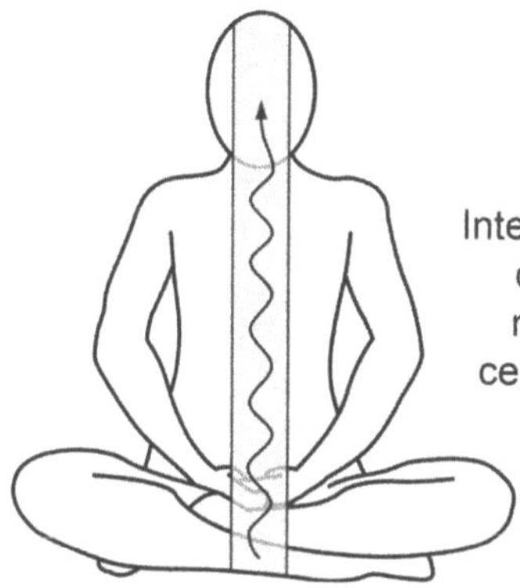

Figure 11.6: The Central Column

This is sometimes known as the 'Central channel' or the 'Taiji Pole' within Daoist traditions. This is a place of very high energetic conduction that will draw the Yang Qi inwards when it is time to move. The result will be a high-frequency vibration running through the centre of your body. It is now time to start leading the Yang Qi towards the lower Dan Tian. Note that this is the absolute earliest point in the Nei Gong process where we begin to lead Qi to the lower Dan Tian for it to be stored. We have previously 'sunk' existing Qi to the Dan Tian, but this has been so that it can circulate into the channels. It is only now, at this advanced stage, that we actually try to 'store' anything. This is contrary to what many schools teach, whereby they try to store Qi in the lower Dan Tian right from the outset of their practice. At best, these methods are useless and so nothing will happen; at worst, they have an effective method and so run the risk of doing themselves harm with this kind of practice.

Filling the Dan Tian

There are three key phrases within Qi Gong society that summarise exactly what we need to do in order to fill the lower Dan Tian with Qi. If we can understand the energetic mechanics behind these phrases, then it is possible to understand how Qi is built up within the lower Dan Tian. These three phrases are discussed below.

Yi Shou Dan Tian (意守丹田): 'Guard the Mind Within the Dan Tian'

Initially, when the Qi needs to be led towards the lower Dan Tian, we need to bring our awareness down to the lower abdomen. In fact, you don't need to be all that exact. Bring your mind down to the lower abdominal cavity and you will find that the Qi begins to move. Here is the key, though: do not 'lead' the Qi with intention; the creation of a mental action in this way will cause the Yang Qi to begin dispersing. Yang Qi is 'fragile' in a way; though it has been built in the Huang of the body, it is quick to disperse. Instead of 'leading' the Qi with intent, simply lower the mind down towards the abdomen. Let it sink under its own 'weight'. The Yang Qi will then be naturally led towards the abdominal cavity with minimal force being used. In this way, the passive action of 'sinking' the mind will be all the effort you require. The result of this will be that the vibrating sensation of the Yang Qi will begin to sink through the body towards your abdomen along with your mind.

This is where the skill now comes in; by moving your mind within the body, it will have a tendency to start generating thought. Do not allow this to happen. This is why it is said that the Yi needs to be Shou, or 'guarded'. The mind needs guarding from invasion by thoughts and mental action. Excessive thinking will disturb the Yang Qi and use it up; guard your mind, keep the senses sealed and maintain the relative stillness and stability of your awareness.

Qi Chen Dan Tian (氣沉丹田): 'Submerge the Qi in the Dan Tian'

The Yang Qi should then be 'submerged' within the Dan Tian. What is the Yang Qi submerged within? Yin Qi is the answer. We have already seen how the field of the lower Dan Tian is formed from Yin Qi, and we shall return to this shortly. We now need to submerge the Yang Qi within the Yin Qi by bringing it into the lower Dan Tian field. This process is indicated within the Yi Jing by the hexagrams Ji Ji (既濟) and Wei Ji (未濟). These two symbols are shown in Figure 11.7.

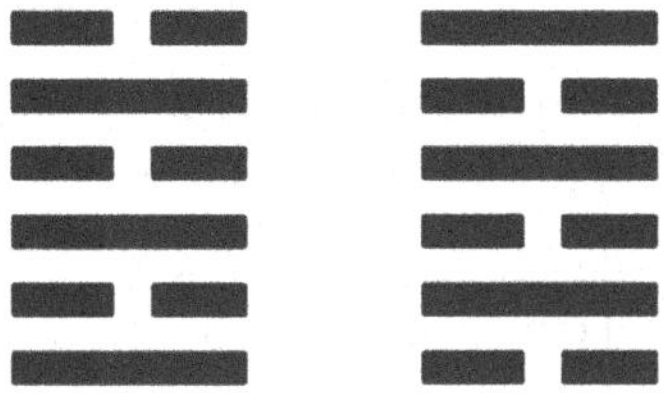

Figure 11.7: Ji Ji and Wei Ji Hexagrams

Ji Ji shows Fire submerged within Water and is named 'after completion'. The Yang Qi has been submerged within the Yin Qi field, and so our work is done with regard to the relationship between the two. Wei Ji shows Fire and Water before this process takes place and is named 'before completion'. In this second symbol, the Fire has not yet been submerged and so they still need work. Remember that the symbols for Fire and Water are used instead of Heaven and Earth (pure Yang and Yin) since our Qi is in an acquired state of being; it is distorted by our acquired mind and mundane thinking.

Dan Tian Xi Qi (丹田吸氣): 'Dan Tian Inhales the Qi'

In order for the Yang Qi to be 'submerged' in Yin Qi, it first has to be drawn towards the lower Dan Tian field. We can begin this process by developing the Yang Qi within our Huang and then sinking the awareness to our abdominal cavity, but still, the lower Dan Tian will not yet take the Yang Qi within its interior. It is a curious thing that even though the Yang Qi will benefit us greatly by entering into the field of the lower Dan Tian, the body is resistant to this happening. This is why, in most cases, the first attempts you make at storing your Yang Qi will be futile. There will be a 'leaking' of the Qi out of the abdominal cavity. It is as frustrating as trying to grasp at clouds.

This is where the character of 'Xi' comes in. This can be translated as 'to inhale', but it also means 'to suck' (a literal breakdown of the character shows the action of 'grabbing' through the mouth).

The Yang Qi is 'Xi' towards the lower Dan Tian because of the way that Yin and Yang relate to one another. Like two magnets, they are drawn to one another. If we wish to draw Yang Qi into the lower Dan Tian or 'inhale' it into the lower Dan Tian space, then we need to develop the Yin Qi qualities of the Dan Tian's 'form'. Through the development of Yin, we draw in the Yang that we have created through our absorbed awareness.

It should be noted here that the alternative phrase of Dan Tian Hu Xi (丹田呼吸) is sometimes used in place of Dan Tian Xi Qi. Dan Tian Hu Xi literally means 'Dan Tian breathing'. Many have mistakenly believed this phrase referred to some kind of Qi Gong exercise whereby the Dan Tian expanded and contracted or something similar, but this is an error in understanding. The Dan Tian 'breathes' the Yang Qi in and out through the action of Yin 'inhaling' Yang towards its core. This is a manifestation of many of the alchemical directions of 'immersing Fire in Water', a common phrase within Daoist classics that has meaning on many levels. In the case of Qi Gong and Nei Gong, this is what it refers to. In the case of consciousness, there are further meanings for Fire and Water. If you wish to read about this, then please refer to *White Moon on the Mountain Peak: The Alchemical Firing Process of Nei Dan* (Singing Dragon, 2016).

Return to Lower Dan Tian (Yin Qi)

We have already looked at the nature of the Dan Tian – the lower Dan Tian more specifically – and how we can develop it. Much of your work with the lower Dan Tian up until this stage has been to help consolidate the existing Qi within your body so that a spherical field can be built. By the time you start working at the level of practice outlined within this chapter, you should already have carried out a lot of development with the lower Dan Tian. The channels should be opened up to a high degree and you should understand the nature of circulating Qi through the lower Dan Tian's action.

It is now, at this stage, that we wish to really further our lower Dan Tian cultivation. We need to learn how to draw the Yang Qi down towards the Dan Tian centre, and to do this, we need to develop its Yin qualities. This can be complex to understand, so let us first look at several factors that characterise Yin Qi.

You already have a certain degree of Yin Qi within your body, just like you have a certain inherent amount of Yang Qi. We work with our existing Yin Qi by developing the lower Dan Tian, just like we work with our existing Yang Qi by stabilising the mind and helping our body to function as efficiently as possible.

To build 'extra' Yang Qi, we need to absorb the awareness into the Huang and stabilise the mind there. This will then, in turn, help the Huang to become a kind of factory for the production of Yang Qi as discussed above. This is difficult but possible if we bring our practice to a high enough level. Yin Qi does not work like this; to build 'extra' Yin Qi is impossible through any method or practice. Existing 'Yin Qi practices' always work with the inherent levels of Yin Qi we already have within our body. This means that we need to find another method for drawing in 'extra' Yin Qi.

We do this by building Yang Qi and drawing it into the field of the lower Dan Tian. Under the natural law of attraction, the build-up of Yang Qi will reach a point of critical mass and so Yin Qi will be drawn into the Dan Tian space as well. This Qi is derived from the environment and is led as a natural response to the level of Yang Qi you have built. This means that your process goes as follows:

- Develop existing Yin Qi within the lower abdominal space by consolidating the lower Dan Tian.
- Build extra Yang Qi through absorption of awareness into the Huang.
- Draw this extra Yang Qi to the Dan Tian under the law of Yin and Yang's attraction.
- Finally, use this extra Yang Qi stored within the lower Dan Tian to draw in extra Yin Qi.

Your level of Yin Qi within the lower Dan Tian structure is dependent upon both the amount of 'field consolidation' you have managed to accomplish at the foundation levels of the training and the strength of your Kidneys. Your Kidneys are esoterically linked to the body's ability to develop and maintain 'magnetic' fields within the body. As your Kidneys decline, then Yin declines and the nature of the various fields within your body starts to diffuse. This leads to leakages of Qi and a deterioration in your health. For this reason, we need to look after our Kidney health according to Chinese medicine principles. The Jing needs to be worked with, developed and stilled to a certain degree, as discussed in Chapter 7.

The Qi that we have been using to engage the Huang up until this point has primarily been the Yang Qi. The Yang Qi moves in a linear fashion through the Huang and causes a reaction along its length as the two meet one another. This is a great deal of the sinew-changing teachings' focus. We now need to start using Yin Qi to do the same. The difference, though, is that Yin Qi forms the Huang into spheres rather than lines. This is very important. All of the bodywork we have completed so far has set the scenes for this stage: the building of internal circles within the body using the influence of Yin Qi upon the Huang.

The building of internal spheres through the action of the lower Dan Tian and the Yin Qi field is the next stage in our development. There are three spheres we need to build: the central sphere of the abdomen and the two outer spheres of the torso.

Central Sphere of the Abdomen

The central sphere of the abdomen is essentially the physical component of the lower Dan Tian. It is often missed that the lower Dan Tian has a very physical aspect to it as well when we reach the higher levels of training. We can develop the Dan Tian beyond the realm of simple energetics and manifest its patterning within our physical body too. To some degree, this will already have begun when the Huang begins to reshape within the abdominal cavity, but we wish to take this further so that our Dan Tian can have a physical form.

The Outer Spheres of the Torso

The two outer spheres of the torso are a 'rounding' of the Huang within the abdominal and thoracic cavities of the body. The diaphragm is the main divider between these two spheres. When the two outer spheres of the body are formed, they will feel as though the body is shaped as shown in Figure 11.8. This is known as 'building the gourd'.

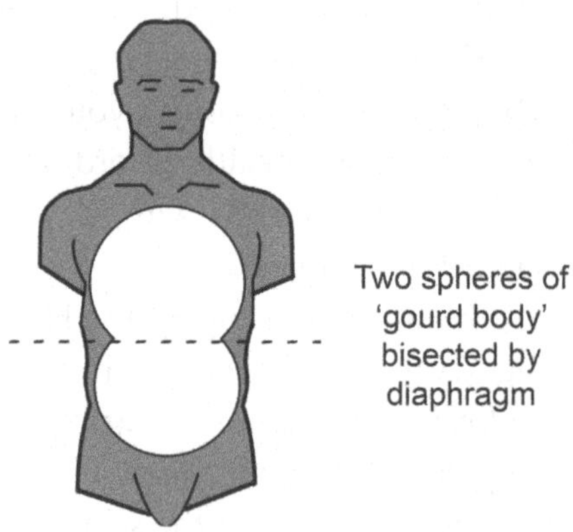

Figure 11.8: The Gourd Body

The Daoist Hu Lu (葫蘆), or 'gourd', has long been an important symbol within the Daoist traditions. If you have not seen a Daoist gourd, it is shaped as shown in Figure 11.9. It is this distinctive shape that we need to build into the two largest cavities of the torso.

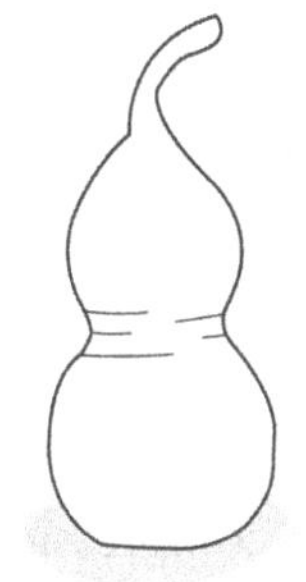

Figure 11.9: Daoist Gourd

The important Daoist immortal Li Tie Guai (李鐵拐) carried his 'immortal medicine' within the gourd and the monkey king Sun Wu Kong (孫悟空) once tricked some demons into believing that he had trapped Heaven and Earth within his gourd! These are, of course, allegorical stories. The 'immortal medicine' contained within Li Tie Guai's gourd is a representation of the various energetic and spiritual substances that are alchemically developed within the body. The 'Heaven and Earth' of Sun Wu Kong's gourd are a demonstration of the coming together of spirit and body that can take place to a very high level within the space of the 'gourd body'. Many Daoist deities and practitioners of alchemy are associated with these gourds and, as always within Daoism, these symbols held a very practical meaning.

Let us look at the building and the function of these various aspects of the internal body in turn.

The 'Form' of the Dan Tian

The lower Dan Tian is Yin in comparison to the upper Dan Tian which is the most Yang of the Dan Tian. Yin is linked to 'form', and so the lower Dan Tian has a physical structure to it at the later stages in its development. The upper Dan Tian is Yang. Yang is linked to more ethereal states; this means that the upper Dan Tian needs to be expanded outwards beyond the limitations of physical structure.

The physical form of the lower Dan Tian is built from the Huang of the abdominal cavity. This initially starts to happen as the Yin Qi field becomes strong enough that it begins to 'grip' and shape the Huang into a rounded pattern. No doubt, by this stage in your practice, you will already have experienced this happening. During some of your practice, the Huang of the abdomen begin to be 'gripped' by the Qi within your abdomen and so they begin to squeeze. The experience is much like something is starting to tighten or engage deep within the centre of your abdominal cavity. It is like a muscular contraction but much deeper within the body. It is normal for these 'squeezings' to come and go during the development of the lower Dan Tian throughout your Nei Gong practice.

We now want to take the mechanic behind the 'gripping' of the Huang and use it to our advantage. To do this, we use a very simple Qi Gong method that many people will already be familiar with. This is the exercise shown in Figure 11.10, the 'Dan Tian compression' exercise.

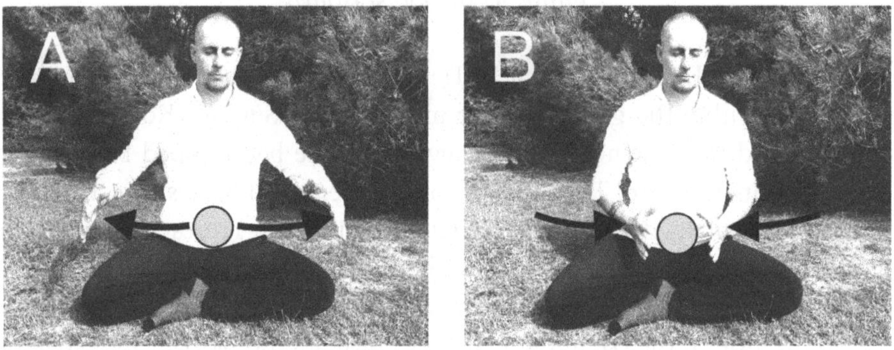

Figure 11.10: Dan Tian Compression

We stay in a seated position, as shown in Figure 11.10, and hold our hands at the side of the lower abdominal cavity. There is no need to connect the movements of our hands with our breathing, but if you prefer to do so, then this is fine as well. We simply move the hands apart, as shown in image A, and then bring them back together, as shown in image B. We repeat this movement very slowly with a high level of absorption of the awareness into the structure of the Huang.

Now, many people will have done similar exercises either standing or sitting, but they will often have missed the most important detail. This is the compression of the lower Dan Tian. Beginners will not be able to do this; it will depend upon how much of the foundation work they have worked through. If the channels are open and the Qi is reaching the hands, then a very important phenomenon will begin to take place – the hands will start to affect the movement of the Yin Qi field and how it interacts with the Huang.

The Hands and Yin Qi

In the centre of the palms are two important acupuncture points known as Lao Gong (劳宫), or the 'palace of toil' points. These are two very large places on the body where the Qi will conduct out into the surrounding environment. These points are important, as they have a magnetic resonance of their own. Many beginners to Qi Gong will stumble across this by accident when they start out in their practice, as they will feel a kind of 'energy ball' between their palms. It is as if you are squeezing some unknown force between the palms. Often, this feeling develops in the earliest stages of your Qi Gong journey but should then vanish after a while, as the body normalises the experience. What you are feeling is the repelling of two identical poles of a magnetic field that is generated by the Lao Gong points of the hands. This practice is often known as 'building the ball' within Qi Gong schools.

The field that is felt in these early stages of Qi Gong training is not strong enough for what we want at this stage in our practice. We need to build it by opening the channels of the arms and delivering more Yang Qi to the palms. The accumulation of Qi in the palms will then serve to build the field in the palms. In most cases, this is accomplished through diligent practice of Qi Gong, but I have also met teachers who opened these points for their students by pushing Qi into their palms. In my early teens, I had a teacher do this for me and it certainly sped the process along. In other cases, some people open the points with so much force and pressure that it actually bursts the blood vessels in the centre of the palms and a stigmata-like bleeding occurs; this is rare, but nothing to worry about if it happens, as it is a normal and temporary reaction.

When the field within the hands is strong enough, they can be used to influence the Yin Qi field of the lower Dan Tian. It should already have been consolidated to a high degree through our prior work, and so the function of the 'Dan Tian compression' exercise should naturally arise out of your practice.

When the hands move close together, they have an influence upon the Yin Qi field of the lower Dan Tian. It is important to understand that it is the field of the lower Dan Tian being 'squeezed' and not the energy between the palms. The energy between the palms is somewhat irrelevant at this stage. Any sensation there should be ignored so that your awareness can remain Shou, or 'guarded', within the lower abdominal space.

As the Yin Qi field of the lower abdomen starts to be distorted by the coming together of your palms, it will start to affect the Huang and they will stretch under the action of your hand motions. As you repeat the movement of the exercise, you should find that you can almost 'pack' the Huang into a spherical shape within the lower abdominal cavity; it is almost as if you are shaping clay.

Once you get a feel for this, you will find the optimum distance for where to bring your hands. Too close together, and there is too much compression within the abdomen; this can be bad for your health as it can lead to stagnation of Qi. You should squeeze the hands and Huang to the point whereby the Yin Qi field only just begins to shape the Huang, and this can tangibly be felt inside the lower abdomen. Once you have this process started, you should be able to move the hands around the lower abdomen as you like, always with Lao Gong facing Lao Gong of the opposite palm, but changing the angle of the palms so that you are shaping the Dan Tian's form in a three-dimensional fashion.

This process should be continued for some time. You will know when it is at a high enough level as the movement and rotation of the lower Dan Tian can now be palpated and felt by another person if they place their hands onto your body. When you rotate or shift the lower Dan Tian field with your intention (not physical muscular contraction), the Huang under the skin will shift and rotate with the field. This gives the feeling of a solid, somewhat inflated ball moving around within the abdomen. In many cases, if you are practised enough, it is also clearly visible.

I should reiterate here, this is not a rotation of the abdomen that is initiated through muscular contraction of any sort. It is not the undulating abdomen of a belly dancer either. It is the turning of the Yin field through the use of intention, Yi. As the Yin Qi field begins to rotate, it 'drags' the Huang with it, and the result is that the soft tissues of the body are curved and moved like an organic sphere beneath the skin and muscles of the abdominal wall. I have seen students and teachers of the internal arts try to emulate this movement 'externally', but if you have felt the real thing, it is very different. Anybody can achieve it, it just takes practice and development of the Yin Qi field.

Building the Gourd

Beyond the building of the lower Dan Tian's physical structure, we also need to generate the spheres of the torso – the gourd body. To do this, we use the same process as described above. We employ the energetic influence of the palms to generate an engagement and shaping of the Huang within the body. This is done through the practice of the exercise shown in Figure 11.11. This exercise is called 'building the gourd'.

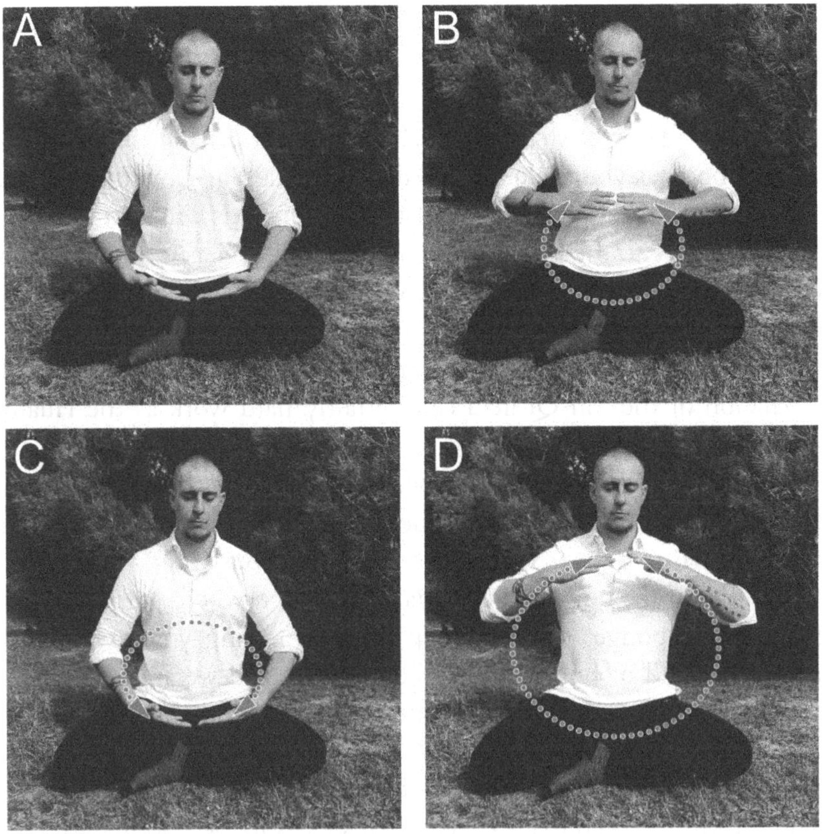

Figure 11.11: Building the Gourd Exercise

The lower circle of the gourd is completed by moving the arms from just above the pubic bone to the height of the diaphragm. The hands begin at the lower position with your palms facing upwards. They then trace around a circle, as shown in Figure 11.11, until they reach the diaphragm. Now, the palms are facing downwards. It is a simple and intuitive movement: simply trace around the edge of a circle that is the same height as your torso from the pubic bone to the diaphragm.

Once you have completed this circle, reverse the process and return to the starting position.

Now, begin the second circle. This time, we move the hands in the same circular fashion, but all the way from just above the pubic bone to the top of the thoracic cavity, up the height of the base of the neck. Once again, when you reach the height of the neck, reverse the process and trace back around the circle with your palms to the starting position.

This too is a very common Qi Gong movement contained within many exercises, but people often miss the rationale behind the movements, as they have not successfully developed the foundations of Yin Qi connecting to the Huang.

If you are managing to connect with this exercise, then you will feel what is a very strong stretching and shaping of the Huang that takes place within the body as your palms begin to distort the Yin Qi within the space of your body. The reaction means that the Yin Qi fields will start to generate a rounded quality to the body's soft tissues. It will feel as if you are shaping a clay vessel into the shape of the gourd body as shown in Figure 11.8. It can be surprising just how much power this takes sometimes. There can be a great deal of resistance, as the Huang is quite strong within the body. The manipulation of the Yin Qi field can be fairly hard work as the Huang is dragged into this spherical shape.

Though it feels like the inside of your body is becoming a gourd (or 'snowman body' as my students sometimes call it), you are obviously not creating two large hollow spheres. As stated previously, the Huang fills all of the cavities of the body and essentially runs everywhere. It is the physical matter of the 'sponge' that soaks up your Qi during your training. The Huang has a kind of honeycomb structure to it, and we are curving all of the fibres of this honeycomb structure within the abdomen. In all of the spaces around the viscera, there is a rounding of the Huang so that your body starts to take on a slightly spherical quality inside. Many people have misunderstood and tried to create 'external' circles in their body during their Qi Gong practice. They do this by rounding the shoulders, back and arms. This is a huge error; it creates stagnation, as it is not natural for the body to do this. The 'rounding' process should be inside of the body, within the Huang. The gourd is inside of you, even if it is not that visibly evident on the outside.

Continue with this exercise for some time until there is a clear feeling of the body having been reshaped in this fashion; most likely, this will take around a year or so of daily practice. You will know when it has been achieved to a high enough level as only now will the Qi really start to move comfortably into the lower Dan Tian.

Filling the Dan Tian

Once the body has been reformed in the way discussed above, you will be able to Dan Tian Xi Qi, to 'inhale' the Qi into the Dan Tian where it shall remain Chen or 'submerged'. The change from linear-type patterning within the Huang to large internal spheres will mean that the Yang Qi will begin to spiral around inside of the body instead of simply being 'discharged' out of the linear channel system. Your body will now function as a combination of circulations within the orbits you have developed and within the torso itself.

When the Yang Qi is generated, then it can be led down to the Dan Tian where it will enter into the spherical Huang and conduct in the way shown in Figure 11.12. This will ensure that the Qi remains within the Dan Tian region.

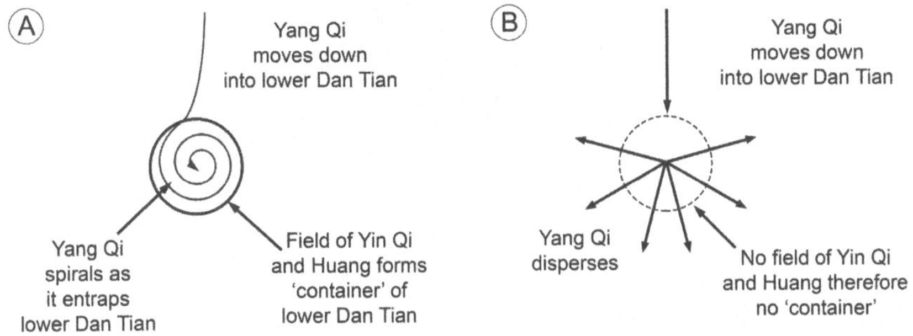

Figure 11.12: Conduction of Yang Qi into Dan Tian

Figure A shows how the Qi will now move through the Dan Tian space, whilst image B shows how it would previously have moved if the Yin Qi field had not been used to reshape the Huang in the right way.

The Yang Qi now only needs to reach the lower abdominal cavity where it will then begin to be drawn into the space within the middle of the Yin Qi field. Yin will draw Yang towards it, and thus the Qi is stored. The shaping of the Huang built the physical shell of the Dan Tian, the 'walls' of the container. If we try to put Qi into a container that does not yet exist, it is like trying to fill a glass that is not there.

Once you have achieved this level of training, you can continue to build Yang Qi and fill the Dan Tian with it. This will begin to take you beyond the inherent levels of Qi that previously were a limit for you. The 'battery' of the Dan Tian can be filled up for a long time, there is plenty of space!

Merging Yin and Yang

It should be noted here that where Yang Qi goes, Yin Qi will also start to follow. This means that now you have the ability to store Yang Qi within the container of the lower Dan Tian, extra Yin Qi will naturally be drawn towards the Yang Qi and enter into the lower Dan Tian as well. The two will react with one another and begin to circulate within the lower Dan Tian in a continuous fashion. Because of the spiralling of Qi that takes place within the Huang 'form' of the lower Dan Tian, it will move the Qi around in a cycle. This was represented with the symbol shown in Figure 11.13, the Taiji Tu (太極圖).

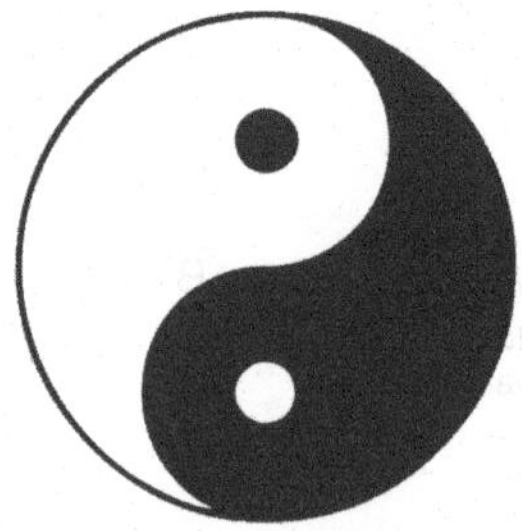

Figure 11.13: Taiji Tu

This symbol was often placed on the lower abdomens of statues and depictions of deities to show both the rotation of the Dan Tian as well as the 'churning' of the Yin and Yang Qi within the Dan Tian vessel. There is a dot of black and white contained within each opposite pole to show the existence of distortions within this Qi; it is still Fire and Water, not pure Yang and Yin at this stage, even though we use the terminology of Yin and Yang Qi within the teachings.

The Qi will build up within the lower Dan Tian, and this is enough for taking you to very high levels of training and development. Beyond this, in the following chapters, we shall look at how this accumulated Qi may be used in the realms of spiritual development and some other areas of practice.

There are also, however, Nei Gong schools that aim to squeeze these two poles together so that the Yin Qi and Yang Qi fully merge with one another. There are various ways in which this can happen, but these methods are rarely shared, and certainly forbidden from being written down or shared publicly. One of the main reasons for this is the sheer level of risk involved in doing this. Yin and Yang may well attract one another, but they do not wish to be squeezed back together and merged into one united entity. To do so takes a lot of power and most certainly careful guidance from a very skilled master. It should never be attempted through guesswork or instructions in written format. This is because it is here, at this level of work, that an error can lead to death. Many reading this will think I am being overly dramatic, but this is not the case. Compression of Yin and Yang in the wrong way, or without the correct safety measures in place within the body, will lead to the development of tumours, possible stroke and heart attack. It is a risk not worth taking unless you are prepared to work very closely with an experienced master of these arts. Even then, it is so difficult an attainment that very few actually manage it. It is better to build the Qi within the lower Dan Tian and use it for health and spiritual development, as we shall discuss in the next couple of chapters.

Signs of Dan Tian Filling

Whilst there are several very forceful methods for filling the Dan Tian, the method outlined in this book is safe, as it is based on passive methods of moving the Qi into the Yin Qi field of the lower Dan Tian. It will take you a long time to do this, so it should keep you busy for a while! As the Dan Tian fills, it will result in improved vitality and general well-being as well as a heightened ability to sense, feel and move Qi. We shall come back to these kinds of abilities in Chapter 13.

As well as this, below are some clear signs of progress for bringing Qi into the lower Dan Tian.

Warmth

In the early stages of Yang Qi moving into the Dan Tian, there will still be a little resistance to the conduction of the Qi. This will result in warmth in the lower abdomen. It can grow very hot when the Yang Qi first enters into the Dan Tian, and it can be a surprise that it is not burning you. This is quite normal and the experience will pass in time as the resistance lessens.

Vibration

As the Qi starts to build, there will be the sensation of a vibration within your lower abdomen. It is as if there is a car engine in there that is ticking over. This is a very positive sign of progress. If you place your hands onto the abdomen of a practitioner who has reached this stage in their training you can feel the Qi within the Dan Tian vibrating out onto the surface of their body.

Shaking

After a long while of vibrating, the Dan Tian will shake from side to side in your practice. There is a clear feeling of a ball within the abdominal cavity as the Qi has filled the Dan Tian to the point of it being inflated. It will shake from side to side very quickly as the Qi reaches a high level. You will clearly feel when the vibration develops to the stage of shaking.

Jerking

It is almost as if the Dan Tian feels a little trapped at some stage and so it starts to suddenly jerk around from side to side. These jerking movements are erratic and will pull the Huang with them. The result of this pulling is that you can find your whole body suddenly jerked to both the left and right. It is quite amazing how powerful these motions can be under the influence of the Yang Qi. You will have no difficulty identifying this reaction!

Bubbling

If the Jing starts to condense to a high level, this can interact with the Qi of the Dan Tian and so this will feel as if the inside of the Dan Tian is bubbling. It is like a soup that is bubbling over on the hob. It is a pleasant feeling, very much as if something is lightly cooking. This is very important within the alchemical meditation processes of Daoism, but only a side-effect of the Nei Gong process that we should expect to move through.

Bouncing

When the lower Dan Tian fills to a very high level, then the 'sphere' of the Dan Tian will be very clear to feel. Though it is really the Qi interacting with the Huang of the abdomen, it can feel as if there is a very solid ball within your abdomen that is about the size of a ping pong ball. It will start to 'bounce' up and down inside of you. As the Huang is dragged up and down, this will create a physical reaction that can clearly be palpated by another person. In some cases, it can be seen; it looks as if there is a ball moving up and down beneath the surface of your skin.

Light

A final phenomenon of the Dan Tian's development is that it can start to radiate light from within. If you 'look' inside your body with your awareness, then there is a light radiating from within the lower abdominal cavity. Those with 'Yin vision' are also able to see this within your body when they look at you, but those with this level of internal development are rare. The experience of light is not necessarily the final stage of development and should not be treated as such. It can come and go along the path of your training.

Radiating the Qi

Once the Dan Tian is built and filled to a high enough level, then there will be a natural reaction whereby the Qi begins to radiate out of you. The pressure from the Dan Tian will have built to such a stage that it begins to 'push' from the inside. The Qi of your body will then begin to conduct out of your entire body and radiate into the space around you. This will build a particular kind of Qi field, as shown in Figure 11.14. This is known as the Dan Yuan (丹元) field within Nei Gong circles.

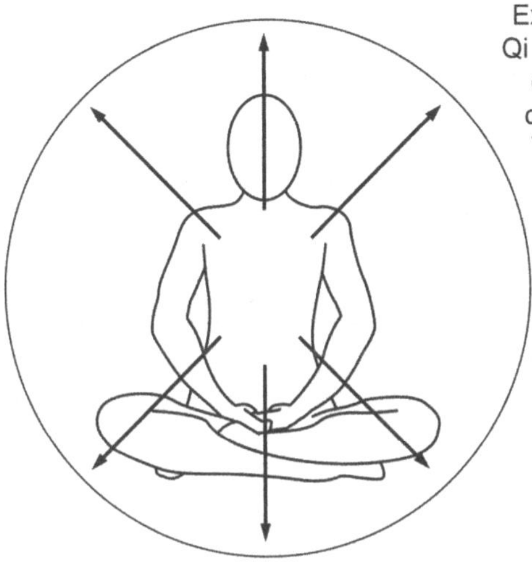

Figure 11.14: The Dan Yuan Field of Radiation

This particular field of Qi is based upon a naturally evolving radiation of energetic information. It is not created in any particular way; instead, the build-up of internal pressure from the Dan Tian pushes the Qi outwards. We all have a certain degree of Qi within the space around us – this is our auric field – but the radiation of Qi and the development of the Dan Yuan field is a more powerful version of this.

When you meet teachers with this kind of field, its influence upon you can vary. Some fields are quite weak, just enough to wash over you with a subtle energetic impact. Other practitioners have a very strong field, so strong that the energy radiating out of the lower Dan Tian is almost tangible. I have known teachers who made the hairs stand up on their students' arms and on the back of their neck when they were in the room with them due to the force being radiated out from their body.

Some teachers use this field consciously, whilst others do not. Those who use their field consciously can generally make it more Yin or more Yang;

essentially, the difference comes down to whether they are emphasising the effect of the electrical discharge of Yang Qi or the magnetism of Yin Qi. Though I use the terms 'electricity' and 'magnetism', remember that I use them loosely; even though these two types of Qi share many of the properties of these two phenomena, the Qi field also carries with it conscious information in the form of a vibratory wave.

A very Yin field can lead you towards greater feats of stillness. Those who develop the Dan Yuan field tend to have this effect. When sitting with these kinds of teachers, you can be lulled into a deep relaxation. When they enter into meditation, it can feel as if you are being drawn into them, as if your energetic field is being sucked into the vacuum of Yin they are creating.

A very Yang field is very stimulating. In the presence of teachers with this kind of field, generally those who practise a lot of very active forms of energy work, you can feel very stimulated. Your Qi will move around the body to a higher level and the tangible experience of the effects of Qi is much higher.

Note that this is a type of energetic influence that is an organic by-product of the practice and the build-up of Qi within the Dan Tian. It is quite separate from other forms of energetic influence such as transmission, Qi emission or empowerments. Let us look at the differences between these abilities.

Radiation of Qi

Radiation of Qi is the natural effect of building up a large reserve of stored energy within the body. The field of Qi is radiated outwards as a result of built-up internal pressure or 'fullness'. This is often a subconscious process. Some with this level of attainment will have control over the nature of the Qi within this field and its effects, whilst others will not. It is often felt the strongest when you are in a teaching situation with these kinds of people.

Qi Emission

To Fa Qi (發氣) or to 'emit Qi' is a process whereby the practitioner consciously directs Qi out of their own body into (generally) the body of another person. This is most commonly done in a therapeutic setting. Rather than being a 'field', this is usually a wave of Qi sent out of the practitioner's hands or fingers. As a process, it does use up the practitioner's Qi (no matter how many systems seem to try to deny this) and consequently can be quite tiring for the practitioner.

The general Qi that is emitted is non-specific to Yin or Yang and has a slightly magnetic quality to it. Some can feel it, whilst others cannot. The effects are variable according to the ability of the therapist, but it is generally used in conjunction with Chinese medical theory. It can be used to push, pull, clear or nourish the Qi of the patient's body.

Very strong emission of Yang Qi is quite different from this and feels like a strong wave of liquid electricity that moves through your channel system. The practitioner delivers an electrical shock out of their body into your own. I remember first feeling it when I was younger and being shocked at how strong it was. After receiving this kind of Yang Qi from several different masters from different systems around the world, it is also interesting to note that the quality of the Qi being emitted feels very different depending upon who is emitting it. Because of Yang Qi's connection to consciousness, you can almost feel the practitioner's personality or nature contained within the Qi. This kind of emission is pretty rare, though; not many manage to cultivate their internal energy to this kind of level.

Beyond this, high-level emission of Qi can also create a whole variety of different reactions and effects depending upon the skill of the practitioner.

Transmission

Transmission is a direct mind-to-mind transference of information. This is a conscious skill that is used by a teacher to impart the deepest aspects of an internal system. It involves the cultivation of Shen to a high level in order for this kind of skill to develop. There are various ways and means for issuing this kind of information. Many of the deeper parts of alchemical training are said to require transmissions from teachers, as they cannot otherwise be learnt; it is through these kinds of teachings that many of the more esoteric aspects of the Daoist tradition have been passed on.

This is a skill that most high-level meditation teachers use within their practice. The role of a teacher of meditation should not be to simply sit there with you; they should, classically, be assisting you through the use of radiated Qi and transmissions that help to bring your Qi and Shen to another level. Generally, this is like a kind of leg-up in the practice; once your mind has experienced that frequency, it has touched upon that state of being, and then it can begin to unfold the process that leads you towards returning to this point.

Empowerments

Empowerments are a form of transmission that have been 'stamped' with the particular frequency of the lineage that the teacher is within. This stamp is like a kind of spiritual fingerprint that makes the empowerment unique to that teacher's particular system of practice. An empowerment is interesting as it serves to 'pull' a student who receives the empowerment closer to the particular frequency of the lineage or tradition.

To understand this, we can think of all the traditions and branches of the spiritual traditions as being like individual radio stations. Daoism is a station, Buddhism is a station, and so on. Even within these frequency bands, there are variations from tradition to tradition. So, for example, the Ling Bao (靈寶) 'Spiritual Treasure', Long Men (龍門) 'Dragon Gate', Zheng Yi (正一) 'Orthodox Unity' lineages and others are various forms and traditions of Daoism. Each was established as a spiritual line by a high-level, realised master, and so each of them could be considered a separate 'radio channel'. Our consciousness is a kind of radio receiver, and if we are new to these arts, we will struggle to tune into the 'stations'; all we get is static! Each empowerment serves to change the radio station a little more until we are fully connected to a lineage and so can pick up the 'channel' with a clear signal. All right, I know this isn't the best analogy, certainly not the most poetic, but it does give you an idea of how empowerments work.

Cautions of Dan Yuan

The reason I am explaining these fields and kinds of energetic transference is to help people gain a better understanding of the mechanics and the nature of these systems. They are not something to strive for. They are just a part of the practice at a certain stage. To strive for such things is an unhealthy attitude towards the journey. Dan Yuan and the radiation of Qi into your auric field is a level of attainment that many will stumble across when they hit a certain stage in their development, and this should be recognised and treated with the respect it deserves; this is because there are a couple of cautions to be aware of when this field starts to develop.

The problem with the manifestation of this field is that it draws people to you. It is almost as if it serves as a kind of energetic charisma that can influence the people around you. There is a subconscious respect that people will develop for you as they begin to pick up on the information contained within the auric field. This is a large part of the reason why many internal practitioners from within various spiritual systems – from Buddhism to Daoism, Hinduism to Christianity and so on – have developed such a following. Perhaps their auric field was fed in a different way? Religious devotion can radiate energy as well as the development of the lower Dan Tian; there are various mechanisms behind the field's development. Whatever the method, the result is the same: when they encounter people, these people often feel drawn to them. A very Yin field can break down barriers for people and automatically instil a great deal of trust within you, a very Yang field can generate the want to initiate change; you may wish to suddenly leave your life and start afresh or do something radical like join the temple/ashram/sangha or whatever.

If a teacher recognises this and treats it with the respect it deserves, then it can be a great teaching tool. It can be used to empower those around them and help them to grow. Sadly, in many cases, the growing following of the teacher stimulates their egoistic side and so they end up taking advantage of people instead. Dealing with the adoration and trust of many people, all seeking for answers and direction in life, can have a very powerful draw upon your acquired self. This is a part of the reason for so many instances of abuse within 'spiritual groups': financial, emotional, sexual, and so on. The radiation of the teacher's Qi has had an influence upon the student or devotee and so they are acting free from their usual defence mechanisms. This is especially going to be the case for people who have actively gone and sought out a teacher; the sheer act of looking for somebody to humble yourself before will create a kind of energetic vacuum that will be filled by the influence of the teacher's auric field.

I think that a few things need to be recognised if you ever reach the stage in your training where this is happening:

- The field is a result of a naturally unfolding energetic process. It is not 'enlightenment' nor an indicator of any particularly high spiritual state; it is the result of an expansion of Qi – it is, at most, a skill and not a cultivated spiritual state. No matter how many devotees look to you for spiritual guidance, you should remember that you are in no higher a place than any other. It is your Qi that is affecting them.
- The nature of teaching others is 'service'. You are there for your students, they are not there for you. This is often forgotten and the results are rarely positive.
- You never have any right to negatively impact on others. Not for personal gain nor as a result of your own imbalances; you should only be there to help others. A great deal of self-examination by all teachers is very important to make sure this is the case.

You should approach these arts and teaching them as if you were a mechanic. Understand the mechanisms behind what you are doing, and help others to understand them as well. This is the safest approach to teaching; be careful of giving yourself the title of 'spiritual teacher', as others will have attachments and associations with this title that can be problematic. Whilst you may call yourself a spiritual teacher with the best of intentions behind what you are doing, it does not always set up the best balance between yourself and your students; the emotional baggage involved in such a relationship can be tricky to work with.

Chapter 12

THE STAGE OF QI TO SHEN

Up until this point in the book we have primarily been exploring the nature of Jing, Qi and the physical components of the body. What has only been looked at in brief is the nature of Shen – spirit. It is here, at the more refined levels of vibrational frequency, that the deepest transformational work can take place. Though much of this stage of the practice crosses over into more meditative training, it is still relevant to the Nei Gong process. It was long understood that the root of many people's conditions lay within their mind and that it was also here, in the more ethereal aspects of human being, that the potential for full transcendence lay.

Before we begin to look at the more spirit-based aspects of the Nei Gong syllabus, we should first clarify some terminology according to the Daoist teachings. We also need to look at the various processes inherent at this stage of our practice. These definitions are important as many terms are used interchangeably within the alternative arts and this can cause confusion.

Spiritual Development

Not everybody will have the same aims for their practice. As stated previously, many will come to the art of Nei Gong simply to improve their health, and this is a wonderful reason for training. Others will aim for the further ends of the spectrum and be seeking enlightenment or immortality, though this is rare; I do not know of many who specifically seek this attainment these days. Those who do look to the further ends of the Nei Gong process will have to look at the processes behind 'spiritual development'. This, quite literally, means to develop the spirit; it really is that simple.

If we look at how people define 'spiritual practice' these days, we will see many philosophical books on how to live your life and how to look the part, but really, these are all just 'trimmings'; spiritual development means to 'develop the spirit'. Within Daoism, this is the Yuan Shen or 'original spirit'. This should be made clear and everybody needs to understand this if they are looking at the Daoist tradition in particular – the Yuan Shen is the 'spirit' that is cultivated if we are going to see our art as a form of 'spiritual development'.

I am making this distinction very clear because there is also the term 'Shen' which, too, is translated as 'spirit' within Daoism. It is this 'spirit' that is said to reside within the Heart. The English translation of the terms is where the confusion lies, as the 'Shen' is not the 'spirit' in its highest sense – it is a distorted aspect of the Yuan Shen, and so, cultivating the 'Shen' and not the 'Yuan Shen' actually lies within the practice of 'self-cultivation' and not 'spiritual development'; even though the two are related, they are not one and the same. Many of the things I had read when I was younger and the assumptions of what 'spiritual development' was ended up being smashed apart by the first high-level masters I encountered. This is because 'self-development' is essentially the practice of 'developing the self', whilst 'spiritual development' is actually the 'ending of self'; in the earliest stages of our training, we need to strike a healthy balance between these two practices, cultivating the 'self' and the 'spirit', but it will reach a stage where they are actually directly conflicting processes.

In order for the higher aspect of spirit – Yuan Shen – to develop, it needs to be 'nourished'. It can be nourished in one of two ways: the first is to nourish it with an abundance of Qi, and the second is to nourish it through residing in stillness. Nourishing the Yuan Shen with Qi is considered the 'lower path' or the 'lesser vehicle' since it can bring somebody only to the development of skill; we shall look at this below. The 'higher path' or the 'greater vehicle' is to reside in stillness so that the Yuan Shen can begin to shine forth under this form of nourishment. In short, it is stillness that is needed for spiritual development and nothing more. If your practice is leading you towards deeper levels of inner stillness, then it is moving towards nourishing the spirit; if it is generating more movement, then it is not. If your practice is on the level of trying to develop your 'self', then it is not at the stage of being a 'spiritual practice' yet in the most literal definition of the term.

Much of the Nei Gong process that involves building, regulating and circulating Qi is not serving to nourish the Yuan Shen; in the same manner, those precepts and guidelines that you choose to follow are also not helping you to develop your Yuan Shen. This means that these kinds of practice are not really a spiritual practice; they may, however, be laying the foundations for progressing into this kind of art further down the line. This is why, to me, Nei Gong is a great foundation for meditative training, but it is the meditative training that is really going to do the 'work' with your spirit.

As a consequence, we can lay out the development of our practice as shown in Figure 12.1. Here, we see a progression from working with the body, the energy system, the mind and then, finally, the spirit.

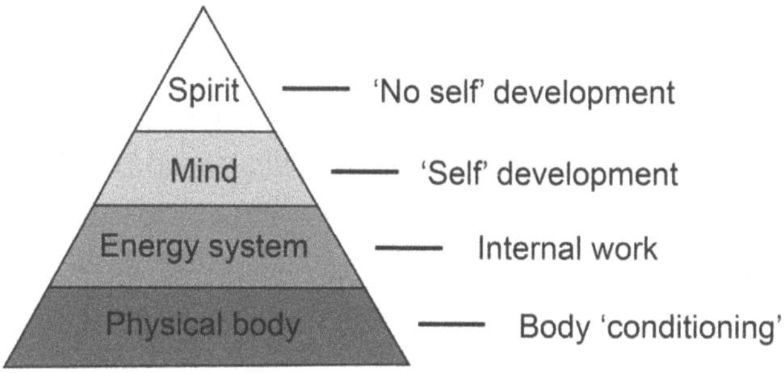

Figure 12.1: Development into Spiritual Training

This may seem like a very exact, black and white way of looking at the term. I apologise for this – yes, it is a very definite way of looking at it, but it is my view that the 'spiritual' community in the wider sense has often struggled to really know what they are doing! Too many woolly definitions and blurred lines between practices has meant that everything becomes a 'spiritual practice', when this may not actually be the case.

The development of Yuan Shen will lead a person to the stage of Shen Ming (神明). This is the Daoist equivalent to the term 'enlightenment'. It is the stage of mergence with the Dao so that a person is 'true'.

Self-Cultivation

Often confused with 'spiritual development' is the concept of 'self-cultivation' or 'self-development'. In my opinion, the majority of people involved in the alternative arts are actually practising a form of 'self-cultivation' rather than a direct 'cultivation of the spirit'; at least, this is the case from a Daoist perspective.

When we look below at the process of how the mind is formed from spirit, we will see that 'spirit' and 'self' are two different things. Our self is what we tend to identify with; it is a built-up aspect of our being that leads us to have a sense of individuality. It is our subjective being that distinguishes us from other people and the part of our being that we will encounter through introspection or contemplative awareness of our habitual behaviours. Our 'self' includes all of our personality traits, memories, desires, moral standpoints, emotions and so on; it is everything we would associate with 'mind'. It is here, with the 'self', that most Eastern traditions identified as the root of all our problems, at least the internally originated ones. It is often said that there are no problems, only problematic reactions to things. Whether you agree with this or not, the reactions being referred to are rooted in the actions of your mind and thus your 'self'.

To cultivate 'spirit' in the higher sense of Yuan Shen means to go beyond 'self'. Enlightenment of spirit means to rise above the subjective experience of separation into the objective experience of union. In this way, practices of 'self-cultivation' can actually become a hurdle to 'spiritual development'. Herein lies the problem, though – we cannot actually rise above the 'self' if it is in a low state. Obviously, 'high' and 'low' are rather subjective terms but, for now, to keep things simple, let us look at this idea on a graph as shown in Figure 12.2.

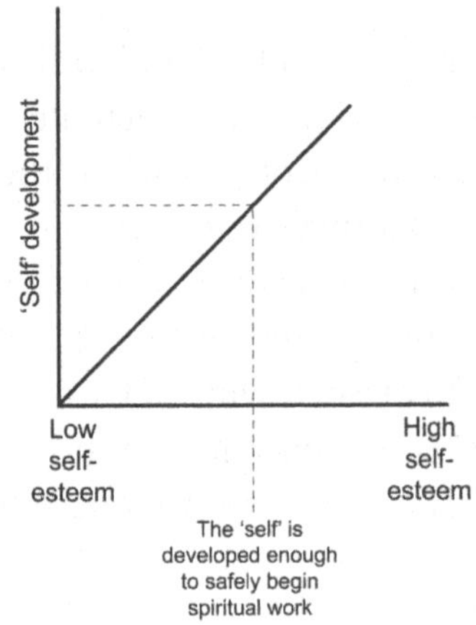

Figure 12.2: Self-Esteem

Again, I apologise for the over-literal way I am looking at these concepts, but hopefully, through doing this, we can start to develop a conceptual framework of various aspects of higher-level internal work and how they relate to one another.

The high- or lowness of a person's 'self' is based in their self-esteem; how worthy do they believe their 'self' to be? Sadly, within modern society, people often have rather low self-esteem. Most people, when they take a subjective emotional evaluation of how they view themselves, will feel pretty bad; this is almost certainly the case for the majority of people who come into arts such as Qi Gong or other internal practices. From what I have seen over the years of teaching, most people come with the idea of needing to be 'fixed' on some level, whether it is a conscious need or not. Of course, this idea of something being 'wrong' is an unhealthy concept in itself, which is why the focus of our practice should never be on this kind of thing, but we should not deny its existence as a background ethos to why people come into these arts.

If a person has a poor sense of 'self', then 'spiritual development' in its most literal sense can actually be quite dangerous. To reside in stillness and try to eradicate the 'self' before it has a certain degree of strength to it can actually lead to chronic depression and other emotional problems. It is for this reason that 'self-cultivation' is a wiser practice for a long time, until a person's self-esteem is sufficiently balanced so that they can progress onto direct work with nourishing the Yuan Shen. This is why, within my own school, I always like people to study the arts in the following sequence:

1. Qi Gong first, with a movement into the Nei Gong process.
2. From this point, we use the process of Nei Gong to make the body and mind function more efficiently. We improve the health, build up Qi and generally strengthen the parts of our being needed for a good level of 'self-cultivation'.
3. From here, we move on to alchemical training and direct 'spiritual development' based in nourishing the Yuan Shen with inner stillness.

Internal Skill

A third definition of what can be sought out at the higher levels of practice is 'internal skill', another way of using the term 'Nei Gong'. Internal skill is quite different from either spiritual development or self-cultivation. The danger is that many people coming into the arts mistake these three for each other. 'Internal skill' is quite literally what it sounds like. It can range from mastery of Qi Gong through to the development of Cheng Jiu (成就), which literally means 'attainments' but can be understood as the equivalent of the Sanskrit term 'Siddhi'. Since most people are familiar with Siddhi, I shall use this term for the remainder of the book.

Siddhi are various paranormal abilities that can be unlocked from within the human mind if we can nourish it in a very specific manner; these abilities range from extrasensory perception through to telekinesis and more extreme abilities such as bilocation. Many will not believe in these kinds of abilities, especially in the West. In Asia, the situation is quite different and it is my personal experience that many practitioners of Qi Gong and Nei Gong train for the sole aim of developing Siddhi. Siddhi will be looked at in greater detail in the next, and final, chapter of the book.

Though the attainment of Siddhi is a very difficult thing, it is far easier than entering into Shen Ming and fully cultivating the Yuan Shen. The attainment of Siddhi is also, on a certain level, somewhat contradictory to true 'spiritual development', though there are some shared qualities to these two paths.

The danger is that teachers who have attained some level of Siddhi then profess to be either awakened or enlightened, and the Siddhi are, of course, the proof that this is the case. I had a teacher of this sort for a while. He could do amazing things with the power of his mind and Qi, but he was not a 'Buddha' as he claimed to be. Unfortunately, others fell for this kind of deception – he had psychic proof after all! Sadly, it is 'red flag' that a teacher has gone down a sorry road when they claim that their Siddhi are the result of being enlightened. Siddhi are developed in a very specific and quite mechanical manner that is separate from nourishing the spirit with inner stillness.

Awakening

'Awakening' is the most obvious English equivalent of the Chinese term Wu (悟). The term 'awakened' and 'self-awakened' are two interchangeable terms with regard to these practices. If a person is awakened, or Wu, then they are able to comprehend and objectively experience the fact that their acquired mind is only an outer layer, and that true self resides at a deeper place. Whilst they are not necessarily enlightened in the sense of having fully developed their Yuan Shen, they have had the clear realisation that they are not their 'self' and that the 'self' is ultimately a transient falsity. This realisation cannot come from reading books or looking at internet memes, it has to be a direct experiential moment of entering into a profound state that is close to spiritual Wuji. Awakening is considered a positive marker on the road to enlightenment, but it is not enlightenment itself.

The term 'self-awakened' essentially refers to having 'woken up' to the truth of the falsity of your 'self'; it should not mean, as it is so often used, that a person was able to achieve some kind of enlightenment without the need of a teacher or system.

When a person is awakened, they are known as a Sheng Ren (聖人) or 'sage' within Daoist terminology; this is a reference to the person who 'understands the inner workings of Heaven', a reference to understanding the true nature of mind and 'self'. It was the Sheng Ren who were the Daoist teachers of old.

Enlightenment

Enlightenment is the nearest English equivalent to entering Shen Ming and becoming a Zhen Ren (真人) or 'true person'. A Zhen Ren is beyond the Sheng Ren in attainment. Whereas a Sheng Ren is awakened to the true nature of 'self', a Zhen Ren has eradicated the 'self' and instead exists as a pure manifestation of Yuan Shen. The Zhen Ren is said to know all and be omnipresent in his awareness. They are essentially deities on the Earth. To the Daoists, the spiritual leaders of old who have had special Siddhi attached to them were Zhen Ren, a term referring to the fact that they are 'true', not operating from the 'false' sense of self. This kind of attainment is only developed out of high levels of spiritual development in the most literal use of the phrase.

Immortality

There is much disagreement within Daoism over the meaning of the word Xian (仙) or 'immortal'. Some say that it is a metaphor for reaching a high level of spiritual attainment, but personally, I understand it in its most literal sense. Whether or not you believe it to be possible is irrelevant. As with the rest of the underlying philosophy of Daoism, it 'belongs' to the people who founded the practices. To understand a tradition, we need to understand the underlying belief structure of the people who lived during its founding. Otherwise, if we change the teachings to suit our own cultural beliefs, then we are carrying out a form of cultural misappropriation. The Daoists referred to the Xian as having magical-type qualities to them that included being able to live forever if they wished or else being able to dissolve into light so that they could forever be apart from the cycle of rebirth; the equivalent of the Xian within the Tibetan Buddhist tradition would be those who attained the 'light' or 'rainbow' body through their inner development. There are further subdivisions of immortals within Daoism and, as usual, it all gets rather complicated when you go deeper into the theory, but it is not very important. I have only included this brief mention of immortality to help with a broader understanding of definitions of terms.

Anchoring of Mind and Spirit

It is a great strength of the Daoist tradition that the mind and body are so inextricably linked. Every facet of human consciousness is manifest and anchored into a different region of the physical body. This 'somatic' way of interpreting human existence means that we can begin to understand the rationale behind many of the alchemical 'mechanics' contained within practices such as Qi Gong and Nei Gong. If we look at this in relation to the above theories, we can see an anchoring of various aspects of consciousness, as shown in Figure 12.3.

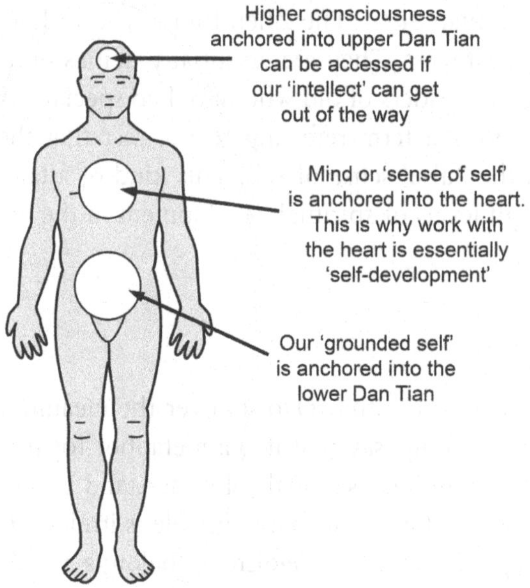

Figure 12.3: Anchoring of Spirit and Mind

As you can see, the upper Dan Tian, residing within the brain, is the seat of 'higher consciousness'. It is here that we can work to develop many of the supernatural abilities associated with high-level internal skill. At the centre of the upper Dan Tian resides the Yuan Shen, though this is not a literal residence. Yuan Shen exists in an all-encompassing fashion, so even though it is said to be anchored into the upper Dan Tian, it is better to see this as the place which we may move through in order to 'access' Yuan Shen. It is only through profound inner stillness that we will reach this place.

The mind, or 'sense of self', is based within the region of the heart; it is a manifestation and aspect of the Heart centre. This is why Xin (心) is used in Chinese to refer to both the 'heart' and the 'mind', often written as 'Heart Mind'. This is the acquired aspect of self that is developed out of the Yuan Shen and the place where our subjective concept of who we are resides. There is then a further anchoring of the five spiritual components of 'mind' into the key organs of the body. Though they are placed within the key viscera, these organs are still always 'expressed', with regard to their machinations, through the heart itself.

Development

Development of the Intellect

There is a type of Qi Gong known as 'scholarly Qi Gong' or 'Wisdom Qi Gong' which is primarily aimed at improving the efficiency of the functioning of the mind and brain. Essentially, its purpose/aim/objective is to raise your intelligence as well as your learning capability and to fend off the decline of mental faculties that so often comes with the ageing process.

Though there are specific Qi Gong systems aimed at this kind of work, it is also an inherent part of all authentic Qi Gong practices that the functioning of the mind will become more efficient. Even in the early stages of practice, we assist this process by regulating our breathing and mind, but then there are deeper aspects to this with regard to the movement of Jing, Qi and Shen. When we discussed the process of marrow washing back in Chapter 7, we looked at how the Jing can be used to improve the mind's functioning, but now we also have the added aspect of Qi.

Essentially, Qi moves through the microcosmic orbit into the head and then travels through the centre of the body, as shown in Figure 12.4.

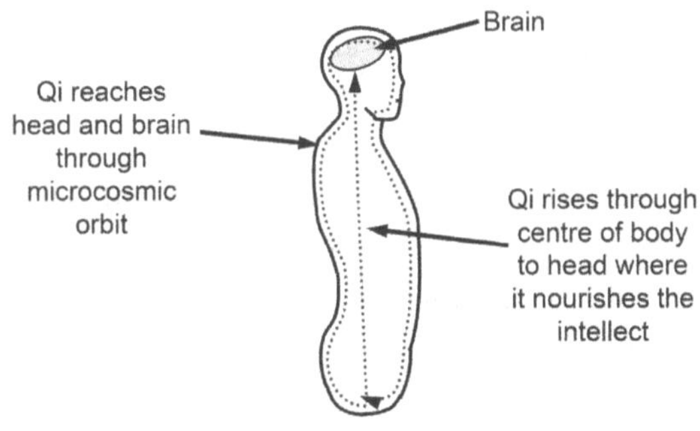

Figure 12.4: Wisdom Qi Gong

This movement of Qi through the body should not specifically be 'helped' in any way as this will lead to a draining of the Jing. What I mean by this is that we do not try to 'draw' the Qi up through the middle of the body with any kind of mental direction. Instead, it will take place of its own accord as the Yang Qi you are accumulating starts to 'fill up' through the body. First, the lower Dan Tian needs to be full, and then, beyond this, the filling will continue into the rest of the body's Huang. With time, the Qi will reach the brain and so begin to nourish your mental faculties. The result is a raising of the intelligence. This is a natural by-product of continuous training; I have only included a discussion of it here so you may see how the mechanics of nourishing the intellect works. All that is taking place is an increase in the efficiency of a naturally occurring internal mechanism. We are simply looking to make it function on a higher level and to slow down the decline of the cognitive processes as we age.

Development of Skills and Abilities

Within the centre of the brain resides the upper Dan Tian. It is here that our dormant higher mental functions reside. Though shut off to the vast majority of us, there is the potential for all sorts of Siddhi residing within the various layers of the upper Dan Tian. We shall explore these in the following chapter. To access these Siddhi, there needs to be enough Qi sent to the upper Dan Tian to fuel its functioning. This Qi can reach the upper Dan Tian through the microcosmic orbit, through the Central channel or through being deliberately guided as in the form of exercises aimed specifically at developing various Siddhi.

Though Qi needs to be sent to the upper Dan Tian to access these kinds of abilities, it doesn't require the kind of stillness work that is needed to access the Yuan Shen or the Shen Ming state. There are exceptions to this, which are the Siddhi that come in the form of milestones to attainment, but generally, 'spiritual development' and the attainment of Siddhi are quite separate things. On top of this there is the added issue that the use of Siddhi often stimulates the acquired mind very strongly, so Siddhi usage can be directly conflicting with attainment of Yuan Shen. This is why many spiritual teachers were wary of Siddhi and many scriptures advised against going down this kind of path in one's practice.

Self-Development

The self resides largely within the heart, and so it is the Heart field that needs adjustment through practice if we wish to develop the self. We shall explore this in greater detail in the next chapter. The self does not necessarily require the same profound stillness that we require for access of Yuan Shen, but a certain degree of inner calm is important for this kind of work. The self is quite separate from the spirit in that it can be adjusted cognitively. What I mean by this is that mental action can actually change the nature of self. Philosophical teachings, ethical guidance and contemplation can all aid in the development of self, but none of these things will aid you in any kind of development of the spirit. Only internally developed stillness can help to nourish the spirit; this can only be achieved through practice. That being said, if the self is not strong enough for high-level inner work, then it will need developing first, prior to moving on to deeper inner development. It was for this reason that precepts and similar teachings were a part of traditions such as Daoism and Buddhism.

Spiritual Development

Though self-cultivation can serve as a platform for spiritual development, it is the ending of self that is needed in order to reach the stage of attaining Yuan Shen. Here lie the deepest aspects of the Daoist path, those parts of the tradition known as the 'greater vehicle'. The rest of this chapter will look at the various teachings involved in developing inner stillness and thus moving towards contact with a higher spirit.

The Creation of Human Mind

To begin working with human consciousness, we first need to understand how it developed into 'mind'. It is always the same; to understand how to work with an element of human existence, we need to first understand how it was developed. Within Daoism, there are very clear generative processes involved in the manifestation of all phenomena; much of the work is then aimed at understanding and, in many cases, returning to the source of this process.

Human consciousness is generated from the singular 'point' of Yuan Shen. Yuan Shen is human consciousness prior to it moving into an acquired state of being. When the mind becomes dominant over the actions of spirit, then a 'refraction' of Yuan Shen takes place and so the Wu Shen (五神) or 'five spirits' come into being. These five aspects of human mind are known as the Hun (魂), the Po (魄), the Yi (意), the Zhi (志) and the Shen (神). These five inter-relate with one another, as shown in Figure 12.5, to give us the movements of human intellect, direction and thought.

The two more Yang of the spirits are the Hun and the Shen which manifest through the elemental energies of Wood and Fire respectively. The more Yin spirits are the Zhi and the Po which manifest through the Water and Metal elemental energies. In the centre of the other four spirits sits the Yi. The Yi fluctuates between various degrees of Yin and Yang, depending upon its interactions and influences from the other spirits. This corresponds with the five element – Wu Xing – theory which places the elements as shown in Figure 12.6.

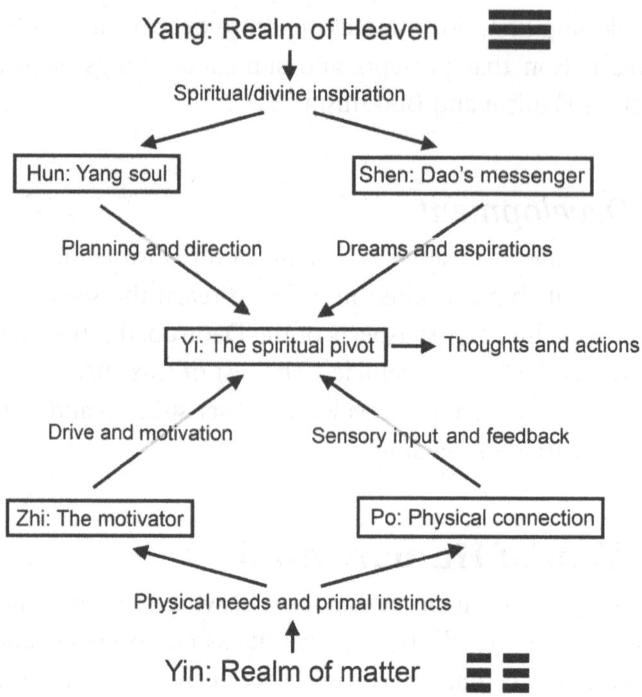

Figure 12.5: The Wu Shen

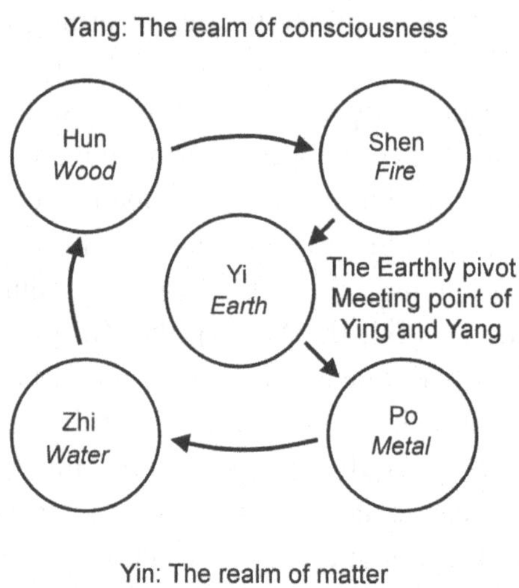

Figure 12.6: The Wu Xing Arrangement

Human beings sit between the two poles of extreme Yang and extreme Yin, which are manifested as Heaven and Earth. In the human mind, these two great poles represent 'divine inspiration', which is said to belong to the realm of Heaven, and 'primal instincts', which are the psychological aspect of the realm of Earth. In order to survive in this world, we require a relationship with these two poles, and it is then the inter-relationship of the five spirits that dictates what exactly the nature of this relationship is.

The Hun

The Hun is considered the Yang aspect of the human soul. There are classically said to be three Hun: the Yang Hun, the Yin Hun and the human Hun or Ren Hun, known respectively as:

- Shuang Ling (爽靈) or 'Clear Divinity'
- Tai Guang (胎光) or 'Shining Embryo'
- You Jing (幽精) or 'Dark Essence'.

The Yang Hun is said to be given to us at birth from the Heavens; it carries with it the collective consciousness of all humanity down through the ages and is the aspect of spirit which, when tapped into, can give access to all human thought and knowledge. This aspect of Hun is considered to be 'on loan' to us for the duration of our lives, and when we die, the Yang Hun 'returns to the source', taking with it all of the experiences we have had during our lives.

The Yin Hun comes from original spirit; it is an aspect of the Yuan Shen and, like the Yang Hun, returns to its place of origin upon death. It is this aspect of the Hun that is said to carry with it the information from previous lives. According to Daoist thought, the Yin Hun is the layer of Hun that transmigrates. Note that in some traditions of Daoism the Yin Hun is also divided into various parts, each coming from the Hun of a previous existence; in these traditions, there is no direct reincarnation from individual to individual but rather a 'composite Yin Hun' made up of various interconnected previous existences.

The third and final aspect of Hun is the Ren Hun; this is given to a person by their parents. The Ren Hun contains a spiritual imprint from the soul of your parents and the family lineage that you are a part of. It is this aspect of Hun which strongly connects family members with each other.

These three aspects of Hun work as one unit to communicate with the realm of Heaven. They inspire us to give plans and direction to the Yi which processes the actions of the Hun. If the Hun is weak, then a person will lack a sense of direction in life. The Hun are rooted in the organ of the Liver and are particularly active during sleep, when they communicate the divine information of the realm of Heaven to us through imagery and symbolic dreams.

The three Hun are portrayed as three deities that carry with them a whole host of heavenly information. They are classically depicted as shown in Figure 12.7, though the personification of the Hun is only to aid people in understanding them.

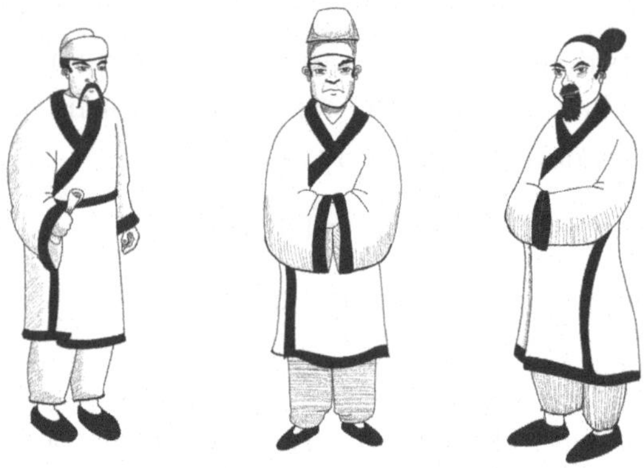

Figure 12.7: The Three Hun

The Shen

It can be quite confusing when first trying to understand the Shen. This is because the term 'Shen' can be used in reference to spirit on two different levels. On one level, Shen is the overall name for the human spirit, but it can also mean a single element of the human mind, as in the case of this model.

The Shen resides within the 'orifices of the Heart' and is said to be the key communicator with the heavenly realm. It is the messenger of Dao which brings aspirations and life dreams into a person's mind. Those with a weak Shen will lack the ability to imagine or have high-minded goals. If the Shen is 'unrooted', then it can result in mania and psychiatric illness; too much information pours into the mind from the heavenly realm without the positive filtering aspect of the Shen protecting the fragile mind.

The Zhi

The Zhi is the spirit of willpower. It is the aspect of human mind which provides the drive and motivation to see a task through. The plans of the Hun and the dreams of the Shen rely upon the motivating force of the Zhi to ensure that they come into being. Those with weak Zhi will find that even though they may have grand schemes, they rarely seem to see them through.

The Zhi is an earthly aspect of spirit rooted in the Yin energies of the planet. Though not directly in communication with the heavenly realm, it does fall under its influence, and a second aspect of the Zhi is that it is, in part, the 'will of Heaven'. The 'will of Heaven' is related to the concept of Ming and its extensions that reach out to affect human life. These paths are manifested from the spirit of Heaven and rooted in the realm of Earth. It is these flows upon which the paths of an individual's life events will run their course. The Zhi exists as a fine balance between the will of the individual and the will of Heaven.

The connection between Ming, Jing and Zhi are absolute and, consequently, all three have a close connection to the strength of the Kidneys as it is the Kidneys that the Zhi is said to be rooted into.

The Po

The seven corporeal Po spirits work together as one to give a person tangible connection to the earthly realm. They are the aspects of spirit which give us an understanding of the impermanence of life and, as such, are also transient in nature. Unlike their Yang counterpart, the seven Po break down upon our death and return to the Yin energies of the Earth, ready to be redistributed to others upon their birth. There is no immortality for the Po, which are acutely aware of their certain demise and their perpetual attachment to the earthly realm; for this reason, they are often depicted as distraught and woe-filled spirits, as shown in Figure 12.8.

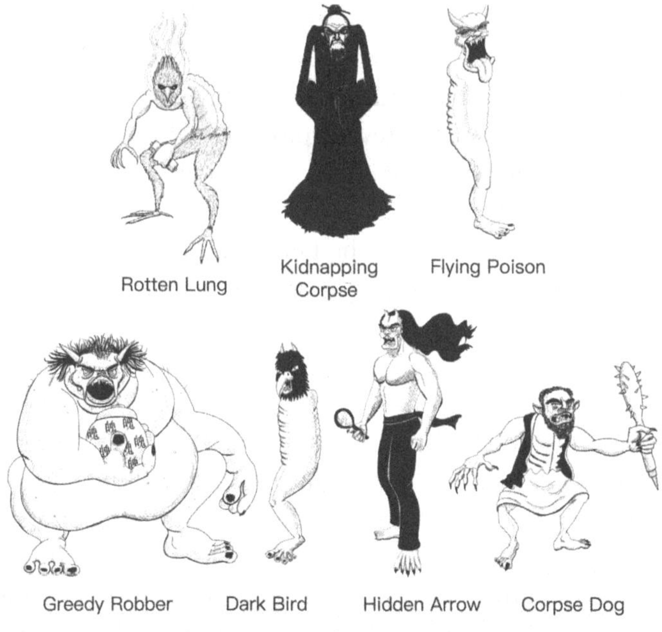
Rotten Lung
Kidnapping Corpse
Flying Poison
Greedy Robber
Dark Bird
Hidden Arrow
Corpse Dog

Figure 12.8: The Seven Po Spirits

Together with the Hun, the Po form the second half of the human soul, the Yin aspect. The Hun attach our soul to the power of Heaven, whilst the Po link us to the power of Earth. Whilst the Hun convey the movements of Heaven to us through dreams and symbols, the Po communicate the realm of Earth to us through tangible sensation and literal meaning. As a part of the soul, the Po may also greatly affect our dreams, but the Po gives us those dreams which are very concrete and down-to-earth in nature. Abstract imagery does not feature within the Po's language, rather they are the more mundane dreams that are not so interesting to recall.

When the Po are divided into seven parts, they are given very interesting names, which are as follows:

- Chou Fei (臭肺) or 'Rotten Lung'
- Shi Gou (尸狗) or 'Corpse Dog'
- Chu Hui (除秽) or 'Kidnapping Corpse'
- Fei Du (飞毒) or 'Flying Poison'
- Tun Zei (吞贼) or 'Greedy Robber'
- Que Yin (雀阴) or 'Dark Bird'
- Fu Shi (伏矢) or 'Hidden Arrow'.

These rather ghastly names were given to the Po because of the belief that, upon death, each of the seven Po leave the human body one day at a time as grief-stricken spirits that, one by one, begin to break down into the Earth. Those who died in great sadness were said to give enough power to the Po that one or more of the seven spirits would remain on the Earth for a prolonged period as a ghostly entity. Such mournful spirits obviously deserve some miserable-sounding names!

The Po are said to be rooted into the Lungs and it is for this reason that lung disorders can arise out of prolonged periods of grief.

The Yi

Sat at the centre of the other four spirits is the Yi. The Yi is a representation of human intellect and manifested thought patterns; it is the 'movement of the mind' under the influence of Yin and Yang, dualistic thinking. The Yi is neither inherently more Yin nor more Yang by nature; instead it is formed from a mixture of the other four spirits. The Yi is the aspect of our mind that processes information from the other four spirits and does something with it. It creates thought patterns which give us a coherent understanding of the information coming to us from Heaven above and Earth below. On its own, the Yi is responsible for very little; it requires interaction with the other spirits to have any real function, and in the same way, without the Yi, the other spirits have no basis within human thought. Table 12.1 shows the main functions of the Yi when it interacts with the other spirits.

Table 12.1: Yi Interactions with the Other Spirits

Yi and Hun	Imagination, dreaming, planning, direction, mental projection
Yi and Shen	Divine insight, faith, belief, comprehension, understanding
Yi and Zhi	Will, drive, concept of purpose, clarity, wisdom
Yi and Po	Feeling, memory, knowledge, learning, logic, reasoning

The strength of a person's Yi is important, as a weakness here will detach one or more of the spirits from their cognitive centre. This will result in an imbalance within their thought processes.

Wu Shen Chao Yuan (五神朝元): Return the Five Spirits to Their Origin

It is a clear instruction within the Daoist alchemical classics that the five spirits need to be 'returned to their original state'. It is here that they can reverse the refraction process and so reunite into Yuan Shen. As much as anything, this is a model of how we should work towards balancing the various aspects of human psyche so that, when they are in harmony with one another, our 'true spirit' will arise. This process is depicted in Figure 12.9. It is the process of 'returning to the source' as it is manifest within the realm of human consciousness.

It is said that there are two major components involved in managing to achieve this. The first is developing a stable and still quality of mind; the second is to understand the Qi of the spirits which, in this case, refers to the manner in which they manifest outwards into the rest of our mental being. We must 'balance the branches' before we can 'recombine the root'. This is why it is said that before we can Wu Shen Chao Yuan (五神朝元), or 'return the five spirits to their origin', we must first Wu Qi Chao Yuan (五氣朝元), or 'return the five Qi to their origin'. Daoism is a tradition based on 'moving in reverse', that is, we look to understand the way in which something is expressed, and then we travel 'against the course' to locate the root of this expression. This is the methodology we use to locate the source of human spirit, the Yuan Shen.

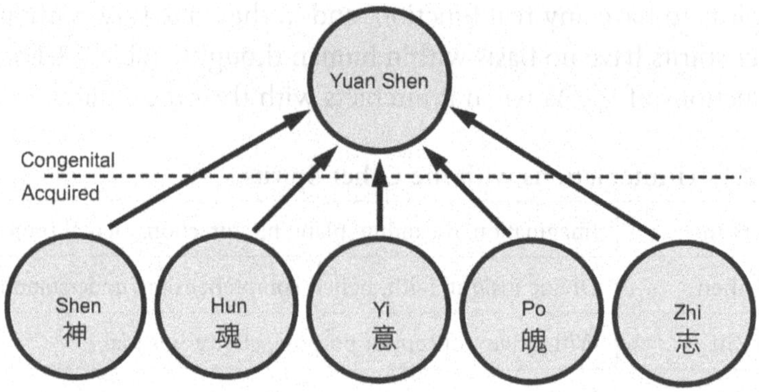

Figure 12.9: Returning the Five Spirits to Their Origin

So, how are the spirits expressed outwards into the mind? This is through a process of distortion that occurs in sequence from our centre to the outer expressions of our nature. It is a sequence or 'layering' within the mind that is generally understood to be built in the order described below.

Original Spirit

At the very centre of our being lies our 'original spirit', the Yuan Shen. This is the very spark of life that was seeded into the potential of our being. It is said that when a person can fully connect with and function from the focal point of Yuan Shen, then they will have attained Shen Ming (神明) or 'spiritual divinity': the Daoist equivalent of what we might call 'enlightened'. The practitioner's experience of the world is now void of acquired and emotionally based attachment to the phenomena of manifestation. Spending time in practice, united with the Yuan Shen, a practitioner will gradually dissolve the acquired layers of mind so that there is no more subjective identification with an erroneous sense of individuality. Expressed 'personality' may still be present, but consciousness has merged with true spirit; the result of this is union with the objective reality.

Though we are generally unaware of the existence of Yuan Shen, its potential lies at the core of all of us. This is why so many Eastern traditions pointed at a state of spiritual transcendence already being within us; we have just forgotten, or else buried its potential beneath layers of distortion.

Wu Shen (五神): The Five Spirits

When the Yuan Shen encounters the realm of manifest mind, it refracts into the five spirits that were discussed above. Curiously, some aspects of these spirits are said to be gifted by Heaven, some by Earth, and others are passed on to us through our family line. No matter their stated origin, they all still originated from within the seed of Yuan Shen; from this, we can understand that, though Yuan Shen is discussed as an entity, it is also an all-encompassing state within which Heaven, Earth and the 'ten thousand things' reside.

The five spirits all exist within the realm of Shen but resonate on different levels. They are each anchored into the vehicle of the body through attachment to an organ system. Whilst Yuan Shen is 'still' in nature, the five spirits are shifting, transient, and go through a process of evolutionary change. It is through the movements of these five spirits that the further expressions of mind are manifest.

Wu Yi (五义): The Five Expressions

The five expressions are the 'baseline' manner in which our five spirits connect into the world. They are the innate functions of the five spirits and the manner with which they connect each of us to the spiritual and material world. The Shen connects us to 'divine insight' and the workings of Heaven. The Hun connects us to the wider 'plans of Heaven' as well as allowing us connection to the 'collective consciousness' of all sentient life. The Zhi connects us to the 'will of Earth', whilst the Po gives us 'untainted awareness' of reality. Sat between these four prime poles, sometimes known as being 'at the centre of the four spiritual directions', is the Yi; the Yi is responsible for our 'original nature'.

It is, in turn, the existence of the five expressions that then enables us to manifest the five De or 'virtues'. This is why, when people move close towards the 'location' of their Yuan Shen, they will find a natural evolution towards a more virtuous state of being.

Wu Zei (五賊): The Five Thieves

The five spirits are anchored into our being, manifest as the five expressions, until we begin to use our five sense faculties which are, as discussed in Chapter 2, known as the 'five thieves'. Note that our senses are known as 'sense faculties' within Daoism, as they are said to contain a separate consciousness of their own. It is through the five thieves that the five spirits then experience the world. It is as if they look out of the 'windows of our mind' in order to view the world. Within some classical forms of Chinese medicine, they even talked of opening the orifices of the mind so that the spirits could be at rest. This was so that the five thieves did not 'steal' from their state and so create emotional turmoil.

Since the five thieves each have their own consciousness, they are subject to acquired distortion, and so it is as the sense faculties bring in 'information' to the five spirits that the start of the psychological distortion process begins. The virtues begin to change and the subjective and emotional mind is formed.

Within Daoist meditative training, one of the first instructions was to seal the senses so that the thieves would not further distort one's mind. The Dao De Jing states that if we 'seal up our windows' and 'stay within our house' then we will begin to truly know the world.

Wu Ai Zhi (五愛執): The Five Attachments

Each of the five spirits has their own attachment which serves to create the acquired mind. The Po then confuses matters by having further attachments of its own, but we shall come to that later. For now, the five overriding attachments of the spirits are an 'attachment to polarities' for the Shen, an 'attachment to position' for the Hun, an 'attachment to subjective individuality' for the Yi, an 'attachment to materialism' for the Po and an 'attachment to need' for the Zhi. If we look at these in turn, we can see how these become the base 'fears' or distorted associations with dualistic existence that arise within the spirits as a result of the influence of the sense faculties.

- The Shen gives us an 'attachment to polarities'. The view of the world that the Shen is now given through its interaction with the realm of manifestation means that it views everything in comparison to its complementary opposite. Up exists because of down, good exists because of bad and so on. The result of this is a sense of separation and division between all phenomena; this is the process which prevents union with the divine source that Shen has the potential to connect with at its deepest level of functioning.

- The Hun gives us an 'attachment to position' as a result of the separation of life into constituent parts by the Shen. If all things are now apart, how do they exist in relation to one another? This is especially apparent when the Hun applies this way of thinking to our sense of self. We now have an attachment to everything from authority and status through to levels of self-worth and importance. Our direction in life is then distorted by this understanding of 'position'.

- The Yi gives us an 'attachment to subjective individuality' which is a further advancement of the attachments of the Shen and the Hun. 'If this is me, then this must be my mind'; this is how we can view the attachment to individual existence that the Yi gives us. As soon as we have a 'mind', then the seeds for identification with a subjective sense of self are planted. This is where we lose sight of the fact that the acquired mind is an 'outer shell' and instead it becomes a form of self-identification.
- The Po is a very Yin spirit and so an 'attachment to materialism' is the result of its distortion. The Po will enjoy attaching to objects and anything that gives us a stronger sense of self according to what we gain. On a very tangible level this can be money and accrued belongings, but on a less tangible level it can be those actions, events or views people have of us that help us to develop a stronger 'sense of self'.
- The Zhi gives us a generally distorted sense of 'attachment to need'. If the Zhi is functioning in a harmonious manner, then it will understand the basic needs of human life which are survival needs – food and shelter. It should keep us aware of what we need to survive on the earthly plane. As this attachment begins to distort, then we can start to think we have 'survival needs' that we do not really need to survive at all.

Wu Ai Bu Ai (五愛不愛): The Five Biases

The five spirits will then act according to the five attachments and start to develop a sense of 'like and dislike'. Preferences like this are what start to develop our conditioned view of the world and so the 'five biases' begin to manifest. These are the preferences of the five spirits according to their attachments. They are quite simply a bias towards good and bad for the Shen, a bias towards those things which are connected to status for the Hun, a bias towards developing an acquired sense of self for the Yi, a bias towards those material possessions that strengthen our sense of self for the Po, and a bias for those things and events that will aid us in our 'survival needs' for the Zhi.

Essentially, this means that the mind will now develop a preferential view of the world based upon 'like and dislike' as a result of the spirits' attachment to the material world. This is because the five thieves have stolen from your consciousness its sole connection to divinity.

It is here, within the realm of bias, that the majority of our mental distortions are developed. Every interaction that we have, every stimulus that reaches us, will come with an unconscious labelling of positive or negative, like or dislike, and this is how we will store our life experiences within the layers of the mind. Our search for more positive stimuli will develop the root of our desires and our need to keep a hold of these positive biases will give us a sense of attachment. Biases will be given to us by people we meet, those who influence us, social programming and, of course, our own distortions. These biases are the substance of our conditioned thinking.

Wu Du (五毒): The Five Poisons

The five biases will be further extrapolated out into the five emotions. This is the way that our Qi is expressed within the body according to the movements of our acquired mind. Each of the five emotions is then a heading, an overriding categorisation for a whole host of emotionally charged experiences. Table 12.2 shows a more complete list of emotional responses, though it could, of course, be added to almost infinitely, such is the complexity of the human mind.

Table 12.2: Human Emotions

Element	Wood	Fire	Earth	Metal	Water
Emotion	Anger	Joy	Worry	Grief	Fear
	Frustration	Excitement	Obsession	Sadness	Panic
	Jealousy	Mania	Pensiveness	Loss	Shock
	Envy	Love	Caring	Defensiveness	Addictions
	Control	Lust	Smothering	Attachment	Wanting
	Rage	Embarrassment	Neediness	Possessiveness	Terror
	Annoyance	Sadness	Empathy	Greed	Perversion

Wu Qi (五氣): The Five Qi

The way that the Qi moves within the body is then categorised according to its emotional quality. These categorisations of Qi are known as Wood, Fire,

Earth, Metal and Water. It is here that the study of Chinese medicine has its place as it is working to try to harmonise the internal Qi that has adapted as a result of the manner in which your emotions have moved.

Wu Xiang (五象): The Five Manifestations

The five manifestations are the way in which the five Qi begin to influence the body's functioning on a physical level. The name 'five manifestations' is rather misleading, as it is actually a series of five headings under which various aspects of human functioning are grouped. These are summarised in Table 12.3.

Table 12.3: The Manifestations of the Five Qi

Element	Wood	Fire	Earth	Metal	Water
Colour	Green	Red	Yellow	White	Blue
Movement	Rising	Expanding	Dividing	Contracting	Sinking
Substance	Qi	Shen	Yuan Shen	Yuan Xi	Jing
Taste	Sour	Bitter	Sweet	Pungent	Salty
Smell	Rancid	Burnt	Fragrant	Rotten	Putrid
Yin organ	Liver	Heart	Spleen	Lungs	Kidneys
Yang organ	Gall Bladder	Small Intestine	Stomach	Large Intestine	Bladder
Tissues	Tendons	Blood Vessels	Muscles	Skin	Bones
Orifice	Eyes	Tongue	Mouth	Nose	Ears
Body	Limbs	Head	Abdomen	Chest	Back

The manifestations are ways in which the various distortions of mind can begin to affect the physical body. This is a more complex way of understanding just how the development of mind serves as the root of internally developed imbalance.

The Five Elemental Movements

The Wu Xing, or 'five elemental movements', of Wood, Fire, Earth, Metal and Water were introduced in Chapter 2. They are a way of categorising and understanding the inter-transformation of phenomena within the acquired world. Some scholars have mistakenly asserted that the Daoists learnt about the nature of reality through observation of the outside world and so decided that everything was created out of five literal elemental substances. This error likely comes about through comparison of the Wu Xing to early Greek thought. The Daoist tradition is based upon observation of the nature of the 'inner universe' and as such is based in the way that spirit, consciousness and energy interact with one another. When it was seen that the singularity of Yuan Shen refracted into five constituent parts, these became the basis for how life developed. The refraction of Yuan Shen into five 'lights' served to form the foundation of the Wu Xing theory. These five lights were then arranged diagrammatically, as shown in Figure 12.10. This is one of two variant arrangements of the Wu Xing used within Daoist theory.

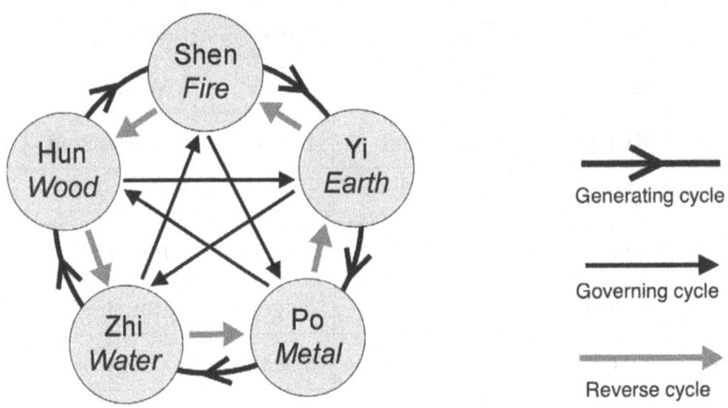

Figure 12.10: The Wu Xing Developmental Arrangement

The five lights of the Wu Xing exist on the level of Shen. Remember that within the Daoist tradition, all life originates within the realm of Shen, essentially condensing downwards into the level of Qi and then further from here into Jing. Jing is the densest of the three, and so if it becomes any denser, it then becomes tangible matter. During the process of our foetal development, the Jing began to form our physical body. This process continues throughout our life with the production of everything from body fluids through to regenerated cells. The brain is an organic 'translator' for the information contained within Jing, Qi and Shen; it converts their vibrational frequencies into a format that we can understand. In this way, Shen is 'read' by the mind and generally converted into a form of light.

Shen as Light

It is said that the doorway to Wu (悟) or 'awakening' is often bathed in light. This light that is discussed is the bright, shining light of Yuan Shen. When the five spirits are reconverged into one singular state, then they will appear within the mind's eye as a bright light. This light is so bright that it feels as if you should be blinded, it brings with it a profound state of expansive consciousness; the effects of this experience can be life-changing, as the light of Yuan Shen 'burns' through the distortions of the acquired mind.

Interestingly, the brain will interpret the information of Yuan Shen in other ways as well. When deeply Christian people experience the merger of Yuan Shen, they often see God or Christ before them. Buddhists will see Buddha, and so on. The deep association we have with spiritual archetypes will mean that the brain will interpret our deepest experience of spirit in the manner that is clearest for us. The problem with this, though, is that any form of personification then ends our connection to spirit. Personification is a 'definition' that is too finite and so the result of this is that the acquired mind becomes involved. The sheer act of the acquired mind's involvement will serve to refract the five 'lights' out of Yuan Shen once more and so the connection is lost. The result is a fleeting glimpse of Yuan Shen that is then lost to us; in this way, our belief system has become a trap.

This is why many Eastern schools talk of 'crushing the deities' when you meet them on your path. They recognise the trap of personification of true spirit. Hence, for me, religion is a fine tool if it speaks to you, but if you go deep enough into your development, then the religion should be stepped out of; the tool has served you well enough, now make the connection to divine spirit your own. One of the most powerful Eastern traditions was knowing when to step away from tradition; curiously, this became a tradition in its own right!

For those who do not hold a strong religious belief or a series of archetypes that have been given to them during their developmental phases, the experience of Yuan Shen will generally arrive as a non-defined bright, shining light. Once again, this is not the aim but simply a by-product of practice; a signpost along the way.

When the five spirits refract out of Yuan Shen, they are manifest within the brain as five coloured lights that lack the sheer brilliance of Yuan Shen but are still quite beautiful in their own right.

The five colours of the Wu Xing are:

- various shades of green and turquoise for Wood
- red through to burgundy and bright orange for Fire

- yellow and earthen tones for Earth
- grey and silver through to white for Metal
- dark through to brilliant blue and purple for Water.

When there are changes within one or more aspects of your elemental makeup, it is common for these colours to show up brightly within your mind's eye. Like most other phenomena, they are to be ignored, as attachment to them will hinder their development. These colours are the basis for the development of the Wu Xing, and it is from here that all of their further manifestations then occur.

Balance of the Wu Xing

If we look back to Figure 12.10, we can see that there are a few ways in which the five elemental movements remain in balance with one another. They each give birth to, govern and are governed by the other elemental movements. This relationship between the five key elemental movements is always changing; it is never still. The nature of existence is transience, nothing is still once it exists beyond the state of Yuan Shen. It is this constant movement of the core elemental foundations of life that keep everything evolving as it should.

This movement and changing balance between the five elemental movements takes place continuously within the core of our being. This process sits at the centre of our consciousness and essentially dictates the manner in which the various distortions of our psychological perception are going to unfold. If the five elemental movements were ever to be fully harmonised with one another – if all of the five elemental sources of Wood, Fire, Earth, Metal and Water were equal in amount and strength – they would reconverge and so Yuan Shen would be reformed; we would experience Wu – 'awakening'.

Within life, this level of balance is not realisable/achievable/feasible. Life events, innate psychological makeup and various other factors will generally mean that we have dominant elements and weaker elements. Though we will experience change in this situation throughout our lives, we will generally have a dominant elemental state that is our most fixed and inherent inner quality. Within Chinese medicine, particularly within the systems more geared towards treatment of psychological conditions, people are categorised according to their elemental 'type'. So, a 'Wood-type' person may have an elemental balance as shown in Figure 12.11. I give this as an example, but you could easily go on to apply this kind of depiction to each of the other four elements.

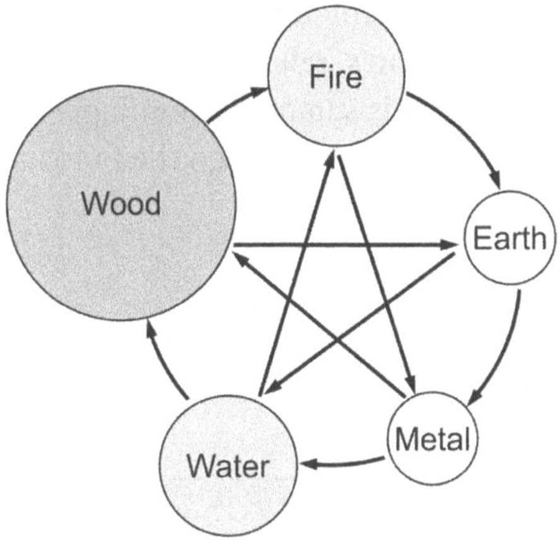

Figure 12.11: Wood-Type Person

The nature of this dominance towards an element will dictate various aspects of your nature; primarily, this is around your 'default perception and reaction' to events or stimuli.

Do not make the mistake of seeing these elemental imbalances as inherently problematic, though; this is not the case. The elemental makeup of a person contains the potential for many strengths as well as weaknesses. For example, a person dominated by their Wood elemental phase can have a tendency towards feelings of frustration and seeing every difficulty as a conflict, but they also have great potential for leadership skills, setting up projects and initiating positive change in their environment. For a full discussion of the nature of these elemental types, I would suggest exploring the theory of Chinese medicine.

Ultimately though, to move towards a state of contacting Yuan Shen, we must move further back towards the source, before the state of division of Shen into these five movements. Though the elemental quality of our makeup may remain, we are able to experience a state deeper than this as well.

The Process of Thought

As already discussed, we can think of the vast ocean of consciousness as sitting at the root of our psychological being. If the ocean becomes truly still, then we will start to experience the nature of our spirit. On top of the surface of the ocean are various waves which are the movements of our mind and these movements are then subject to the 'wind' of our thoughts. By stilling the wind, the idea is that the waves begin to subside and so the ocean returns to stillness. Daoist metaphorical parlance states that when the ocean is still enough, it will reflect the moon upon its surface; it is only the waves that are preventing the ocean's 'reflective' qualities. The 'moon' is the light of the Yuan Shen. This idea is summarised in Figure 12.12. Although a metaphor, if we can understand this idea, then the fundamentals of stilling the mind can be comprehended.

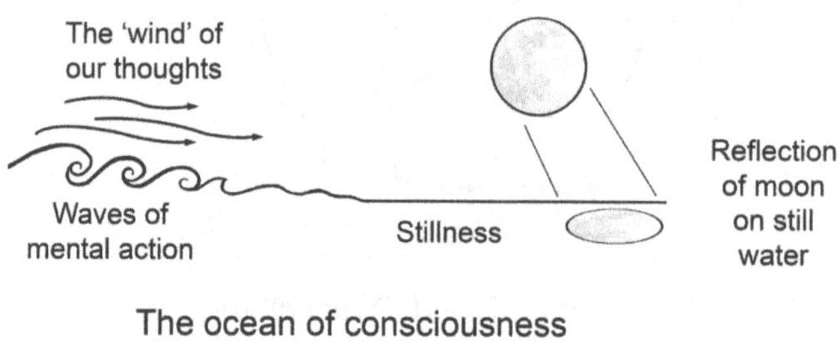

Figure 12.12: The Ocean of Consciousness

Within Daoist practice, there are said to be three main ways of training for the mind. These are three types of training which are an inherent part of the Daoist tradition. It is through these three main methods that the 'five spirits return to their origin'. These three methods of training are described below.

Nei Guan (內觀): Inner Looking

The first aspect of stilling the mind is Nei Guan or 'inner looking'. The mind is used to 'looking outwards'. When we interact with the world it is in this manner; our sense faculties will want to interact with those things that create a form of stimulation. This then serves to develop and grow the acquired mind in accordance with our experiences. Whilst this is important for being able to function on a daily basis, we need to learn the skill of 'inner looking' if we are to begin any kind of developmental process that moves us closer to Yuan Shen.

We begin to look inwards as soon as we begin our training of Qi Gong and/or meditation. By sealing off the senses and allowing our awareness to move inside, we will begin to develop the skill of Nei Guan. At first, it is very difficult to do – do not fall into the trap of thinking 'looking inside' is going to be easy; it will not be. The main reason for this is that the acquired mind is accustomed to seeking its nourishment from the outside world. As soon as it is starved of this process, it will start to 'rebel'; this is what we talked of when we discussed the 'monkey-mind' in Chapter 6. This rebellion will begin with a hyperactivity of the mind as it starts to produce a stream of random thoughts; it can be surprising just how crazy your mind can become during silent sitting practice. From here, if the stream of thoughts is not enough to cause your mind to become disturbed from its stillness, then it will find memories and emotionally charged events to bring to the front of your mind; this is when old arguments or heartbreaks can come to the surface of your mind.

A major trick that the mind will produce is the manifestation of boredom. Boredom is rarely discussed as a hurdle to your development but it can be a major issue within the internal arts. Boredom is the acquired mind's primary way of forcing you to seek out extra forms of stimulation. If you are not using your various sense faculties to bring nourishment to the acquired mind, then it can bring you almost torturous levels of boredom as a way to force you to stop your practice and seek stimulation; in fact, in many cases, there doesn't even have to be very much boredom to overcome many practitioners' will! Figure 12.13 summarises some of the mind's tricks.

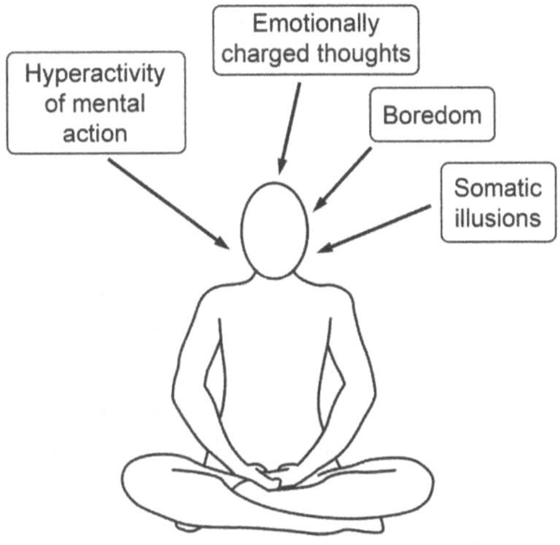

Figure 12.13: Tricks of the Mind

If none of these tricks of the mind are working, then the acquired mind can even create somatic experiences to disturb your peace. These often take the form of an intense itch right on the end of your nose! If you end your practice to scratch that itch, then the acquired mind has what it wants: you have stimulated the sense faculties through your involvement in the experience and so, once again, the mind's peace is disturbed. Such are the levels of rebellion that the mind will go to when you first start to 'look inside'.

Once you have broken through all of those barriers by spending enough time letting go of the arising experiences, you will finally begin to 'see' inside. This is not a literal visual form of seeing. This is quite different from some of the abilities that can come from Nei Gong training whereby you can see Qi within the visual spectrum; this, instead, is the start of an awareness of how your mind functions.

Nei Guan will generally bring with it a stark realisation of how you are psychologically aligned. Many of us suffer from the affliction of not being able to see ourselves clearly. It is a bit of a cliché to say that none of us truly know ourselves, but it is also true. The first step towards understanding the wider reality is first understanding exactly who you are and why you think and act in certain ways. A key aspect of this is understanding exactly what the motives and root reasons are for the way you think, react to and process thoughts and events.

As well as this, when the rebellion of the stimulus-seeking acquired mind has slowed a little, you can begin to see just how your thoughts arise and how they are either fed or starved by your awareness. This kind of Gong is required for further development into the realm of balancing the five spirits and it will arise out of regular practice of patiently sitting and 'looking inwards'.

Xin Zhai (心齋): Heart Mind Fasting

When there is a movement of the mind, then a thought arises. These thoughts can range from completely mundane through to deeply profound. They can have an obvious emotional root to them or else they can appear absurd in quality. Many of these thoughts are based in attachment to memories, whilst others are rooted in projected desires and fears. Whatever their nature, the emergence of thoughts serves as the root for the actions of the acquired mind. This is where the application of Xin Zhai, or Heart Mind Fasting, comes into play.

The 'food' that the mind is 'fasting' from is our conscious attention. Basically, it comes down to the idea that where we give our attention, we also give our Qi. On top of this, the quality of our attention also dictates what that Qi will do. What this means is that when thoughts arise, those that are given our attention will become a 'thought stream', a linear evolution of a thought, that then turns into a mental process.

Think of it like this: if I have a thought of something seemingly irrelevant, say a cactus, then it is nothing important. It is the fleeting image of a spiky plant that has popped into my head. Even though there is no major emotional attachment to this image, if I give my attention to this image, then it will be 'fed'; the 'fast' is over. My Qi will now become involved and so the thought of a cactus can begin to take seed and unfold for me as a stream of thoughts. What was simply a random image will now be processed by my emotional mind, my biases, my conditioned thinking, my desires and my attachments. The image of the cactus will stay within my head and my mind will start to race through all of the associations I have with a cactus; I will see images of cowboy movies, unwanted Christmas presents, pain I once experienced when I touched the spike on a cactus and so on. I may decide that I want a cactus and so my mind will start plotting a path and time to the garden centre where I can obtain one. The mind also works on association and so the thought of going out shopping will then lead me to think of other shops I may want to visit, people I may meet and so on and so on. This process will then continue until it is replaced by a new and more pressing thought stream. This is the process of how a thought 'seed' is fed by our attention, given Qi and then becomes a 'thought stream'. It is through the development of these streams that further distortion of the acquired mind takes place, and so the Yuan Shen is buried further beneath the mire of built-up layers of mind. Figure 12.14 summarises the process of thoughts becoming thought streams.

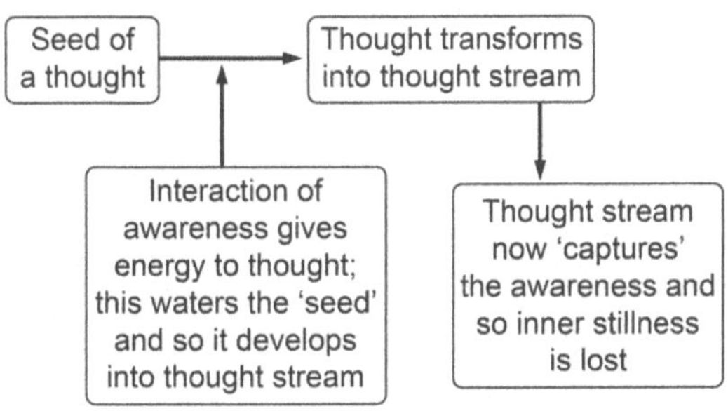

Figure 12.14: Thought to Thought Streams

The example above may seem like a rather random one – why cactuses? I have just chosen a simple example, a random thought that appeared in my head whilst I am sat here typing. But this process will be taking place all of the time in your mind, every second of your life. When awake, these thoughts are largely dependent upon the influence of the sense faculties, and whilst you are asleep, these images are drawn from your subconscious mind. In times of 'dullness', when the mind is not receiving stimulating information, then it will be your memories and mental projections that form the seeds of these thought streams. If a person is very prone to this kind of mental movement, then we may call them a daydreamer, since it is closer to the psychological mechanism used by the mind when we are asleep.

Major issues develop when a person goes through this process involving a very emotionally charged thought. Perhaps you suffered an awful trauma and this trauma has stayed with you as a memory. Maybe your mother died in a dreadful accident involving that cactus? Now, whenever you see a cactus, it brings back all of the terrible associations you have with them. Feelings of sadness, loss and grieving may manifest within you and a whole stream of thoughts will unfold that causes a chronic shift in your emotional makeup. It is these kinds of experiences that leave the most lasting effects on us and also, sadly, these kinds of thoughts that are the most difficult to deal with and let go of. This is because there is a part of the acquired mind that is above all concepts of good and bad. Although you may recall your trauma as being terrible, to the mind it is just another form of nourishment, and a particularly strong one at that. With regard to mental nourishment, the stronger the better, and so these kinds of thoughts can stick within your head and repeat themselves over and over. This is why many people get caught up in very negative-seeming thought patterns that can engulf their life.

To make the mind 'fast', we need to 'starve' it of our Qi. To do this, we do not give it our attention. This is the root of why so many traditions tell you to simply observe what is taking place within your mind without becoming involved. Whilst this is a very difficult instruction, it really is the way to retrain the mind's actions. Within our methods, we have a way to assist in this process, which is why we look to develop conscious absorption into the processes of our practice, starting with our breath and developing through into the actions and movements of Yin Qi and Yang Qi. These are the 'bananas' for the 'monkey-mind', something not based in the movements of thoughts and emotions so that the mind can start to be trained. With time, it will realise that you will not give it the attention it desires. No matter how many thoughts are produced within your mind, your awareness is not getting involved; it is busy elsewhere.

This use of a process as a kind of 'banana' is obviously a stop-gap. It is a temporary measure until you have attained a certain quality of mind, the Gong of being able to stabilise your awareness into the inner universe of your consciousness without feeding the mind. In my experience, this takes place in five clear stages. You will note that I have stuck to the Chinese tradition of using 'five' when I discuss the mind; it seemed appropriate somehow!

1. Your mind is always in movement. Every single second of your life, the mind is generating waves.

2. The mind is in movement whilst you are practising, but you can be absorbed into something else. With time, the movements will fade away into the distance and your thoughts start to become like distant echoes.

3. Now you can take your mind off any distracting processes. The 'banana' is no longer required and so now you can simply sit and practise Xin Zhai for protracted periods of time. When you end your practice and return to daily life, the movements of the mind will restart.

4. At this stage of development, after you end your practice, the stillness of mind will stay for an extended period of time. You can now manage 'stillness within movement', meaning that you can carry out your daily life whilst still practising Xin Zhai.

5. At this final stage, you have practised Xin Zhai to such a level that there is never any unnecessary movement of mind, no matter what you are doing. This is the level of 'no mind' that hardly any will ever reach. It is a state of inner stillness that is a precursor to full awakening.

Movement brings you closer to 'mind', whilst stillness is the realm of 'Yuan Shen'. This is the basis of Xin Zhai teachings.

Zuo Wang (坐忘): Sitting and Forgetting

The principle of Zuo Wang, or 'sitting and forgetting', is an aspect of Daoist meditative training that will arise from developing the mind to a point of profound stillness. What is 'forgotten' is the overriding control of the acquired mind. Although the acquired mind is required by all living people, it needs to be recognised for the 'tool' that it is. It is the part of our mind that recalls, remembers and understands how to deal with the outside world. This makes it a rather important part of our being!

The issue comes when we start to overidentify with the acquired mind and believe it to be who we really are. This is how we build up a 'false sense of self'. Who are we? To the Daoists, we are an integral part of the wider universe, a drop in the ocean of the wider cosmos and an expression of the ruminations of Dao. When we attain union with this state of being, then we are said to have found the gateway into an awakening experience. When we identify with the acquired mind, and the distortions have become our point of reference, then we have developed a sense of separation from existence that is considered 'false' by the Daoists. We need to 'sit and forget' this sense of self so that we can merge with the state of higher spirit that sits at the centre of all being. The subjective has become the objective.

As with the other 'chains' of Chinese concepts outlined in this book, Nei Guan will lead to Xin Zhai if we go deep enough. The result of a deep practice of Xin Zhai is the development of Zuo Wang.

Wu Yao (五藥): The Five Cures

Continuing with the theme of 'fives', here are the Wu Yao or 'five cures', sometimes known as the Xian Yao (仙藥) or 'immortal medicines' within alchemical traditions. It is these 'cures' that are required to begin the returning of the five spirits back to their original state of Yuan Shen. The cures are described below.

Harmonious Qi

When the Qi of the body has been worked and developed to a state of harmony, then the foundation of cultivating the five spirits has been established. The Daoists often talk of regulating the 'five Qi', and in this sense they are actually referring to the five elemental qualities of Qi as they are expressed in the body; these essentially become the elemental categorisations of the channel system and associated organ and tissue systems. This stage also relates to the foundation of 'good health' that we should aim to build within the Daoist tradition if we wish to start moving towards 'self' or 'spiritual' cultivation. As stated at the start of this book, all of this, the health of the body and the development of mind, is based in the same idea – improving the efficiency of the body's functioning. The start point for this is the Nei Gong process and the harmonising of the body's Qi.

Still Mind

The processes discussed here involving Nei Guan, Xin Zhai and Zuo Wang are all concerned with the stilling of the mind; the ending of the waves on the ocean of consciousness. The foundations for these qualities should already be established in the fundamental Qi Gong skills of regulating the breath and regulating the mind. In this way, Qi Gong practice and the Nei Gong process are a precursor to meditative training.

Tranquil Nature

The expression of your inner state is manifest to your nature, the way that your persona is shown to others as well as how you experience the world. When the heart is 'light', the mind 'quiet' and your demeanour 'content', then your nature will be tranquil. This process is worked on internally through our cultivation process as well as externally through the application of precepts and philosophical teachings.

Forgotten Emotions

Whilst our emotions are a wonderful thing – they give us a rich experience of the world and serve as the root for all the creative aspects of our being – they should not be overidentified with. Remember that this is what the term Wang (忘) or 'forget' refers to within Daoism: a movement away from an overidentification with the objective sense of self that we have a tendency towards. If the emotions can be there, but not overidentified with, then we can start to still the mind's actions and so move closer towards a state of inner harmony.

Spirits in Harmony

With the mind still, the five spirits can begin their process of 'self-purification', the shedding of deep inherent distortions. This will happen as a by-product of being freed from the machinations of mind. As they begin to settle, the 'dust is cleaned from the mirror' and so they move into a more harmonious state. This will help them to start reconverging and so here the light of Yuan Shen can be re-experienced.

The Five Collections

When the 'five cures' have been put in place, then this will, in turn, help to take you back through the Wu Yun (五蘊) or 'five collections'. Don't worry, this is the final 'five' of the chapter! We have already looked at how each of the spirits has individual expressions, biases, attachments and so on. These are further broken down into the Wu Yun, and it is through harmonising the spirits that the Wu Yun begin to reverse themselves. The Wu Yun are:

- Se (色) Appearance
- Shou (受) Reception

- Xiang (想) Wanting
- Xing (行) Preference
- Zhi (識) Storing.

I have included the Wu Yun as they are a nice, simple model for explaining the process of interacting with the world that has been discussed in this chapter. In short, they are a way that the five thieves serve to develop the acquired mind. We go through the Wu Yun in sequence when we interact with the world. Initially, we encounter the Se, or outer 'appearance', of a phenomenon or event. From here we Shou, or 'receive', our false perception of this experience into the mind. There is then a process of mental cognition that involves Xiang, or 'wanting'; do we want this experience or not? This is the level of bias; it leads us to Xing, or 'preference'. In many cases, this is based on previous experiences and learnt behaviour. Finally, we Zhi, or 'store', the outcome of this process in the mind as an acquired layer of the mind. It is this process which is reversed when the five spirits can reconverge. It is said that when we reach this level, we begin to perceive the world as a child, free from preconceived ideas.

White Moon on the Mountain Peak

From the above discussion, I hope it will have become clear that, ultimately, it is the inner stillness that brings us closer to a state of Yuan Shen. Through bringing the five spirits to a state of stillness, we can begin to reconverge them and so begin to enter into deeper spiritual development. The result of this generally comes with the experience of the bright shining light of Yuan Shen. This is a good sign of progress, though obviously not the goal in its own right. The shining light can come and go, it will flicker, appear hazy, sometimes extend out into your life outside of meditation and sometimes not appear for months on end; such is the nature of internal training. The variables involved in these practices and how they develop for you mean that we can do our best, but there will always be unknown aspects of the practice for us.

The longer we can reside within stillness and nourish the Yuan Shen in this manner, the more developed our spirit will be. The analogy for this that I always found the most poetic was attaining the 'white moon on the mountain peak'.

At this stage in your practice, it is really advanced alchemical training that you should seek out. Your Nei Gong has established a solid foundation for you, but you now need to study the alchemical meditative traditions of Daoism in greater detail.

In the final chapter, I will summarise many of the aspects of the Nei Gong tradition that bring up questions for people; these will include the Heart centre field or 'middle Dan Tian', the attainment and function of Siddhi, the macrocosmic orbit and the Ling. I hope you will forgive me for the final chapter being something of a mixture of pieces of information; I simply wish to make sure I have covered as many of the bases as I can when outlining this enigmatic process to you!

Chapter 13

EXTRA ASPECTS

The process I have discussed within this book has, up until this point, been a very direct and linear path that will lead you through the classical alchemical stages of Jing to Qi, Qi to Shen and then Shen to Dao. The basic premise of this is that the Jing needs to be cultivated, understood and then stilled. From here, the Qi is awakened, circulated and then, at much later stages, increased and stored in the body. The foundations developed in the Jing and Qi aspect of the training are then used to build an efficient platform upon which to cultivate the Shen. Ultimately, it is the level of stillness within the mind that will serve to move a person towards direct cultivation of Shen. When the Shen has reached a stage of spiritual development, then it will lead to union with the non-dual state known as Dao. This is the basis of Daoist practice; from here, the various lineages and systems have their own slant on the process and their own methods for cultivating along this path.

Much of the above process is outlined within classical teachings such as the Sinew-Changing Classic and the marrow-washing teachings. On top of this, these 'energetic mechanics' were then combined with the philosophical and alchemical scripture of Daoism; the fruit of this merger was the basis of all the arts we practise today that are associated with the Daoist tradition.

In addition to this very clear and direct path of progression through the system, there are also various side branches that are a part of internal training. These extra aspects to the practice are somewhat difficult to put into a linear path as they are not necessarily on the route from Jing to Qi to Shen and so on. On top of this, not every tradition embraces these aspects of the arts. Major examples of this would be 'heart work', an area of practice that most alchemical traditions placed little importance upon, and practice focusing on the Central channel, which is a more prominent aspect of training within the more 'magical' Daoist schools.

Because of the difficulty in identifying the exact position of these areas of training on the path of Nei Gong, I have put them here as a series of short sections in the final chapter of the book.

The Central Channel

The first aspect of the training I wish to look at is practice focusing on the 'Central channel'. The Central channel is a tube-like pole of conductivity that runs through the core of the body, as shown in Figure 13.1. It is not dependent upon any particular physical structure and is considered to be an aspect of the Thrusting channel network.

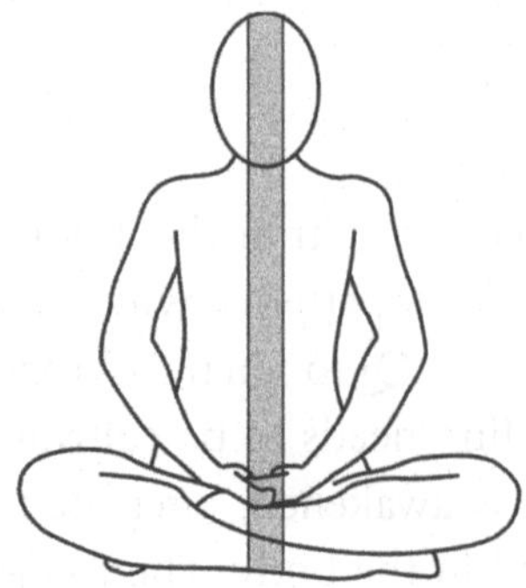

Figure 13.1: The Central Channel

The Central channel is an interesting part of the body because it is linked to so many aspects of our internal makeup. Although it conducts Qi in the same manner as other channels, it also conducts Jing and Shen along its length. On a physiological level, it is very closely linked to the function of the endocrine system as well as the health of our blood. In women, it is the prime channel that governs the health of their menstrual cycle and, as such, it is used heavily in Chinese medical treatments.

It is important in Nei Gong, as it is the channel that connects the three core Dan Tian together, as shown in Figure 13.1. Communication between the three Dan Tian takes place along the length of this deep, internal pathway and much of the conversion of alchemical substances relies on the functioning of this channel.

When there is enough Qi within the body, then there is often a process of expansion of energy away from the Dan Tian into the length of the Central channel. It generally initiates from the base of the body, around the region of the lower Dan Tian, as shown in Figure 13.2.

This idea of Qi radiating out of the lower Dan Tian is a vital part of advanced energetic work. It is through this radiation that Qi can be moved from its storage location in the body and used for various reasons. An example of this would be to issue Qi within a Chinese medical setting, where Qi is emitted from the therapist into their patient's body so that their own internal Qi can be adjusted. This is a principle known as Wai Qi Liao Fa

(外氣療法) or 'Qi Gong healing' as it is more commonly known. There are two main ways of doing this; one is to 'push' the Qi out with intention. This method generally has a detrimental effect upon the practitioner if they do this regularly over a long period of time.

The second way to emit the Qi is to build up the level of energy within your body through Nei Gong training until it is already on the verge of 'spilling over' out of your body. At this stage, the Qi will radiate out through the body's Huang, so to emit the Qi is actually very simple: you are simply doing what the Qi already wants to do. Much of the strength of this emission will then depend upon how well the Qi within the lower Dan Tian has radiated through into the Central channel, as shown in Figure 13.2. When the Qi fills up the Central channel, then it can reach right through to the top of the head as shown.

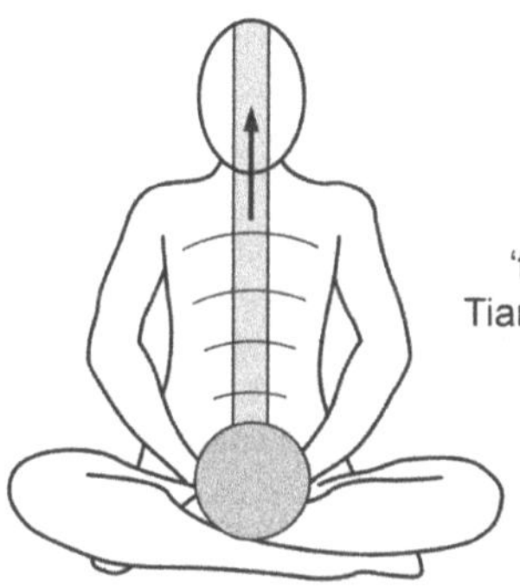

Figure 13.2: Expansion of Lower Dan Tian

There are then two places where the Qi can begin to 'leak' from the body. The first is at the level of the Heart field. This leakage will take place as a result of emotional upset; we shall explore this below when we look at the Heart field in more detail. The second place that the Qi can leak from is in the head, around the region of the upper Dan Tian, if there are strong psychological issues.

It is not my intention to go into great detail about the subject of Wai Qi Liao Fa – it is a big area and the kind of topic that could easily fill a very detailed volume; what should be understood, though, is that if this Qi 'leaks' into the radiated field of a therapist, then they can unwittingly transfer this information to their patient. Qi is also a form of information, remember, especially Yang Qi. This is why there needs to be a solid level of internal development for any practitioner of energy work that involves healing another person in some way.

When the Qi begins to enter into the Central channel, then it will start to lead your awareness very deep into your body. Here, within the centre of the body, is also an aspect of Shen. This is what makes the Central channel so interesting and so powerful. There are whole meditation systems based around working with the length of the Central channel rather than with the Shen that is anchored into the upper Dan Tian or with the mind at the level of the Heart field (as is the case with some Tantric Buddhist systems). The Shen within the Central channel is an extension of the wider spirit of the cosmos and this is a part of the reason why Daoist schools based in magical or environmental practice use it to such an extent. It is a literal pillar of spirit that extends through us, between Heaven and Earth. This is shown in Figure 13.3.

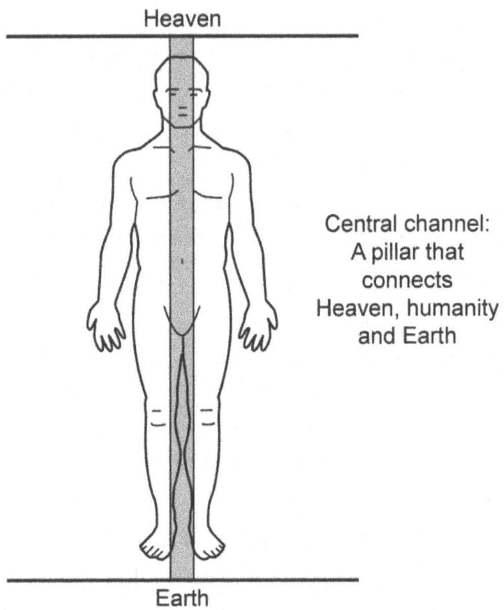

Figure 13.3: Extension of Central Channel Through the Body

Although the methods I have outlined within this book are not directly aimed at the Central channel (these systems often use mantra, mudra and transmission heavily), it is possible to open the Central channel naturally as a by-product of your wider practice. When your awareness becomes absorbed into the Central channel, then there is often a series of unfolding processes which can lead you off on a different path of practice for quite some time. In my personal experience, the process within the Central channel tends to unfold in the following sequence:

- Mental ease
- Emotional release
- Contacting trauma
- Realisation of Xing
- Elemental shift
- The bliss stage
- Encountering Shen
- The trap of emptiness
- Convergence

Within myself and the people I have taught – those who have entered into this kind of process – I have seen a common pattern of moving through this sequence. Whilst there has been a little variation in the way that the experience has manifested from student to student, this is the general pattern that work with the Central channel entails. Let us look briefly at each phase of the work.

Mental Ease

When the Shen of the Central channel is first experienced, it can be very calming. When the awareness soaks into the core of the body, there is a real feeling of ease. This is then generally followed by a clear feeling of the Central channel starting to fill up with Yang Qi. As the vibrating sensation of the channel filling reaches a certain level, this Qi begins to spread through the body. This is a very pleasant stage and certainly one of the nicest parts of the Nei Gong process as far as somatic experiences go.

Emotional Release

The emotional release that we discussed in Chapter 9 can start to manifest here. If there has already been a lot of previous work with 'surface' emotional issues, then this phase can be quite brief and painless. If not, then expect anything from tears and shouting through to hysterical laughing. The body will really want to express the emotional information stored within the structure of this channel.

Contacting Trauma

Stored deep within the Central channel are your most powerful traumas: those experiences which root themselves right into your centre and influence many of your thoughts and actions. These are generally experiences from childhood, as the issues faced during your developmental years are generally your deepest.

This can be a difficult phase of the process and is certainly something of a double-edged sword. With the right teacher and mindset, you can be led through this process rather swiftly and in a 'clean' fashion. If you enter into this phase with little in the way of guidance, then it can be psychologically very scarring. Though suppression of emotional trauma is not a positive way to deal with issues, it does take place for a reason – burying a trauma is often the mind's way of protecting you from continuously reliving the emotional information contained within that trauma. When we start to access these issues, then they will usually resurface. I have had students enter this stage and suddenly recall deeply suppressed memories that they had forgotten about.

Proceed with caution with this kind of work. We wish for the root of the trauma to be cleared, but in a safe and smooth fashion; it is possible to do yourself harm if trauma is 'wrenched' from the body – something I have seen happen, and I often wince at the effects that the process is having. Slowly and carefully is often the best way to proceed with this kind of work.

Realisation of Xing

Beneath our trauma and most influential issues lies the root cause for our nature, our Xing. When we have delved deep enough, then it is often the case that we suddenly realise why it is that we think, act and behave in a certain way. If I had to choose one aspect of our 'self' that can be realised at this stage, it is our motives. Our motives are powerful things, they are a huge influence upon our nature and yet, at the same time, we are generally completely unaware of them. The mind is a complex thing and many people will either subconsciously hide their motives or else lie to themselves about what their innermost motives are. Do we operate from a place of compassion or fear? Are we trying to help or hinder others? Is this due to our own insecurities? These are the kinds of questions that many are unwilling to ask of themselves and, to be honest, they are almost impossible questions to answer in an intellectually honest fashion. We generally need to absorb our awareness into the root of our Xing to experience what these motives are.

I can personally attest to the fact that when you confront the root of your own Xing, it can be highly uncomfortable; it is amazing just how much of our own nature is based upon a foundation of emotional imbalance. There is an old maxim – 'know yourself and then know others'. This is certainly very true for this kind of work. Once you have experienced the root of your own nature, you will find that you are often able to penetrate through to the core of other people's nature as well. A window into your own 'workings' often serves to build a window into others'.

Elemental Shift

Once the realisation of Xing is there the intention of positive change is required. Knowing something and changing something are often two very different things. There may be actions we need to take on an external basis. These are simple enough, but what about our inner nature? It is here that we need to make the biggest changes. If our intention is true and we can reside in non-judgemental observation of the root of our Xing, then this change will come.

It is here that the biggest switches to your personality will take place. These can often be major changes to your likes, dislikes and world views. External behaviours will change and often there will need to be a major shift in your life course. This is the stage where many practitioners suddenly make drastic changes to their lives and careers. Just be aware that even though these changes are positive changes that you need to make, those around you have a set view of who you are. When this view is challenged, then it can be very difficult for them. Just remember to take those closest to you into account and make any required transitions as smoothly as you can. Do it in a far smoother way than I did when I reached this stage in my practice; I caused a great deal of disruption during my greatest 'change period' and, with hindsight, I wish I had tried to make my transition period more pleasant for those around me!

The Bliss Stage

When the changes come, it can be a major relief. Essentially, you have made a large shift in your Ming. Ming has an energy to it and this energy is expressed through the Jing. The Jing will then move through your body and bring with it a strong sense of bliss. This feeling can hit you in a very physiological fashion and then also on a more psychological level.

The physiological reaction to this stage is often a kind of 'post-orgasmic' pleasure. The kind of blissed-out state that makes you want to lay back, relax and check out of life! In some cases, it can actually generate feelings of sexual pleasure within the nervous system that come and go like waves through your system.

The mental aspect of this is a kind of mental bliss that most deep meditators go through at some stage. It can last for a period of time that varies between a few months through to the rest of your life. If it lasts this long, then you have gone wrong. Both physiological and psychological bliss are considered traps on the path. As with all experiences, we need to move through them if we wish to keep developing. The problem is that the very pleasant sensations that come at this stage are very addictive, especially for those who have previously been living in a state of mental disharmony.

Some systems have focused heavily on this feeling of bliss and they will do anything to stay there. The result is the development of deviant systems where the hunt for bliss is the goal of the practice. Whilst there is nothing inherently wrong with this, it is a glass ceiling to your spiritual development that dedicated practitioners should seek to move past. Those stuck in this stage will often appear as if they are stoned and will generally say very 'blissed out' but nonsensical things in conversation. I have encountered lots of people stuck in this trap through my involvement in the alternative scene. Though this is fine, and it's hardly the worst place to be stuck, I always had an interest in moving past it.

Encountering Shen

Beyond the bliss stage, those who can apply the principle of letting go and maintaining absorption of awareness into the process will start to discover the Shen contained within the Central channel. This is another way, a more Tantric method, to locate and work with the Yuan Shen. It is accompanied by a white light that expands through the length of the Central channel. When you look inside, the pillar of light is there and the feeling of bliss is no more; what is left is a feeling of mental and emotional stillness. Those with the 'Yin Eyes' skill can also see this pillar of light within you; it is a positive sign with regard to your progress, but just a sign, nothing more. As with all signs, it should neither be sought nor attached to as this will prevent your development.

The Trap of Emptiness

The experience of mental and emotional stillness that results from going this deep into your centre can often lead a person into the trap of emptiness. It is said within Daoism that Jing or stillness will lead a person to Xu or emptiness. This emptiness is extreme Yin and, as such, it will lead to the emergence of Yang, and so something 'new' will fill this emptiness. This will generally be the effects of Yuan Shen and then the final stages of opening for the Central channel, the macrocosmic orbit.

There is, however, a difficulty here. Modern people are very 'heart centred'. That is to say, we are very emotionally driven. The quality and state of our emotions and feelings are very important to us and to society as a whole. We often ask and are asked 'How do you feel?' and whether we are all right, meaning 'Are you emotionally okay?' Our society is very focused on exploring our emotions, and yet, many people struggle with a deep sense of emotional unhappiness.

This situation has started to influence the teachings of the spiritual arts which nowadays often are focused on the emotions. We have spiritual arts to make us feel happy or loved, to help us express love and so on. Whilst I am not against this kind of development in any way, we should note that this was not how the traditions were expressed in their original format.

Take Daoism as an example. Modern writings and internet memes on 'the Dao' seem to focus on how to be happy, loving, and so on. It is all about the emotions and how you feel. If you then take some time out of modern writings and actually look at the classics – go for it, read some of the translations of the writings of Liu Yi Ming (劉一明) and his contemporaries – you will see that there has been a major shift in the way that these arts are being represented. None of the detailed exploration of your emotional state or 'how to be happy' appears within them. Instead, the focus was on moving beyond your emotions as these were an aspect of 'self'. Beneath the emotions lies stillness, a stability of the mind that leads to emptiness; this is where the real change can take place.

Clearly, there has been a shift in focus for many of these practices and this is why most writings that purport to be about Daoism are actually related to the tradition in only the vaguest of senses. The result of this is that when people, through their practice, actually touch upon the state discussed within Daoism – the state of Jing that leads to Xu – it can be a real shock. Even though the states discussed are not negative in any way – actually, they are completely neutral, they can only exist because of the fact that they are undivided into the poles of positive and negative – the lack of emotional highs and lows can seem like a deep state of depression has manifested. This is what is often called the 'long dark night' in meditation communities. It is like going cold turkey from your emotions and so entering into a kind of psychological withdrawal.

I have known many who have fallen into this trap. So attached to their emotional states were they that when they encountered a state free from emotions, it sent them into a downward spiral! This is how attached we are to our emotions. I am sure that some of you reading this are already baulking on the inside; perhaps you feel that emotions are a good thing and that we should have them? Well, I agree with you, emotions make life interesting. The point is, though, that true spiritual development exists 'behind' these emotions; it can only take place when they are stilled and are no longer a factor for us. It is the difference between feeling good and spiritual growth.

Convergence

Convergence is the final stage of the sequence. This is a rather secretive part of the process that I will not be elaborating on, in respect to the sect I am part of.

The Macrocosmic Orbit

I refer you back to a line from the Dao De Jing: 'Heaven treats the people as if they were straw dogs.' We discussed this phrase in the context of Ming back in Chapter 7. Now, within the context of our mind, 'Heaven' is our consciousness. The 'people' in this instance are the myriad thoughts and emotions that spring up within the ocean of our consciousness. Though they should be recognised and enjoyed, as with the 'straw dog piñata', they are ultimately disposable and so should be allowed to fade away. If we can continue to reside within the Central channel with our awareness, then we can move beyond the 'trauma' of experiencing a state of no emotions and so the Central channel will begin to extend outwards into the macrocosmic orbit.

The microcosmic orbit is a circulation of Qi or other vital substances that takes place within the Governing and Conception channels. It exists within the microcosm of the body. The macrocosmic orbit is a circulation of Shen and Qi that takes place outside of your body within the macrocosm of the external environment. Some disagree with this and state that the macrocosmic orbit is a circulation of Qi within the arms and legs but, to me, these are still just extensions of the microcosmic orbit. The macrocosm is the space around us, the 'large Heaven', if we translate the Chinese directly.

The macrocosmic orbit grows out of the Central channel when enough 'work' has been done. It takes the form of the circulations shown in Figure 13.4.

There is a very distinct pulling of the Qi through the middle of the body. It reaches the crown of the head and the base of the perineum and then starts to extend outwards as shown. It comes with a very clear stretching of the body from these two points that is very strong whilst it is taking place. This then serves to extend a line of vibrational connection out into the environment above you as well as down into the planet. This is accompanied by an extension and strengthening of the natural field of energetic information that extends out into the space; this is an aspect of the auric field. This strengthening of the auric field serves to connect you more strongly into the environment, to turn you into a 'conduit between Heaven and Earth' as shown in Figure 13.5.

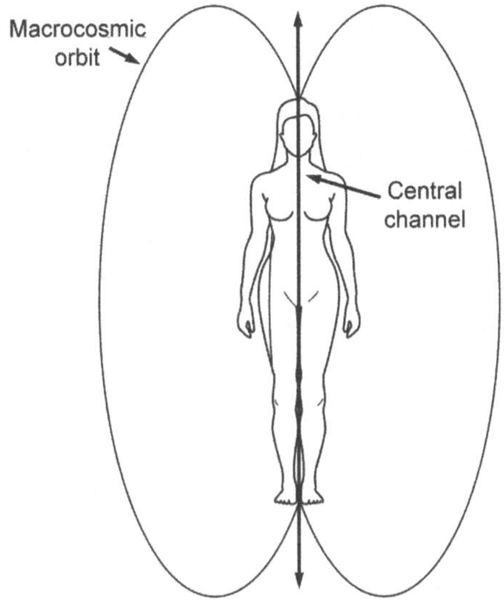

Figure 13.4: The Macrocosmic Orbit

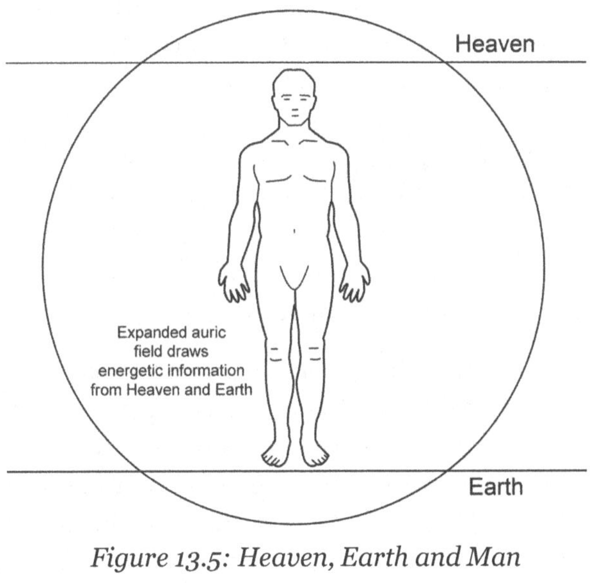

Figure 13.5: Heaven, Earth and Man

This energetic connection is already there for all of us; the macrocosmic orbit only serves to strengthen the efficiency of this process. The field around us is very important as it has the ability to send, receive or store information. As the body stores energetic information, so does the field of energy around us. This field of information can be read by skilled practitioners of Shen- and Qi-based therapies. This is a skill known as Gan Ying (感應) or 'sensory echoes', a poetic term that refers to the ability to be able to read the nature of a person's Qi. This can be done through 'off the body' palpation or through directed energetic resonance. This 'reading' is generally taken from the patient's auric field rather than the channels of Qi themselves.

A similar skill is Gan Zhi (感知) or 'sensory knowing'; at this level, the therapist will 'know' the nature and root of a disharmony as soon as they are in your presence. This high-level form of diagnosis is based upon absorbing information via the macrocosmic orbit mechanism. Though it can be very effective in the hands of skilled practitioners, it should be noted that the biggest enemy will always be self-delusion with regard to the development of these kinds of skills!

When the macrocosmic orbit is opened up, then the exchange of information with the environment can be very great indeed, and a practitioner will develop all kinds of understandings about their environment and the people around them. A skill known as the 'magical knowing' may manifest out of this whereby the reading of energetic information is now much greater than information drawn in from the senses. A person with this skill will seem to know a great deal about you, even on your first meeting.

As the skill develops, both the receiving of information from higher realms and connection with spiritual entities become possible. The scope of this skill is only limited by the strength of the practitioner's spiritual development.

According to the Daoists, the sign of a fully established macrocosmic orbit was the Wu Tong (五通) or 'five communications'. These were five ways that the practitioner's auric field would be able to communicate with the surrounding environment once they had fully merged with the Qi of Heaven and Earth. These five communications are:

- *Communicating with the present:* The practitioner will be able to understand exactly what is happening at any given moment. Initially, this will be in the immediate environment but, with time, it can be anywhere they place their awareness, even in other parts of the world. They will be able to read the truth behind any event, as the information being absorbed into their auric field is free from distortion.

- *Communicating with the past:* The practitioner will know about a person's past as soon as they meet. They will understand the cause-and-effect influences that have had an impact upon a person's current state.
- *Communicating with the future:* Since time is not a linear entity, the practitioner will know what will happen in the future. This can be the future of a person or what events will take place in the time ahead. The accuracy of these predictions will then vary depending upon the level of spiritual development of the practitioner. The concept is that all information, including potential information, is already there to read if we are able to.
- *Communicating with Heaven:* The 'Heaven' discussed here means the abode of the deities, immortals and higher-level spiritual entities. At a high level of macrocosmic orbit development, it is possible to communicate with these kinds of spirits. They can bring guidance, support and teachings if a person knows how to work with them.
- *Communicating with Ming:* An understanding of a person's Ming and their relationship to it will come as a result of the full macrocosmic orbit being opened up. For therapists, this can bring with it the deepest level of information regarding the nature of why illnesses are developing.

The above five communications are a kind of Siddhi that naturally evolve out of the opening of the Central channel and the macrocosmic orbit. They are a by-product of the practice and not to be aimed for in any way. It is through moving through the above-mentioned processes that they will likely arise.

The Use of Imagination

If you have read through this book, you will have noted that there is little in the way of use of the imagination. At no point are there any instructions based in imagining colours and visualising lights, deities, flowers, crystals or any other number of other exotic images. There is a reason for this: imagination and the use of generated visual practice has no place within Nei Gong. In fact, it has little to do with the vast majority of authentic practices. I have travelled to many countries and trained with many high-level practitioners of the Daoist arts, and none of the authentic teachers ever asked me to use my imagination in any way at all. Despite this, when looking at what many people practise in the West, there are many systems that involve imagining colours swirling around inside of the body, guardian animal spirits looking over you, and so on and so forth.

The use of imagination in these practices is based upon a major misunderstanding. Within classical teachings, there are clear descriptions of the visual phenomena that may arise out of your practice. There are discussions of white lights, coloured patterns, geometric symbols and many other visually striking experiences that may arise within your training. The point is, though, that these visual experiences should manifest naturally as a result of what you are doing and serve as a kind of confirmation that you are on the right path. The classical texts were written as a way of helping to confirm what you were doing rather than giving you direct instruction on what to do. If you look at classical texts, there are actually very few practical instructions at all; these were supposed to be passed on to you by your teacher. People have mistaken the 'confirmatory symbols' as 'instructions' and so are now imagining colours and lights and falsely believing that this is Qi Gong practice.

Imagination goes hand in hand with mental action as well as delusion. We cannot allow the awareness to become passive and 'listen' as it is supposed to if it is engaged in generating various fanciful visual constructs. The quality of the mind must not be based in picturing results.

The Heart Field

The second component that should be looked at is the nature of the Heart field. This is the expanse of Qi that exists around the middle Dan Tian region of the body, as shown in Figure 13.6. The inner layers of this field exist within the body, whilst the outermost layers expand out into the area around you. This distance will vary a great deal from person to person.

It is interesting to note that the field of the middle Dan Tian was only given cursory mentions within the oldest Daoist texts; since it is considered the seat of the 'mind' and thus the 'self', it was not seen as a part of the energetic matrix that should be greatly involved in alchemical training. Instead, the focus was on the lower Dan Tian (the driving force and alchemical crucible), the upper Dan Tian (the seat of Yuan Shen) and the yellow court region of the solar plexus, as there was a lot of alchemical work that could be carried out at this point. The use of the yellow court is more prominent within alchemical meditation practice than it is in Nei Gong training.

This situation most likely changed with the absorption of Buddhist ideas and teachings into the tradition. Many Chinese Buddhist methods use the Heart field and, as Daoism integrated the Chen (禪) Buddhist teachings into its practice, they also started to recognise the Heart field as an important energetic centre.

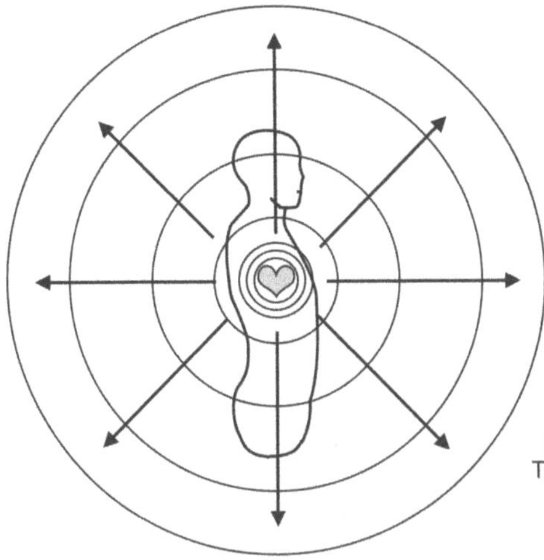

Figure 13.6: The Heart Field

The Heart field has a number of important qualities to be aware of:

- It is understood within Daoism to be the place where the mind is rooted. It is here that our emotional self is most strongly experienced and here that the Shen, the Fire elemental aspect of our 'fragmented original spirit', resides.
- Although the various emotions are linked to different organs of the body, they are all expressed through the Heart and its associated field. This means that the quality and nature of your Heart field is greatly affected by the state of your emotional mind.
- The Heart is recognised as being the electromagnetic focal point for the body. It processes thousands of times more electrical and magnetic energy than the brain on a daily basis. The level of this power is then felt within the body's Yang Qi and Yin Qi. An imbalanced Heart field can 'leak' the Yang Qi through a kind of static discharge and cause Yin Qi fields to become dispersed.

- The brain and the Heart communicate in a very clear way. The brain interprets vibrational information so that you can understand it intellectually, whilst the Heart filters it in an emotional manner.
- The Heart's 'memory' means that it will develop a kind of stored resonance for emotionally charged events. This is partially why a person can start to find themselves interpreting many events through a kind of 'remembered filter'. This level of distortion can be one of the trickiest to clear from a person's stored energetic quality.

With regard to our practice, the Heart field is related to the following factors: how we feel emotionally and how we process and move Qi through the region of the chest.

How We Feel Emotionally

Returning to statements made earlier in this book, even though these internal practices are a great form of medicine, it is not really ideal to focus on this aspect of the practices. In the same way, the practice of Qi Gong and Nei Gong can be a great way to help harmonise your emotional state, but we should still not focus on this area of the practice. What I mean by this is that we should simply focus on practising the art for the sake of the art; the benefits will then unfold of their own accord as we go deeper into the process. By focusing on a perceived 'damage' or 'weakness' that we may see ourselves as having, we develop an attachment to this condition. Once the attachment is there, the problem is more difficult for the body to deal with.

This is most certainly the case for work with the Heart centre. As a teacher, I do not spend a great deal of time teaching about or working with the Heart field; that being said, students who move into the Nei Gong process will strengthen the Heart field to a high degree. This can be aided with transmission and there are various exercises designed to work specifically with the Qi of the middle Dan Tian, but essentially, our focus is rarely there. This is because, as an energy centre, it is best if it is built as a by-product of the Qi that moves from the lower Dan Tian, out through the channel system, into the rest of the body. In the vast majority of cases, students will find that, with practice, their emotional state improves, they are less prone to more negative mental states like depression or sadness, and they find that they are able to connect with people and life to a far higher degree. These are all aspects related (mechanically) to a strengthening of the Heart field and its Qi.

The Density of Emotions

All emotions and feelings carry with them a certain degree of energetic 'density'. Those emotions with a higher degree of density will attach to the mind, through the Heart, to a far higher degree. Those emotions that lack density, that are lighter in nature, will not so easily attach to the Heart; they lack the Qi to anchor into our system. As much as anything, learning how to let go and not hold on to emotional baggage is learning how to energetically lighten the experience of an emotion as it enters into our field. These kinds of ideas are suggested within the Western expressions 'light-hearted' or having a 'heavy heart'. In Chinese medicine, this issue is also recognised, as the Heart Qi can 'sink' if it becomes too dense. Many of us will have felt this when we have experienced some of those emotions that really attack the Heart's energy: betrayal, the sudden death of a family member or the broken heart of failed romantic relationships. The result is often a pressure or tightness in the chest; it is as if something is stuck there. This is a kind of psychosomatic response to the energy of the emotion; it is the strongest experience you can have of the density that can come from a heavy emotional reaction.

This is why one of the greatest forms of medicine is laughter. We all know this instinctively, and I have even heard of laughter being prescribed as medicine for some people! This can obviously be difficult when you are very depressed, though, and, to be honest, we can't just go around laughing at everything; I am not sure that it is socially acceptable. Let us look at how this is relevant to the Heart centre, though. Laughter has an energetic mechanic to it within Daoist thought. When we are happy, the Qi is light; within Chinese medical thought, it is said that the feeling of joy actually slackens the Qi. 'Slackening' implies a loosening and a movement away from density. If you watch the Qi of somebody who moves from sadness into feelings of joy, their Qi begins to spread and, in some cases, disperse. The result of this is that the Heart can heat up a little due to the extra energetic movement through its region of the body. The heat of the Heart will need to be vented – it is like the steam coming out of the chimney of an old steam train – and the result is that we laugh – the body's natural way of venting heat from the Heart. So, when we feel joy, the Qi is less dense; when we laugh, we vent excess Qi from the Heart. This process is summarised in Figure 13.7.

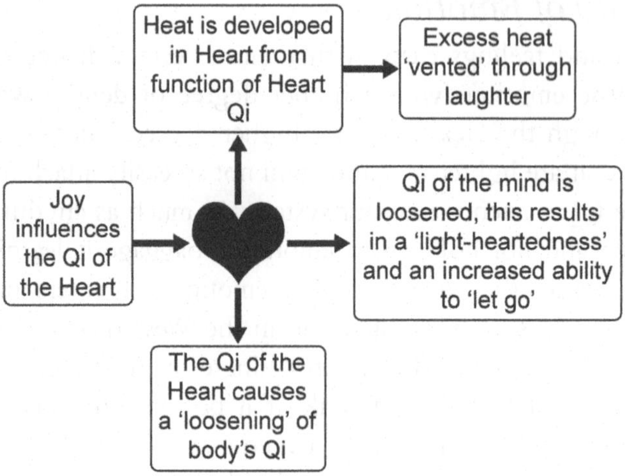

Figure 13.7: The Energetics of Joy and Laughter

Now, this process is obviously a very acute form of energetic release. Many people find it difficult to be in a joyful state all of the time; life brings with it a whole plethora of emotional experiences. On top of this, we can't go around laughing all the time, and those who carry a lot of sadness will obviously not feel like laughing anyway. But we can match the energetic mechanic of joy in our practice.

Let us look at this mechanic – it is essentially a loosening and lightening of the Qi. Anger and frustration create tightness, depression creates a chronic heaviness of the Qi; we want these qualities to be replaced by a lightness and looseness of our energy. This is essentially what we are doing all the time throughout the Nei Gong process. We learn how to awaken our Qi in the earliest stages of the practice. Then we learn how to move the Qi through our body using the channel system. On top of this, the work we carry out with our breath and mind helps to teach us how to let go. As our passive abdominal breathing method begins to evolve onto new levels, we start to develop the ability to 'Song' through our breathing as we discussed in Chapter 5. All of these methods are changing the overall quality of our Qi so that it is no longer so heavy/dense. The work that we do to change the nature of our Qi will start to affect the nature of the Heart centre in the way described above. The Heart field will change in quality, as the Qi within your Heart is a reflection of the Qi within your body and vice versa. This is how Daoist body-based practices work: they create a change within the densest and the most tangible place, and that change is then effected 'upwards' along the spectrum of Jing–Qi–Shen towards the mind. The result of this is that, as you practise, your developing Qi will start to change your emotional makeup; it really is that simple.

Remember that the Daoists were originally a very practical bunch. Their pragmatism was based around looking at how they could best develop a person through training. Their aim was, ultimately, to develop into spiritual immortals. Whether this is your aim as well, or if you even believe in this, is not the point. This was the aim of those who developed these practices. As with any goal, it is essentially a kind of 'problem' that needs a 'solution'.

So, how to become an immortal? The Daoists' answer to this was the path of inner development that is inherent to the Daoist tradition. Every aspect of this path was simply to help them reach the place they were aiming for. When they looked at one's emotional makeup, they realised that this was an issue that needed dealing with, as were one's physical and energetic health. They recognised that harmony of the body's state was required in order to take one to the state they sought out within their arts. They took a look at the nature of mind and realised that it was a pretty confusing thing to work with; the complexity of mind makes direct work with one's emotions quite a tricky practice. We only have to look at the complexity around the subject of psychology to see just how much of a quagmire we are going to get involved in if we delve into the mind directly. So, they took a different route, and worked with the Qi instead. Change the Qi, and there will be a transferred alteration to the quality of the mind.

This was the inner work of the mind, an aim for adjusting the quality of Qi. The tradition, like many others, then combined this process with 'outer work' that was primarily focused upon one's behaviour. When the two parts came together, it would result in a deep and lasting change for the Heart. Figure 13.8 shows how the inner and outer work for the Heart Mind work as one unit.

We looked at the outer work of Daoism back in Chapter 6. These are the precepts and the qualities that the Daoists were trying to establish within a person when they first became initiated into the tradition. The precepts listed there are repeated here for your convenience:

- Be mindful of the cause and effect of dealing with people
- Do not commit any sexual misconduct
- Do not steal nor deal with those who do
- Tell only truth and do not mislead others with your speech
- Avoid intoxication and conduct yourself with purity

- Honour your family, hereditary line and ancestors
- Carry out kind actions and support those who do
- Assist those who are less fortunate in regaining their dignity and fortune
- Carry out your actions in accordance with the Dao, yet don't expect the same of others
- Place others' attainment of Dao above your own

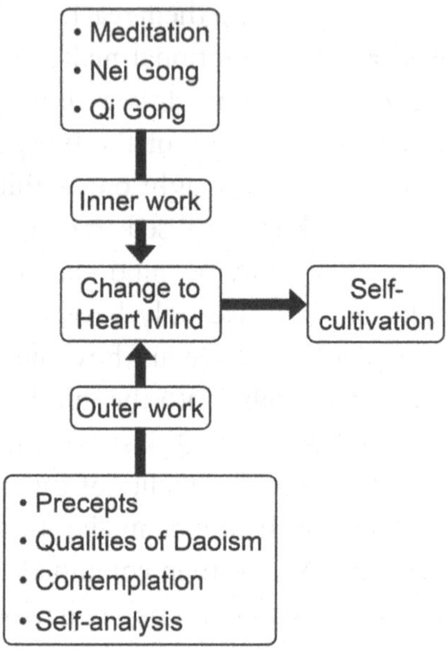

Figure 13.8: Inner and Outer Heart Work

If a person's mind could be transformed from the inner work as well as the outer work, then it would start to move into a state of harmony. This would then help to lead a person towards a more balanced way of being, make their system function at a higher level and also ensure that they moved closer to the 'frequency' of the tradition of Daoism itself.

It is also understood that the field of the Heart is where a great deal of our ability to 'connect' comes from. When two people encounter one another, there is a degree of merging of the Heart fields. Before there has been any verbal or body-language exchanges of information, there is an energetic transference that takes place. A great deal of subconscious information is received in this way. A person's Heart field can be open to the reception of information in this way, or else it can be closed off to it.

In some cases, there is a lack of strength to the Qi which causes a person to absorb information from another with no protection. This can result in taking on others' emotional states to your own detriment; sometimes this happens simply by being in another's vicinity.

By strengthening the nature of the Qi within the middle Dan Tian and developing the loose and light qualities inherent within Qi Gong practice, we will give the Heart a degree of supporting strength as well as help its ability to process emotional experiences in a healthy way – a way that does not involve a high degree of attachment to negativity. Energetic movements and disturbances in the Qi of the Heart can lead to a 'leaking' of the Qi and so, from this standpoint, these are all very practical changes to make if we wish to progress in our training.

Qi and the Chest Region

When Qi moves through the body, it inevitably has to move through the region of the chest. This happens on a medical level, as Qi moves from the heart region into the channel system, and also on a training level when we raise Qi through the body. One major expression of our energy is through our emotions, and it was for this reason that a stilling of the emotions was advised within the Daoist tradition. The Heart field must be strong and the emotional mind balanced. If this is not the case, then there will be a leakage of Qi from the heart region, as shown in Figure 13.9.

Our emotions use up a massive amount of energy. This takes place through the previously discussed process of 'giving' Qi to our mind so that it then transforms into a 'thought stream'. When the Heart is in a state of flux, all of the energy running through this part of the body (thousands of times more than the brain, remember) will be fed into our emotional reactions and so our Qi is 'used up' here. For a tradition that was focused upon developing their Qi to higher levels, this was obviously an issue. As the Heart grew more still and the emotions moved towards a central point, then the Qi leakage was blocked up and you no longer had a large 'hole' in your energetic system that would impair your cultivation practice.

This is especially important for women as they have an extra location for the storehouse of their Jing within the region of the chest. Men have Jing that moves from the kidney region down to the perineum and lower Dan Tian; women have an extra movement of Jing that takes place from the lower part of the body upwards into the chest. The close proximity of the Jing to the emotional centre of the Heart means that an excessive leaking of Qi from the region of the middle Dan Tian will drain the Jing as well.

This is why inner stillness is a vital part of all women's cultivation practice and indeed should be a part of all women's lives if they wish to be healthy. Since this book serves as an overview of the non-gender-specific aspects of Daoist training, you should refer to the book *Daoist Nei Gong for Women: The Art of the Lotus and the Moon* (Singing Dragon, 2016) as this has a great deal of information regarding the more unique aspects of female alchemical cultivation.

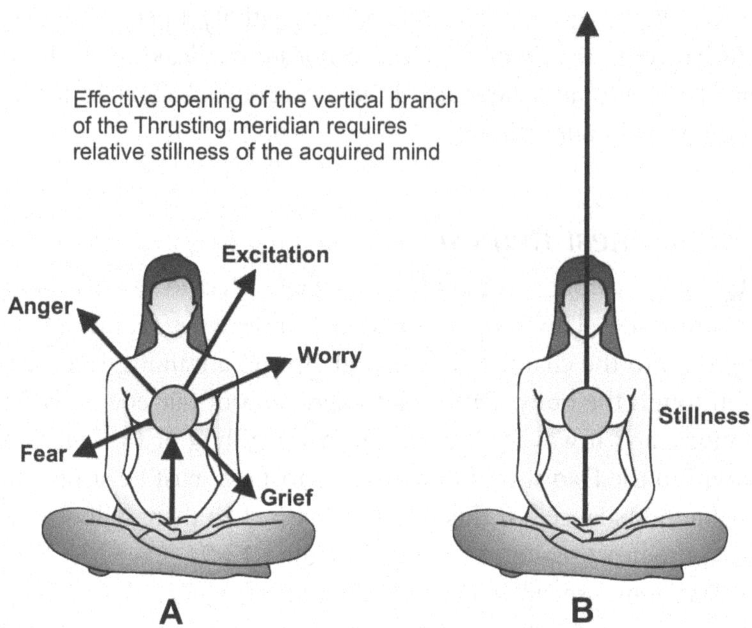

Figure 13.9: Leakage of Qi from the Heart

A final aspect of the Heart's functioning is linked to its expression of either the emotions or their converted form, the virtues.

The Emergence of De

It was understood that the five spirits, the fragmented aspects of Yuan Shen, lie at the root of our emotional movements. It is a facet of the way our mind works that if the five spirits are in a state of movement, they will manifest the emotionally charged energies of the acquired mind. If they grow still, then they can actually start to express themselves in a healthier manner, as the five De or 'virtues' of Daoism. Table 13.1 shows the connection between the spirits, the emotions and the virtues.

Table 13.1: The Spirits, the Emotions and the Virtues

Spirit	Emotion	Virtue
Shen	Excitation	Contentment
Hun	Anger	Patience/understanding
Yi	Worry	Empathy/compassion
Po	Sadness	Bravery/conviction
Zhi	Fear	Wisdom/clarity

To understand the place of the De and virtuous action, we should look at the teachings of the Dao De Jing. Within the text, it is made very clear that 'when Dao is lost, De arises, when De is gone, then decency manifests, when decency is gone, then justice is required, when justice is gone, then we are left with only ceremony'.

What this implies is that De is a higher state of functioning than that of the emotions, but it is still not close to Dao. Dao is attained through spiritual cultivation, whilst De is still an expression of self-development. That does not mean we should not be virtuous, of course not, we still need to function within the outside world on a daily basis and virtuous expression will make the world a much better place. But it is not going to lead you towards development of Dao – only through eradication of the 'self' will Yuan Shen lead you to Dao. This is why I make the distinction between 'spirit' and 'self' so clear. Both may be needed, but they should not be confused with one another.

The Dao De Jing goes on to say that when De is lost, then decency arises, or rather, the need for it. Now, when a person is not operating from an innate place of virtuous expression, they need to understand what decency is. In the majority of cases, this is a learnt behaviour. Societal and family norms will tell you what is a 'decent' way to behave to others. If you operated from Dao, then your 'non-action' would result in everything being as it should be; it would be 'just right'. If you operate from De, then your innate nature will cause you to do the right thing and carry out kind actions. If you do not have an innate virtuous state, then the emotions are ruling you; instead, we need decency to make sure we all get along and do each other no harm. This is where external rules such as precepts and guidance from teachers were required.

When decency is gone, then we need justice instead; forms of punishment and law to make sure that people do what they should. The fear of retribution is required to keep people in check since they will not act decently of their own accord. The Dao De Jing then goes further to state that even justice can break down and all we are left with is 'ceremony', an empty reflection of justice to keep people happy. Although this is a comment on societal structure, it is also a series of teachings on the progression of our inner state as we move from a congenital to an acquired state of mental functioning.

If the Heart can grow still and the emotional mind can be brought closer to a state of harmony, then the emotions will begin their natural conversion to De and so the 'self' will function in a more altruistic fashion.

Excitation to Contentment

The spirit of the Shen resides within the Heart. It is the spiritual manifestation of the element of Fire. Excitation and manic outbursts are the most extreme manners in which this spirit will express itself when it is in a state of excess. During these times, the Shen is at a high and often completely out of control. This would be considered to be like the flames of the fire burning high. Like a burning flame it cannot burn so brightly forever, and so this state of heightened emotional activity must come to an end. The high turns into a low and so we experience the opposite of excitation: a low time where emotions such as sadness come to the fore.

Also contained within the range of the Shen's emotional bandwidth are the emotions of joy, happiness, pleasure, love, connection and even lust. All a natural part of human life, it is the Heart and its spirit, the Shen, which produce the emotions which so many place great importance upon. Of course, there is nothing wrong with these emotions in themselves; it is their transience which is more of an issue. Joy cannot be permanent by its nature, pleasure cannot be such for too long without ceasing to be pleasurable, lust is often easily sated and, sadly, even love all too often fades away. This is the nature of emotions, they are fleeting experiences which we only register because of the existence of their opposites. We require the entire range of emotions to register even one of them, and so no matter how much we seek to remain within the positive emotional highs of the Shen and the Heart, we will undoubtedly also be subject to the movement of the other spirits as well. Excessive, prolonged states of excitation cause the Qi of the Heart to flicker and 'burn'. If this becomes a constant pattern, then it will cause the Qi of the Heart to become deficient.

The virtuous expression of the Shen is an experience of contentment. This is a more constant feeling of satisfaction with the situation you find yourself in. Unlike the flickering flames of the emotions of the Shen, contentment is more stable. This satisfaction begins to stir the Heart towards stronger manifestations of connection, and so this satisfaction pulls you into a more powerful relationship with your life.

Anger to Patience and Understanding

The spirit of the Hun is rooted into the Liver. It is the spiritual manifestation of the element of Wood. Wood energy flows out of the Hun and through the body with a driving force that generates the potential for growth and energy. When directed into something positive, Wood energy can generate huge amounts of creative power. It is the energetic basis upon which a great deal of ethical and political movements are built. Wood energy gives us the power to stand up for our own rights and what we believe in.

This potential for taking action is important for human existence, but unfortunately it also has the opposite characteristic of being responsible for all of the destructive aspects of human nature. In its most extreme or undirected manifestation, Wood energy produces outbursts of anger and rage along with feelings of jealousy, placing importance upon status, a need for power and a number of other negative personality traits; though quick to flare up, these feelings often leave a stain upon the acquired nature that makes them easy to return to time and time again.

If Wood energy is not able to flow freely, it often has the opposite effect of moving inwards and becoming trapped inside a person. The result is a feeling of inner frustration which can cause a person to become angry at themselves. In interactions with people who make you feel angry, if you cannot express this anger, then it often contributes to feelings of frustration which can be very self-destructive. Often, the only way this energy can be expressed is through manipulative or passive-aggressive-type behaviour patterns.

When the spirit of the Hun is able to express itself in a virtuous state, it produces the quality of patience. Patience in this case is largely concerned with your ability to deal with others. It is the patience to interact with the rest of your life without allowing it to lead to anger or frustration.

The other virtue often listed as being related to the Hun is understanding. A great deal of conflict within the world is related to people's inability to relate to or understand each other. Confusion due to distorted information passing between two people has been the root of many conflicts throughout history. As the Hun starts to express itself in a virtuous manner, it raises a person's ability to apply understanding to life's situations.

Worry to Empathy and Compassion

The spirit of the Yi is rooted within the Spleen. It is the spiritual manifestation of the element of Earth. Classically connected to the emotion of worry as well as chronic overthinking, the spirit of the Yi is often overly concerned with possible future outcomes and perceived problems. In an increasingly fast-paced world which is set up to draw people's awareness out of themselves towards external concerns, the Yi is often existing in a state of constant tension. For many people, a practice such as meditation would be the most positive activity they could introduce into their lives. Even if the lofty aims of enlightenment of immortality are stripped out of the practice, sitting with the awareness gently inside of the body would help to calm the Yi.

On top of this, the Yi is intimately connected to the rest of the five spirits, meaning that its health is a reflection of the whole spectrum of human emotions. Any emotional disturbances are going to throw a person's Yi into a state of overthinking. This has the effect of draining the acquired Qi, which will then affect the rest of a person's health.

An interesting facet which appears within people with an imbalance in their Yi is their need to either receive support from others, or to be overly sensitive to the idea of sympathy. Character traits such as neediness will appear in somebody with an imbalance in the Yi. The need for extreme amounts of sympathy from those in their lives goes hand in hand with an oversensitivity to perceived insults from others. The Yi can also lead a person to being overly smothering when dealing with close family or friends. If none of these needs are met, then the Yi can feel undernourished and a deep sense of loneliness can set in.

The virtuous expression of the Yi is empathy and compassion towards all beings. These are virtues based in healthy levels of connection and awareness of the needs and inner nature of those around them. Possibly the most important of the virtues with regard to dealing with others, the Yi constructs compassion from the combined spiritual information of the other virtues.

Sadness to Bravery and Conviction

The spirit of the Po resides within the Lungs. It is the spiritual manifestation of the element Metal. The emotions resulting from the movement of the Po are almost heavy in nature. When they move into a state of extreme imbalance, they can cause a person to feel as if they have a tight ball constricting their insides. These are the emotions of sadness, grief, an awareness of loss or depression. These emotions are heavy and binding. A person who has suffered for a long time with them will generally start to develop a very closed-up posture within their body. The chest will close up as if the Heart itself is attempting to hide itself away from the world. In extreme cases of emotional hurt derived from the spirit of the Po, the Metal elemental energy will actually begin to separate a person from the outside world. This results in feelings of emotional numbness or symptoms of shock. Rather unfairly, to the outside world this can appear as if this person is emotionally cold or aloof, when in fact their Po is simply seeking to protect them from any more emotional damage.

The virtuous expression of the Po spirit is classically listed as bravery, though in modern times perhaps 'conviction' is a more appropriate term. Like the finely forged blade of a steel sword, these virtues which develop from within the Heart of the spirit of Metal serve to enable a person to cut through any feelings of sadness and grief, as well as many perceived problems within life. The virtue of courage is important for those walking the internal path of Daoism as there are always many challenges put in a person's way. Daoism long recognised this fact, which is why Daoists placed such importance upon this character trait within their discussions of virtuous behaviour.

Fear to Wisdom and Clarity

The Zhi is the spirit which resides within the Kidneys. It is the spiritual manifestation of the element Water and responsible for the emotions of fear and anxiety. In extreme cases, this spirit will manifest through feelings of chronic perceived threats, a psychological trait which is practically crippling as it prevents a person from seeing any life event in an undistorted manner.

Fear is often a subtle emotion which, like water seeping through the cracks in a rock face, permeates into a person's being. Though these small pockets of fear-based energy may go unnoticed for a while, they begin to increase in amount until they are the basis for almost all of a person's thought processes. Just as the Kidneys are seen as the foundation of a person's health within Chinese thought, so the emotion of fear is often seen as the foundation of all emotional imbalances.

In its virtuous state, the spirit of the Zhi has the potential to manifest in pure wisdom, the ability to see the nature of the world and its underlying phenomena with a high degree of clarity. Zhi is often considered the most difficult of the spirits to convert into its higher state, which is why the virtue of wisdom was so highly prized within the Eastern traditions.

Siddhi

I will start to bring this book to a close now by looking at one of the most controversial aspects of internal training: that of Siddhi, the abilities that are gained from internal training when it reaches a certain level. These are recognised internal skills such as Ban Yun (搬運) or telekinesis, Tou Shi (透视) or 'X-ray vision', Kan Qi (看氣) or 'seeing the energetic realm' and many more. There are higher-level skills which involve perception of Xing and Ming as well as lower-level Siddhi to do with the ability to emit Qi and Shen. When you begin to explore the teachings of Nei Gong and Daoism, it is incredible just how many different abilities and skills have been recorded. Some of the Nei Gong sects even have closely guarded texts that list the various Siddhi alongside the mechanical qualities the practitioner would need to have achieved at the level of Qi and Shen in order to manifest them.

Many of the higher-level abilities require the development of Ling or 'magical spirit'. Though 'magical spirit' is maybe a slightly woolly translation of the term, it can bring us closer to understanding what the Ling is seen as being. If Yuan Shen is worked with and evolved to a high enough level, then it can bring us to two places: to Dao and to Ling. Figure 13.10 shows how these two develop out of Shen.

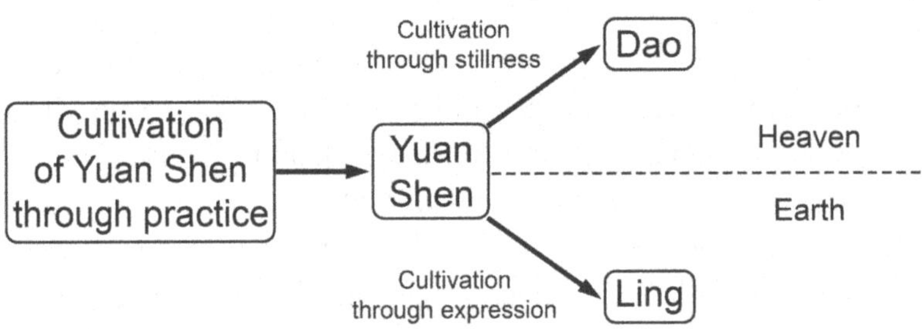

Figure 13.10: Ling and Dao

As you can see, on the level of Heaven, the evolved Yuan Shen brings us to Dao. On the level of Earth, the realm of manifestation, the Yuan Shen can act as Ling. This means that, in the grand scheme of spiritual cultivation, the path of Ling is seen as a lower path. Though the Ling should manifest, it should then be risen above and moved past in order to continue the path of progression, otherwise we will be held back in attaining the true jewels of the Daoist tradition.

That being said, let us look at what Ling is. Ling is considered an expression of the more evolved aspects of spirit when it functions in the realm of manifestation. It is said that Ling Shen (靈神) – 'magical spirit manifest through human mind' – produces Ling Qi (靈氣), the 'expressed energy of the Ling'. This Qi then results in the production of Siddhi which may manifest within a practitioner.

It is said very clearly that a person should not strive for the attainment of Siddhi, and this is certainly true as it can cause all sorts of distortions. Mentally striving for these kinds of abilities will generate distortions in the mind and this can lead to sickness as well as imbalances in your psychological makeup. Also, once developed, if they are used extensively, then they can burn up the energies you have accumulated. There is also a deep Ming aspect to Siddhi, meaning that striving for them and using them actually distorts the cause-and-effect resonances of your life path. It is for these kinds of reasons that Siddhi were seen as something to not strive for and to rise above in your practice. That being said, please remember that you generally cannot rise above something you cannot do! What I mean by this is that I see practitioners of these arts, especially in the West, saying things like 'don't strive for abilities' when, generally, it is because they don't have any. That would essentially be like me, tomorrow, going into a dance class (I can't dance) and telling the world that I have risen above high-level dance and I shall not strive to become an amazing dancer as that is a form of attachment. Whilst there may be some aspects of truth in this (at least the part where I said I could not dance), it is also something of a cop-out.

The fact is that almost every high-level master of these arts has some kind of Siddhi. In many cases, this is comparatively low-level stuff such as emission of Qi, transmission of Shen or heightened sense functions, but they are still a present part of their practice. I have also met a number of teachers with very high-level Siddhi, the kinds of abilities that many people reading this won't believe in anyway. From what I have seen, those teachers who use their Ling repeatedly and to a great extent tend to suffer some kind of health consequence. Generally, these are related to problems with the liver, heart or prostate. This also seems to be the case for teachers who use their skills for fame; there is a Karmic mechanic I don't quite understand, but it is clearly present. Those teachers who have attained some kind of Siddhi, but use them sparingly, especially in the context of teaching or medicine, do not suffer the same problems.

It is not the abilities gained that are the issue, but rather the way that they are seen and used. Within the tradition of alchemical Daoism, they are seen as a signpost of attainment, not a goal. If they are seen in this way, then a practitioner's relationship with them tends to be much healthier. This is the same with all of the signposts within these arts, some of which I have highlighted in this book. If we take the signpost of the channels opening, for example, these are not a Siddhi: they are physiological changes that take place within the body as a by-product of the training. We don't try to create these changes, we just practise our art. The result of our practice is that, at some stage, these changes will take place. We don't then fixate on these changes; instead, we continue our practice with an acknowledgement that we are moving in the right direction. The abilities gained from the practice of Nei Gong are exactly the same. When skills such as emission of Qi and transmission arise, then great, it shows that we are on the right track; our body is converting in function in the right way – the direction we want to take it. If, on the other hand, we strive for the abilities of Qi emission and transmission, then, whilst there are indeed methods to attain these skills, they generally end up being forced and bad for the body overall.

Even the higher-level skills listed above, such as being able to see the energetic realm and even to see through physical matter (a skill used in classical Chinese medical diagnosis), are just signposts along the way; they are exactly the same. Let them arise, let them be, move on; this is the idea. But do not demonise them as a sign that you are going down the wrong path as is so often said these days.

Some Siddhi are related to elements of your body moving into balance. I describe below the elemental Siddhi of Daoism.

Fire Elemental Balancing

When the elemental energy of Fire has begun to harmonise within your body, then your ability to regulate your own body temperature will arise of its own accord. You will be able to walk around in the snow with only a pair of shorts or walk around in the tropics with many layers of clothing on and you will not suffer as a result. Note, the skill works both ways: you need to stay at a central state of temperature in both climes. This is a sign that the Qi of Fire, the energy rooted into the Heart and the Shen, is starting to move towards a central, harmonised state.

Teachers will test you for this by making you practise your meditation in the snow or high up in cold mountains. They might also make you practise Nei Gong in extremely hot places. In this way, they are not testing for the ability itself, if you get what I mean, but they are observing a practitioner making use of the ability, the Gong, to see how harmonised their internal state has become.

Earth Elemental Balancing

When the elemental energy of Earth has begun to harmonise, you will develop a kind of tangible sensitivity to others' feelings and somatic experiences. Essentially, it is a type of energetic empathy, called Gan Zhi in the Qi Gong community. This happens when the energy of Yi and the Spleen is starting to become more harmonised. Teachers will test this (and check it is not imagination or self-delusion) by changing the quality of their own Qi using their intention and then asking you to feed back to them what they are doing.

Metal Elemental Balancing

The elemental energy of Metal will forge your focus into a very strong state when it begins to harmonise. It will become unwavering in its attention if you require it to be. The stability of the focus is still based on a kind of inner passivity, but it is able to hold its stability without becoming distracted. Teachers will test this by getting you to meditate in difficult places – places that are very loud or very unappealing to practise in. If you can ignore the distractions, not just externally, but internally as well by maintaining a stable mind, then the element of Metal is starting to harmonise. This Gong is based in the energy of the Po and Lungs.

Water Elemental Balancing

The elemental energy of Water will bring a kind of wisdom with it that is often referred to as just 'knowing'. It is a sign that the energy of the Kidneys and Zhi is becoming harmonised. Teachers will test it by teaching you only part of a practice, a few aspects of the art, but then seeing if you know the rest of the practice. It is something quite different from 'figuring it out'. It is a literal knowing of the rest of what you are being shown. Generally, this test becomes a major part of a student's training when they are in an esoteric lineage tradition. This is why high-level teachers will often only show half of an exercise or half-explain a concept.

Wood Elemental Balancing

The elemental energy of Wood will bring a kind of 'time suspension' with it when it moves into a state of harmony. This becomes especially clear during seated practice whereby a feeling of a few minutes' practice in your subjective experience can actually equate to a few hours or more in 'real time'. Many people will stumble across this kind of experience when they start out in meditation as the Wood elemental energy and the associated Hun start to shift according to your practice. With time and a high degree of balance developing within the Wood element, this then will become a permanent Gong. This is often tested by teachers who will ask you to spend extraordinary lengths of time in meditation practice. These times can often be for entire days without moving.

I know that, to some reading this, it will sound fantastic and unreal, but it really is the case. If the Wood element starts to find its centre, then time takes on a different quality. When you are functioning on a daily basis, the Wood is subject to all kinds of movement, but when still, during meditation, time does not have the same effect upon you. You will occasionally have experienced this when sleeping: the Hun leaves your body when you sleep, and the Wood elemental energy is no longer affecting you in the same way. You wake up in the morning and it feels as if you have only just gone to sleep. The night feels like it has only been moments and yet you have been in bed for eight or nine hours! This is not quite the same thing, but it is a related mechanic involving similar aspects of the energetic system.

Signposts, Not Goals

There are a huge number of skills or Gong that can manifest out of your practice. I have just shared some of the lower-level skills here so that you can understand how they are used in the Daoist arts: as signposts, and not as goals that are strived for. That being said, in my experience, high-level teachers of Nei Gong and Daoism will often test their senior students to see if they can manifest these skills. It is a clear way of seeing how a student is developing as it leaves very little chance of uncertainty. It is all about the quality of your Jing, Qi, Shen and Ling.

Concluding Thoughts

I shall leave the main part of the book here, with these final sections that seemed to be a little apart from the rest of the Nei Gong process. Over the years, I have trained with a number of different teachers and now teach my own students in various locations around the world. The process outlined here is the path I take my own students through so that they may experience the nature and benefits of Nei Gong.

The key messages I have wanted to convey in this book are that there is a clear path of progression within these arts and that there are generally clear and tangible signs of progression to be had along the way. For those of you reading this book, those who have managed to stick with me all the way to the end, I hope there have been at least one or two things you can take away from the text. Obviously, each system of practice is different. You will have variations within what you do, and the process may be different from the one that I am describing here; that is fine, variety is the spice of life! I never wish to 'convert' anybody or convince them of my way of doing things. Instead, I hope that looking into the particular methods outlined within this book has enabled even a little light to be shone on what you yourself are doing.

The process outlined in this book has been focused on the Nei Gong side of the tradition. There is also the Nei Dan or 'internal alchemy' aspect to the practice. It is here that practitioners of Nei Gong generally progress onto once they have built a solid enough foundation in the levels of Jing and Qi. If you are interested to see how deep the rabbit-hole of Daoism can go, I would suggest looking into alchemical meditation methods.

I am not really a 'writer' as such, I find it difficult and I am aware that my writing style can sometimes lack finesse; I can only apologise for this and for anything I have failed to make clear in the book. I wish you all the best in your own practice and hope that the traditions of Daoism, whatever form it may take for you, will continue to help you along your own path.

Appendix

Qi Gong Deviation

It is a fact of the internal arts that they will always carry with them a certain degree of risk. You are, in essence, engaging in a practice that involves going inside of your mind and body, often within the energetic blueprints for your entire makeup, and making various adjustments to all of this. No matter how skilled you are, how proficient your teacher or how traditional your system of training, there is still always a slight risk. Some teachers of Qi Gong would deny this and adamantly disagree with me, but I believe that this is a slightly risky attitude to take towards a complex internal practice. No practice is without risk. That being said, the chances of danger are slim. Only a very small percentage of people actually develop problems with their practice – far less than people who engage in football, rugby or martial arts, and there is even a much smaller chance of health damage than for those who do no exercise whatsoever!

Over the past decade of teaching, I have encountered quite a number of people with problems caused by their Qi Gong training. I don't, however, feel that the number of people I see is a reflection of a mass epidemic or Qi Gong disharmonies. I feel that I see so many of these people because they seek me out for assistance. I am not sure where exactly, but somewhere my name must have got out as a 'treater of Qi Gong sickness'! These people have come to me from around the world and from numerous other systems of practice. In many cases, I have been able to help them, and in other cases, I have not; every therapist has their limitations, and in the case of Qi Gong sicknesses many of the symptoms can be quite complex. Also, if you don't know the ins and outs of the Qi Gong method that the patient was practising to lead to these problems, then that makes treating them difficult. The more you understand about the mechanics of what they have done, the more likely it is that you will succeed in helping them.

I generally find that those who fall ill that I have treated for Qi Gong-related problems fall within one of the following categories:

- People who already had a disposition towards some kind of psychiatric imbalance. Qi Gong, especially advanced methods, is never advised for those who struggle with an obvious psychiatric illness. It is also a bad idea for those on strong anti-psychotic medications, as the movement of Shen that can come from Qi Gong training does not go well with these kinds of drugs.
- People who are of a very obsessive type tend to run the risk of developing problems with their practice. These types of people can tend to overdo things in their training and make their body far too Yang in nature. They can burn out the Yin essence of their body; without this support, they run the risk of developing conditions linked to too much rising of Yang.
- People who use recreational drugs alongside their practice; in particular those who use hallucinogenic drugs are at risk. It's worth mentioning that this includes mushrooms and ayahuasca, since I have seen that many alternative arts practitioners don't seem to class these as drugs when I speak with them. To make it clear: I am including these two natural substances in the category of hallucinogenic drugs.
- People who don't follow the instructions of their teacher closely enough. I have had several people come for treatment who had decided that they would 'experiment' with the methods given to them.
- People who have been practising a 'made-up' system that has been developed in modern times. No matter what the good intentions of a modern system's creator, they can never, in their lifetime, hope to compare to the generations of masters who have been involved in the founding of the traditional systems. This means that many modern-created systems have the potential to do harm.
- People who have had poor teachers run the risk of doing themselves harm.
- There are some systems that do not blend together well and so when they are mixed they run the risk of causing harm for the practitioner. Though the modern fashion is for 'fusions', this can actually be harmful within the internal arts especially, as some systems work from the 'top down' and some from the 'bottom upwards'. If systems of these types are trained simultaneously, then they run the risk of creating Qi deviations.

Types of Condition

Generally, when problems arise, I divide them into three main types and treat them accordingly. These are: minor issues, serious conditions and critical issues.

Minor Issues

Minor issues are mild imbalances that manifest as a result of errors in Qi Gong practice. In the majority of cases, these are temporary feelings of nausea, dizziness or other short-lived symptoms. Many practitioners will experience these at different times in their practice, and the problem will generally subside if they take a day or so off their practice. If, when resuming practice, the issue persists, then generally a visit to any well-trained Chinese medical doctor will solve the issue.

Serious Conditions

In the case of more serious conditions, the practitioner should immediately stop all Qi Gong practice. The reason I make this very clear is because the biggest danger would be an unskilled teacher stating that the symptoms are actually signs of 'clearing out' and that the student should persist in their practice. I have also known of practitioners who developed serious issues through incorrect Qi Gong practice who then went and tried a different system of Qi Gong to help deal with the issue. This rarely works, because once an energetic 'patterning' has been built into the body, any energy work will reinforce this pattern, no matter what that practice is. So, if I have reversed my Qi and sent it the wrong way up to my head, if I start a Qi Gong regime, even if it is a system aimed at sinking the Qi, the Qi will generally continue to rise. This is because the pattern is now in place, and so any practice will become a form of fuel for the problem.

Generally, serious conditions can be helped by seeking out a skilled Chinese medical practitioner who has an understanding of Qi Gong-related imbalances. You should only return to Qi Gong if the condition has been rectified and only under close supervision from a skilled practitioner who you trust.

Critical Issues

Without meaning to sound overly dramatic, some issues are so problematic that they can be life-threatening. Though rare, I have known of people who caused themselves such damage through internal practice that it cost them their lives. I am not exaggerating here. If you have not experienced the nature of deep Qi Gong or 'heavy-ended' Nei Gong training, then this will sound kind of crazy, but it is not. Some practices are so risky that if you make an error, it can lead to the development of tumours and suchlike. The heads of some internal practice systems have died very young, from either cancer, heart disease, stroke or something similar as a result of their practice. In almost every case it is somewhat of a scandal, since the deceased master was previously touting their system as a means to health and longevity.

Sadly, these kinds of critical issues are difficult, if not impossible, to treat.

Though only a brief introduction, I have listed some main categories of Qi Gong-based illnesses that can develop from incorrect practice of these arts. I wish to reiterate once more, though, that I am not trying to scaremonger! These conditions are, on the whole, very rare. You are highly unlikely to encounter these issues in your training if you follow the guidelines of the practice and your teachers' instructions.

Chinese Medical Conditions

Many of the more minor issues that can develop through Qi Gong practice are the kinds of imbalances that are discussed and taught within Chinese medicine. These are conditions such as Liver Qi Stagnation, Lung Qi Deficiency, Liver Blood Deficiency and so on. These are the result of either a minor reversal of Qi that has been caused through making an error in your training or else was already there inside of your body but has been brought to the surface through your practice. In the majority of cases, these conditions are not such an issue, provided they are recognised and dealt with before they become long-term chronic conditions.

These kinds of conditions can normally be helped by visiting a skilled Chinese medical practitioner and receiving treatment from them. I would say, though, for these kinds of imbalances, make sure you find a practitioner who adheres to the traditional view of imbalance rather than a 'Western model' acupuncturist. The reason for this is simple: the condition has been caused by an energetic error; it is an illness based in a problem with your Qi. It needs a treatment from a practitioner who views the problem in this light – an energetic diagnosis and treatment for an energetic issue.

It is also for this reason, in my opinion, that all sincere Qi Gong or Nei Gong teachers should also be qualified in Chinese medicine or at least have a thorough knowledge of Chinese medicine theory if they ever wish to teach anything more than the absolute foundations of these arts. If you are a teacher without this knowledge, then at least make sure you make good connections with a local, trusted Chinese medical practitioner to whom you can refer any students who may need help. Even if a student has a pre-existing imbalance, it can be helpful for them if you can identify the presence of an imbalance and refer them for treatment. This will help with their training as well as with their overall health.

For students of Qi Gong and Nei Gong, you can find out about these kinds of conditions yourself by getting hold of any in-depth Chinese medical textbook. This can actually be helpful on a number of levels: it can help you understand the nature of your own imbalances, it can help you identify if a problem is arising, and it can also help you to understand more fully the way that Qi moves and manifests within the body. The more you understand Qi, the more you will move towards attainment of Gong.

Qi Gong Deviation

Qi Gong Chu Pian (氣功出偏) or 'Qi Gong deviation' is the overriding term for Qi that has been caused to reverse its flow within one or more of your channels. This can result from an inherent condition being brought to the surface through your training or else as a result of incorrect movement of Qi, often through forced use of willpower or excessive use of visualisation in your practice. It can also come as a result of excessive use of Zi Fa Gong in your training with no understanding of grounding the experience safely.

Those with a knowledge of Chinese medicine should note that the kinds of reversals that fall under the heading of Qi Gong Chu Pian are quite different from the kinds of Qi counterflow that can cause acute bouts of vomiting or acid reflux. These kinds of deviations are literal reversals of energetic flow within a channel. Each channel has a core directional flow that is considered healthy. Though there will always be a degree of two-directional flow within all channels, there is a key direction that the Qi should be moving in for the majority of your life. If Qi reverses in one or more of the channels, then it can lead to problems developing.

When Qi reverses within a channel, it generally leads to pain and aching feelings that distend along the length of the channel. There are generally also muscular shakes and twitches along the length of the channel. Note that the experience of shaking can be Zi Fa Gong and thus quite normal for Qi Gong development, but would be considered Qi Gong Chu Pian if they persist outside of your practice time. If, during your daily life, there are shakes and tremors in the muscles of the body accompanied by pain, then you should really consult with your teacher about the chance of having developed a deviation that needs treatment.

To treat the condition, there will likely be some adjustments that need to be made to your practice. You will need to learn how to 'ground' the Qi to a better level, and your teacher will have to help you with this. Also, look at the strength of the intention you are using and consider revisiting some of the foundational steps for regulating the mind as discussed in this book.

Chinese Medical Protocol

If you are a Chinese medical practitioner and you are looking to aid a person who is suffering with a condition related to Qi Gong deviation, then first seek out underlying deficiencies. The tremors are a manifestation of pathogenic Wind and, as such, look to the Liver and Blood as a good starting point. From here, seek out the channels affected by using sensation along the channels as well as presenting symptoms of channel blockages.

From here, the length of the channel will need to be opened over the course of several treatments. I generally find that using the Jing (井) Well points to initially open the channels will help with alleviating the discomfort, and if you add in the Xi (郤) Cleft point of the channel, it will help to stabilise the Qi in the channel. From here, a couple of treatments in, begin to restore the correct flow of Qi to the channel with the point combinations shown in Table A1.

Table A1: Channel Qi Deviation Points

Channel with deviation	Point selection
Lung	Tai Bai (太白) (Sp 3) & Tai Yuan (太淵) (Lu 9)
Large Intestine	Zu San Li (足三里) (St 36) & Qu Chi (曲池) (Li 11)
Stomach	Yang Gu (陽谷) (SI 5) & Jie Xi (解谿) (St 41)
Spleen	Shao Fu (少府) (Ht 8) & Qian Gu (前谷) (Sp 2)
Heart	Da Dun (大敦) (Lv 1) & Zhong Chong (中衝) (Pc 9)
Small Intestine	Zu Lin Qi (足臨泣) (GB 41) & Hou Xi (後谿) (SI 3)
Bladder	Shang Yang (商陽) (Li 1) & Zhi Yin (至陰) (Bl 67)
Kidneys	Jing Qu (經渠) (Lu 8) & Fu Liu (復溜) (Kd 7)
Pericardium	Da Dun (大敦) (Lv 1) & Zhong Chong (中衝) (Pc 9)

Triple Heater	Zu Lin Qi (足臨泣) (GB 41) & Zhong Zhu (中渚) (SJ 3)
Gall Bladder	Zu Tong Gu (足通谷) (Bl 66) & Xia Xi (俠谿) (GB 43)
Liver	Yin Gu (陰谷) (Kd 10) & Qu Quan (曲泉) (Lv 8)
Governing	Bai Hui (百會) (Du 20) & Qi Hai (氣海) (CV 6)
Conception	Zhong Wan (中脘) (CV 12) & Qi Hai (氣海) (CV 6)

The points listed above should be needled bilaterally and the needles retained for a longer time than many use in their practice; around the thirty-minute mark is usually a good length of time.

Of course, these are only starting points for your treatments; all point prescriptions should be individually tailored to the patient according to their presenting conditions, but at least the above table will help to guide you when presented with a deviation of Qi as a result of Qi Gong practice.

Entering the Fire to Invite Demons

Zou Huo Ru Mo (走火入魔) or 'entering the fire to invite demons' is a rather grand name for a Qi Gong deviation that is of a more serious nature. Unlike the previous condition of Qi Gong Chu Pian, all practice of Qi Gong should immediately be stopped. When practice has been ended, some cases will begin to clear up of their own accord over a period of time whilst others will require assistance from a skilled medical professional. In the cases that improve of their own accord with a cessation of practice, I would still suggest never returning to Qi Gong practice; it really is not a wise choice for you as a practice. This is because many cases of Zou Huo Ru Mo develop as the increased flow of Qi causes a latent psychological condition to manifest. Many people live with the potential psychiatric imbalance their whole lives without being aware of it, but the practice of Qi Gong brings this condition on and makes it an issue.

The condition is the result of the body becoming too Yang in nature. This is often due to blockages within key channels deep within the congenital energetic matrix. When there is an increased flow of Qi through this area of the body, it leads to resistance, as it cannot pass the blockage. The result is heat that can be felt deep inside of the body. This is what they call 'entering the fire'. If I ever see a student sweating profusely in their practice and going red in the face, then I keep a close eye on them. In most cases, they are actually fine and the issue is a temporary reaction, but in some cases, it can be the start of 'entering the fire'. It is a part of the role of the teacher to be able to identify the nature of what is taking place for a student and keeping them safe. Generally, if the heat is short-lived and fades almost immediately after the student ends their practice, then it is fine; it is a temporary result of increased Qi flow. If the heat persists, however, then there is the risk that a deep channel is being taken into a state of imbalance.

Following the stage of 'entering the fire' is the stage of 'inviting the demons'; this is the result of long-term building up of the 'fire'. The 'demons' that have been invited are mood swings that can range from mania and anger outbursts through to long-term depression and feelings of worthlessness. If the imbalance hits this stage, then it can be very difficult to treat with conventional Chinese medical treatment.

Chinese Medical Protocol

Blockages within the deeper channels of the body are generally the result of a deep trauma that occurred during the developmental years. To locate these blockages, it is generally required that you explore and treat the congenital channels (eight extraordinary channels) to locate the imbalance. As well as this, the pathogenic Heat will need clearing from the body. Due to the large amount of variation in where this Heat can reside within the body, I cannot suggest specific points. It will really come down to the diagnostic process to identify its location and clear the correct region of the channel system. 'Entering the fire' rarely, if ever, takes place in the organ channels, though, so you must look to the congenital channels for the source of the issue.

Once the 'demons' have entered and there are psychological imbalances present, then things become a lot trickier. Clearing Heat from channels is one thing, but helping to alleviate mental issues as a result of pathogenic Heat within the body is quite another. Though the Shen can be calmed in the conventional manner, there will generally need to be some Qi emission from a practitioner with this ability. In this case, you will need to use a Yin Qi-type field to lead the pathogenic Heat from the congenital channels out towards a clear exit point from the body. This will need to be followed by the drawing of Yuan Qi down from the upper regions of the body to the lower Dan Tian and Ming Men area before it is drawn out and cleared. The techniques of Ping Zhang Shi (平掌式) or 'horizontal palm method', and Shi Jue Jian (式訣劍) or 'secret sword method', are the most suitable for this level of Yin Qi movement. Doing this requires having built your Yin Qi connection to a high enough level that it can be projected into the patient's body.

Steaming Bones

Gu Zheng (骨蒸) or 'steaming bones' is a condition discussed within Chinese medicine. However, it is not really a common condition that is seen on a regular basis in clinic. It is possible for this condition to show up as a result of incorrect Qi Gong practice whereby the practitioner has caused a strong deficiency of the body's Yin through excessive forcing of Qi flow or due to extreme blockages within the body. The excessive movement of Qi has caused the foundation of Yin to become damaged, and the result is 'steaming bones' disorder.

I have seen this condition arise in those who have practised incorrect alchemical meditation as well as in those who have forced the microcosmic orbit to manifest too early in their training. It manifests as a chronic feeling of heat that is coming from the centre of the bones themselves; it is as though the bone marrow itself is burning. It is very uncomfortable and comes with feelings of irritability, restlessness, insomnia and, generally, night-sweating. It can be very serious if left untreated, as the foundation of your essence is being detrimentally affected. If the condition is caused by the microcosmic orbit being forced or being generated through excessive visualisation, then continued practice of the orbit will serve to exacerbate the condition. As the condition then develops, it will drain the Jing at a very fast rate.

Chinese Medical Protocol

'Steaming bones' can become a very serious condition indeed, so the immediate intervention should be that the person ends all Qi Gong practice. They may well be able to return to their training at a later date, but they will need the imbalance rectified first. Upon returning to Qi Gong, they will have to spend a lengthy period in very Yin practices, building up the strength of their essence. They should then only return to practice once they have found a competent teacher who can guide them safely into internal work.

The first step in the treatment of this disorder should be the nourishing of Yin. Realistically, the level of Yin deficiency that the patient has suffered will be best supported through herbal formulae. A detailed diagnostic process should inform the therapist as to which herbs are prescribed but examples may be:

- Zhi Bai Di Huang Tang (知柏地黄汤)
- Da Bu Yin Tang (大补阴汤)
- Tian Wang Bu Xin Dan (天王补心丹): this formula is more suitable if the condition has also disturbed the functioning of the Shen.

The formula will need to be taken until there are clear signs that the Yin of the patient is beginning to be replenished. From here, the Heat will need to be purged from the body in the usual fashion, and then there will need to be a 'lowering' of the Qi that will, no doubt, have gathered in the upper regions of the body due to the overly Yang state of the patient. This is most easily done from the emission of a Yin Qi field and the use of the Ping Zhang Shi 'horizontal palm' method or the Long Xian Shi (龍啣式) 'holding with dragon mouth' method to lead the Heat downwards and then pluck it from the body. A high level of internal development is needed in order to be able to pluck from the depth of the marrow.

Poison Fire Tainting the Heart

Du Huo Gong Xin (毒火攻心) or 'poison fire tainting the heart' is a condition whereby there has been too much lifting and extraction of sexual energy upwards towards the heart in Qi Gong practice. It is a common problem for those who practise strong internal methods aimed at building power from their sexual energy. It can also result from excessive use of lifting the perineum, especially during orgasm, in the case of males. Poison fire can also develop from those who use 'dual cultivation' sexual methods in the wrong manner, or in those who seek a life of complete sexual abstinence but do not know how to deal with the energy of sexual desire that can arise. I have seen this deviation develop quite a few times in practitioners of contemporary Qi Gong schools who mistakenly believe that they should build their internal development upon a base of sexual energy.

The perineum is the place where your Jing moves towards as one of the first stages in its cycle around the channels of the body. This is a place named Hui Yin (會陰). It is here that the foundations of your sexual drive are based. There are many safe methods for recycling or developing this energy and many that are risky. Most of the riskier methods involve powerfully contracting the perineum and drawing the sexual energy from Hui Yin upwards into the body. This is a misunderstanding of the methods, as it shows a lack of understanding of alchemical conversion of Jing that needs to take place according to the marrow-washing teachings. When this sexual energy moves upwards, it can start to meet the Qi of the Heart centre. The result of this is the generation of 'poison fire'.

Poison fire is a form of Qi that distorts your psychological state. Essentially, it means that the part of your mind based in sexual and base desires begins to distort the part of your mind that feels empathy and connection to others. It can also begin to change the way you understand the romantic aspect of your being, and this can become distorted by the poison fire, too. Essentially, the person suffering with this condition has drawn the Qi of their base desires up into the Qi of their view of others and the world. This can lead to issues ranging from an excessive thirst for power through to the desire to sexually manipulate and use others. In the more extreme cases, the poison fire starts to distort your nature so much that it can lead to paedophilic tendencies; the poison fire has perverted how your mind sees the most innocent and vulnerable.

This is a condition that has affected a great many practitioners of the arts to varying degrees and, sadly, shows up amongst many teachers of the arts.

Chinese Medical Protocol

Unfortunately, this is a very difficult condition to treat with Chinese medicine. The first thing that is needed is that the person ends all Qi Gong practice immediately, especially if they are in a position of potential power, such as a teacher. After this, the cycling of Jing must be changed so that it does not transfer upwards towards the Heart but instead moves backwards into the Governing channel. This will be a challenging adjustment to make, as the route of poison fire is often very ingrained into the patient's system.

Points around the base of the Governing channel need to be opened, such as Yao Yang Guan (腰陽關) (Du 2) and Ming Men (命門) (Du 4). These are then coupled with Guan Yuan (關元) (CV 4) in order to get the Qi to move through the correct regions of the lower abdominal space. There then needs to be 'pulling' and 'plucking' adjustments made to the Jing's path of travel using the Ping Zhang Shi 'horizontal palm' method or the Long Xian Shi 'holding with dragon mouth' method. A strong field of Yin Qi may be needed to draw the Jing into a new line of circulation, and then emission of Yang Qi into the region of the lower Dan Tian and Lu may be needed to anchor this new pattern of Jing movement into the body.

A second branch of the treatment needs to be focused on removing the poison fire from the Heart itself. First, the Shen will need to be calmed in the usual fashion, and then the channel of the Heart will need opening. Classically, it was always the Pericardium channel that was used in place of the Heart due to the fragility of the Heart system but, in the case of poison fire, we need the Heart channel itself.

Open the Heart channel with the combination of Da Dun (大敦) (Lv 1), Zhong Chong (中衝) (Pc 9), Yin Gu (陰谷) (Kd 10) and Qu Ze (曲澤) (Pc 3). Now draw the Heat out of the channel either using the Jing Well points or 'plucking' once more with Qi emission methods.

This protocol should help you to work with this kind of condition, but remember that there will need to be a lot of counselling-type intervention taking place at the same time. Though the treatment will change the energetic mechanics of the condition, direct intervention with the patient's thought patterns will be helpful, too. I have found, more with this condition than any of the other forms of Qi deviation, that it is the willpower of the patient to change that really makes a difference. On top of the treatments, there needs to be a real desire to deal with the issue from the person suffering with it.

Possession

Possession within Chinese medicine falls into one of two categories: internal and external types. Both of these types of possession can result from incorrect and dangerous Qi Gong practice. Internally based possession is essentially the result of an excess of Qi causing an extreme emotional disturbance within your own mind. Externally based possession is invasion of your mind and body by an external spirit – a Gui (鬼).

Internally Based Possession

Internally based possession tends to affect those who cannot let go of an emotionally charged event. For example, maybe a person is angry over an argument that they had with another person five years prior to starting Qi Gong. This anger is so all-consuming that it has turned into an obsession; their entire life is impacted on every level by this problem. When they then start to increase the amount of Qi within their body through practice, they begin to feed this emotional obsession. If this aspect of mind is fed to a high enough degree, then it can actually start to develop a kind of sentience. It becomes an entity in its own right that exists within the afflicted person's mind as a kind of schizophrenic fragment of their own persona. They will then begin to be 'haunted' by this internally developed 'ghost'. These ghosts can be based in any emotional extreme, not just anger. Grief and a sense of loss are another common basis for this kind of possession.

Symptoms can include extreme mood swings, obsessive-compulsive tendencies, as well as hearing the voices of the internal 'ghost'. You would expect to see signs of psychiatric illness that are made worse by the practice. Often, this comes with extreme bouts of paranoia that are exacerbated whenever the person starts to go through their Qi Gong exercises; unfortunately, the ghost itself likes to be fed, and so they tend to develop an obsession with practising very hard. This obviously perpetuates the cycle of disharmony.

Externally Based Possession

Externally based possession is possession in the more literal sense. There has been an invasion of the body by an external spirit or ghost. Sometimes these ghosts are neutral in their behaviour, whilst others are malevolent in nature. I am aware that many of you reading this may not believe in such occurrences, but this was the belief system of those who developed these practices. It is also very real for those who are experiencing such an affliction.

It is said that the world of ghosts cannot see the world of the living very easily; it is as if they are peering at us through the dark. Only in times of emotional difficulty or heightened spiritual states can we be seen by those denizens of the spirit world; it is as if a lamp has been put on, and suddenly we are exposed to the influence of Gui. It is for this reason that people may contract an external possession during traumatic times or during practices such as meditation whereby a 'lamp' has been put on.

On the top of the head are four points known as the Si Shen Cong (四神聰) or 'four alert spirits'. They are a group of points gathered around the crown of the head. These four points are said to guard us against the intentions of the spirit world and, as such, they cover the 'lamp' from view. When we experience a trauma or spiritual surging of Qi, then these four points can become damaged and so their protection is weakened; it is during these times that external ghosts are said to be able to invade us.

Symptoms include extreme psychological imbalance and mood swings, along with extreme paranoia and similar traits to internally based possession. The symptoms may come on very quickly and the patient may also give the invading ghost a name. They may have open conversations with them and, at other times, express themselves as the ghost, meaning that their behaviour and even voice may change. People have been known to speak in 'tongues' and recall memories that are not their own.

Generally, the spirit will drain its host, and the result of this is a depletion of the Jing and Qi; this will happen to a very serious level, meaning that they often have a sunken look to their eyes which are surrounded with dark rings.

Chinese Medical Protocol

Obviously, the first thing the person should do is end all internal practice of any sort. Even after treatment, they should probably never do any form of Qi Gong practice again. They are likely to be susceptible to this kind of issue recurring.

Treatment should be focused around the expulsion of the spirit; the classical points suggested for this kind of treatment were the 'internal and external dragons'. The internal dragons were used for internally based possession and the external dragons for externally based possession. The internal dragons are Tian Shu (天樞) (St 25), Fu Tu (伏兔) (St 32), Jie Xi (解谿) (St 41) and a point a quarter finger's thickness below Jiu Wei (鳩尾) (CV 15). The external dragons are Bai Hui (百會) (Du 20), Da Zhu (大杼) (Bl 11), Shen Shu (腎俞) (Bl 23) and Pu Can (僕參) (Bl 61).

These points are used to help with the expulsion of the energy associated with a possessing entity, and then from here, a field of Yin Qi should be utilised, focusing on plucking the entity with the use of the Long Xian Shi 'holding with dragon mouth' method and the Jian Jue Shi or 'secret sword' method. After this, the Si Shen Cong points will require sealing through strong tonification methods.

As well as the above protocol, there will be a whole host of associated signs and symptoms that will need dealing with. These will involve a lengthy diagnostic and treatment process using standard Chinese medical protocols. It is generally very draining to remove a possessing entity and so do not be surprised if the patient is left very deficient. They will need guidance on diet and possible supporting herbs to bring them back to a state of good health.

On top of these advised points, there are also the 'ghost points' which are indicated in the case of possession and invasion by ghosts. Since the protocol for their use is quite unique, we shall look at the ghost points in a separate section below.

Kundalini Sickness

Though obviously not a Chinese term, 'Kundalini sickness' is a phrase you will often hear within the internal arts scene. In many cases, it is incorrectly used as a general term for sickness arising from internal practice. It is actually a very specific condition that arises as a result of sending too much Qi upwards within the body too quickly. The Sanskrit term 'Kundalini' means 'coiled primal one' and it refers to a form of energy that lies dormant at the base of the spine.

Within many Yogic traditions, it is the aim of the practice to awaken this dormant energy and bring it up through the body to open all of the Chakras and, ultimately, the spiritual centres of the head.

Classically, practitioners of these arts would prepare for a long time, go through a series of developmental stages (not too dissimilar to Nei Gong in some ways) and start to work with the Kundalini energy under the strict guidance of a qualified master. Nowadays, people can do online courses to find out the methods without having to go to all that effort! This, coupled with the widespread popularity of all things 'Yogic', has meant that many people are engaging with Kundalini-type exercises without the proper guidance, understanding or foundations. In the majority of cases, this is not really that much of an issue; the lack of training essentially means that people are stuck in the realm of imagination. But there are also those people who already have a leaning towards this energy awakening anyway. This is the nature of life: some people are safe with practices, whilst others are not. We now have many cases of people practising the internal arts of Asia and accidentally sending the Kundalini energy up through their body without there being any safety or foundations in place.

Within Qi Gong, the arising of this energy takes place very slowly and only after there has been enough preparation of the microcosmic orbit. Essentially, the Kundalini energy comprises congenital fluid, Yin Qi and Yang Qi. The various stages of circulation inherent within Nei Gong training gradually shift all of these energies through the body. Problems arise when people mistakenly send all of this energy upwards at the same time, with little regard for the need to send it back down again or to still the Jing so that there is a foundation of Yin to ground the reactions.

I am aware that I am mixing Yogic and Qi Gong terminology here. This is something I don't usually like to do; I prefer to keep terminologies and practices separate. The only reason I am mixing the terms here is so that Qi Gong practitioners and Chinese medical therapists will have some kind of working model that they can understand when confronted with Kundalini sickness patients.

The symptoms of Kundalini sickness tend to involve hyperactivity of the nervous system combined with a patient who seems to be 'wired'. The Shen is generally disturbed and there is the feeling of Qi rushing upwards very quickly through the person's body. It can actually be quite disturbing to be in the patient's presence, as their hyperactive Qi field will drain your own.

It is common for there to be sharp headaches, eye pain, flickering lights in the eyes, electrical shock-type feelings in the spine, neck and head, extreme tendon tightness in the neck and shoulders, and mood swings. The senses will be heightened and it is normal for the sickness to bring with it huge 'downloads' of gibberish-type information that the brain cannot process fast enough; the result is that the person suffering with the sickness often has a twofold-type condition: on the one hand, they know they are suffering and in pain, but on the other hand, they often feel that their experience has elevated them spiritually.

This is a very Yang condition that is uprooting, hyperactive in quality and mentally disturbing.

Chinese Medical Protocol

The first thing that the patient should do is stop all practice, especially anything based around either meditation or breathing practices. Many cases of Kundalini sickness are the result of forced breathing methods combined with complex visualisations, and so these should all be ended immediately. Gentle moving practices are much better for the patient, along with brisk walks and physical endeavours. The more they can 'get out of their mind' and into their physical body the better.

Initial treatments with acupuncture want to be calming but should not aim to treat the Shen directly. This means that the commonly used Heart points such as Shen Men (神門) (Ht 7) should not be used. This is because the spirit is very fragile at this time and therefore we wish to simply take some of the energetic pressure out of the system rather than dealing directly with the spirit.

Consider the use of points on the channels of the legs, distal to the Qi that is rising into the head, to help bring everything down. The Liver channel is going to be particularly important, as it is highly likely that the patient's pulse will show tightness in this channel and many of the symptoms related to Kundalini sickness are similar to Liver Yang rising and Liver Fire-type conditions. In many Chinese medical systems, the Liver is linked to the nervous system anyway, so this will be helpful to keep in mind during the first few treatments you give. Initially, for the first few times you see the patient, you will use a conventional TCM-type treatment to ground them. Points such as Tai Chong (太沖) (Lv 3), Xing Jian (行間) (Lv 2) and Tai Xi (太谿) (Kd 3) are going to be good starting points. Beyond this, you will need to carry out a full diagnosis and rely heavily on the pulses to tell you how to help calm the body down.

Continue with these kinds of treatments for a few visits, until you start to see a soothing of the body's Qi. Most important are changes in the presenting symptoms around the region of the patient's head as well as a clear progression of the quality of the pulses.

To tackle the root of the condition, look to the Qian Chuang (乾窗) or Celestial Window points. These are important points, as they relate to the way in which Qi rises into a patient's head as well as the Jing Bie (經別) 'divergent channels'. These channels connect the interior and the exterior of the body and have an important function in clearing spiritual problems: they essentially purge pathogens stuck deep inside the congenital channel system as well as the nervous system. Their natural function is, at night, to 'breathe out' many of our emotional tensions, and consequently, the points are often used in an emotional context. Because of their connection to the nervous system, though, we can also use them to deal with the tricky condition of Kundalini sickness. The Qian Chuang points are:

- Tian Fu (天府) (Lu 3) mansion of Heaven
- Tian Chi (天池) (Pc 1) pool of Heaven
- Tian You (天牖) (TH 16) window of Heaven
- Tian Chuang (天窗) (SI 16) heavenly window
- Tian Rong (天窗) (SI 17) heavenly manifestation
- Fu Tu (扶突) (LI 18) supporting prominence
- Tian Zhu (天柱) (Bl 10) Heaven's pillar
- Ren Ying (人迎) (St 9) humanities welcome
- Tian Tu (天突) (CV 22) heavenly crevice
- Feng Fu (風府) (Du 16) wind palace

These points can be used alongside selected points aimed at tackling emotional disturbances for the patient, but should not be used in conjunction with any 'physical-type' points in a single treatment. So, if you were also treating frozen shoulder (which seems like an odd concern when the patient comes with Kundalini sickness, though), this would have to be in a separate treatment. This is because you wish to keep the body focused upon a single level of treatment – that of the mind and divergent channel system.

To select the points, palpate the patient's neck (with the exception of Tian Chi, all of these points sit on the neck). When the Qian Chuang points are blocked, then there will be tightness or aching at the point when you push it. Insert the needles at the blocked points and retain them for some time, around thirty minutes or more, to help the Qi move out of the body. With a few treatments, this should begin to take the pressure off the nervous system and so begin to alleviate the condition.

The Chakras

There is a common error within the Qi Gong community whereby the three Dan Tian are believed to be the same thing as the seven chakras, albeit three of them. This is not the case. The three Dan Tian exist as an aspect of the energetic matrix with associated physiological components, as discussed within this book. The seven chakras exist within the spiritual range of frequencies with some associated tethers into the energetic realm. Though they have no literal form, the seven chakras are experienced as being much smaller than the Dan Tian and have a very clear quality to them that can only really be experienced when at the stage of harmonising the Shen. Within Qi Gong, they are known under three sets of names: either the Qi Huo (七火) 'seven fires', Qi Ding (七鼎) 'seven cauldrons', or the Qi Lun (七輪) 'seven wheels'. The seven fires, cauldrons or wheels reside within the spiritual aspect of the channel running through our spine. They serve as a way to unlock various aspects of the Yuan Shen with regard to how it is tethered into the realm of manifestation.

Though I have not included any real information on the chakras within this book, they are indeed a part of the Daoist tradition. I decided to omit them from the text as they are not generally used within Nei Gong training; instead, they form a larger part of the practice of Shen Gong (神功) 'spirit skill', Xin Ling Li (心靈力) 'psychic ability development', or Guan Chan (觀禪) 'realised perception'. These systems of practice develop refinement of Shen through Tantric meditation methods, directed development of Siddhi and enlightenment, respectively. Although they have a relation to Nei Gong, they are distinct systems of practice in their own right and would require separate books to fully do them justice.

That being said, for interest, those who would like to understand the place of the chakra system within Daoism may be interested in the general functions of each of these spiritual centres and so I have listed them below:

- Chun Zhen Lun (純真輪) Wheel of genuine truth
- Zhen Zhi Lun (真知輪) Wheel of genuine knowledge
- Zheng Dao Lun (正道輪) Wheel of the upright path
- Ren Ai Lun (仁愛輪) Wheel of benevolent love
- Da Tong Lun (大同輪) Wheel of great harmony
- Kuan Shu Lun (寬恕輪) Wheel of expressive compassion
- Zi Jue Lun (自覺輪) Wheel of self-awakening

Wheel of genuine truth: This Lun, or wheel, sits at the base of the spine, or sometimes it is described as being in the region of the perineum.

It is the equivalent of the Muladhara Chakra, as it is generally known within Yogic systems, and the 'sacral fire' of alchemical traditions. The Chun Zhen Lun governs the base desires of the mind; when it is open, base desires are transmuted into supreme will that is aligned with the will of Heaven. There is a recognised trap here: if the Lun in this location of the body opens prematurely, with a lack of spiritual refinement, then a practitioner will be left with a deep, nihilistic dislike of life.

Wheel of genuine knowledge: This Lun sits at the level of the lower lumbar region of the spine. It is the equivalent of the Svadhisthana Chakra, as it is generally known within Yogic systems, and the Ming Men fire of alchemical systems. The Zhen Zhi Lun governs your emotional programming; when it is open, a higher degree of emotional intelligence unfolds within you. There is a recognised trap here: if the Lun in this location of the body opens prematurely, with a lack of spiritual refinement, then a practitioner will become driven by power and dominance.

Wheel of the upright path: This Lun sits at the level of the solar plexus. It is the equivalent of the Manipura Chakra, as it is generally known within Yogic systems, and the Zhong Shu (中樞) fire of alchemical traditions. The Zheng Dao Lun governs your spiritual sense of 'self'; when it is open, the knowledge of 'right action' and 'right practice' as is required to first build and then dissolve the sense of self is innately understood. There is a recognised trap here: if the Lun in this location of the body opens prematurely, with a lack of spiritual refinement, then it is possible to become overly attached to the sense of self; the materialistic side of your nature can become an overwhelming drive.

Wheel of benevolent love: This Lun sits at the level of the Heart centre. It is the equivalent of the Anahata Chakra, as it is generally known within Yogic systems, and the Shen Dao (神道) fire of alchemical traditions. The Ren Ai Lun governs your sense of connection to others as well as the way in which you relate with them. When this Lun is opened, it brings with it a great sense of peace and loving connection to all life forms. There is a recognised trap here: if the Lun in this location of the body opens prematurely, with a lack of spiritual refinement, then a deep feeling of disconnection from all others can be experienced. This results in loneliness and depression which permeates through the Shen of the practitioner.

Wheel of great harmony: This Lun sits at the level of the occiput or, sometimes, it is linked to the throat. It is the equivalent of the Vishuddha Chakra, as it is generally known within Yogic systems, and the Ya Men (啞門) fire of alchemical traditions. The Da Tong Lun governs your ability to communicate the deeper truths of your spiritual being. When this Lun is opened, it brings forth the ability to express yourself with honesty and truth in a way that permeates through to the core of the 'self' of others. It is the important Lun centre of spiritual teachers within the esoteric Daoist traditions. There is a recognised trap here: if the Lun in this location of the body opens prematurely, with a lack of spiritual refinement, then feelings of mistrust and resentment can arise in a person. This often comes with a feeling of constriction of the throat that is worsened when in the company of other people.

Wheel of expressive compassion: This Lun sits within the centre of the head. It is the equivalent of the Ajna Chakra, as it is generally known within Yogic systems, and the Yin Tang (印堂) fire of alchemical traditions. The Kuan Shu Lun governs your ability to experience the true nature of reality as well as the complexities of Ming as it is experienced by all living beings. When this Lun is opened, it gives the ability to perceive the nature of reality as well as a deep understanding of the spiritual needs of others. There is a recognised trap here: if the Lun in this location of the body opens prematurely, with a lack of spiritual refinement, then delusion, madness and great mental anguish will arise.

Wheel of self-awakening: This Lun sits upon the crown of the head. It is the equivalent of the Sahasrara Chakra, as it is generally known within Yogic systems, and the Bai Hui (百會) fire of alchemical traditions. The Zi Jue Lun controls your connection to the heavenly realms and Dao itself. When this Lun is opened, it brings with it an awakening to the delusion of your false sense of self; it is the precursor to enlightenment within esoteric systems utilising the Lun system. There is a recognised trap here: if the Lun in this location of the body opens prematurely, with a lack of spiritual refinement, then there will be insanity, a tendency towards demonic influence and a great level of inner suffering that will arise from being still attached to the earthly realm.

Extreme Stagnation of Yin and Yang Energies

This condition is included as a warning rather than as a condition that can be treated. If this level of Yin and Yang stagnation occurs, then there is very little that can be done; you are pretty much guaranteed to die from this imbalance.

This kind of problem develops from overly forceful squeezing of Qi into various parts of the body, a practice that is very common with many of the more intense Nei Gong traditions. These systems often aim to build large amounts of Qi within the region of the abdomen and perineum. Qi is consolidated to a very high level and then pushed down towards the perineum. This is generally done with the aim of developing supernatural powers or great strength.

To do these kinds of practices, you require very open channels and a high level of internal circulation of Qi. If you do not have these qualities, and you begin to compress your Qi to a high level, then you run the risk of developing an extreme level of stagnation of Yin and/or Yang. This will almost certainly turn into cancerous tumours that are very difficult to treat. These tumours generally develop in either the brain, the liver or the prostate. They develop very quickly and spread around the body with the Qi as it moves through your channel system.

There is also the issue of too much Dao Yin whereby practitioners aim to constantly expel Qi from their body using forceful methods and guided intention. This puts a great degree of strain upon the body and generally causes either a stroke, heart disease or liver failure; once again, these are very difficult, if not impossible, conditions to treat.

The basic rules to protect against this kind of error are to work slowly, carefully, gently and under the guidance of a qualified teacher. Do not try to build and squeeze Qi anywhere within the body until you have ensured that a very strong foundation has been built within your channels, and make sure you understand the correct balance of nourishing and purging Qi through Dao Yin. Those who push and push with their practice are the ones who will suffer.

A Mention of the Ghost Points

An extra mention should be made of the thirteen ghost points (十三鬼穴) of Sun Si Miao, a famous Chinese doctor who lived during the Tang dynasty.

The ghost points are thirteen points on the channel system that are associated with complex spiritual disorders and the invasion of the body by ghosts. They are listed below along with their Chinese names. The original names of the ghost points have been changed in contemporary TCM, so some names may differ from what many acupuncturists are accustomed to.

- Gui Gong (鬼宫) (Du 26) ghost palace
- Gui Xin (鬼信) (Lu 11) ghost purity
- Gui Lei (鬼壘) (Sp 1) ghost heap
- Gui Xin (鬼心) (Pc 7) ghost in the Heart Mind
- Gui Lu (鬼路) (Bl 62) ghost road
- Gui Zhen (鬼枕) (Du 16) ghost pillow
- Gui Chuang (鬼床) (St 6) ghost bed
- Gui Shi (鬼市) (CV 24) ghost market
- Gui Ku (鬼窟) (Pc 8) ghost hideout
- Gui Tang (鬼堂) (Du 23) ghost hall
- Gui Cang (鬼藏) (CV 1) ghost preserve
- Gui Chen (鬼臣) (LI 11) ghost official
- Gui Feng (鬼風) (Extra Point) wind ghost

In modern Chinese medicine ghost points are seen as treatments for mood disorders and other emotional imbalances. They were originally seen as treating a literal invasion by ghosts. They were essentially the most basic of the ways in which exorcisms could be carried out within Chinese medicine.

Though we have already discussed the two main types of possession above, along with treatment protocols, the ghost points are included here for extra information. It seems relevant to include them as they can be used to treat many of the more confusing symptoms that can arise from errors in Qi Gong or other internal practices.

Gui Gong (鬼宫) (Du 26) ghost palace: This point is listed for manic behaviour, depression, suicidal tendencies, obsessions and fears originating in possession by malevolent spirits. It is also the point generally indicated for the treatment of spirits that cause night paralysis and demons that haunt you both in your sleep and waking. If the demons can be heard speaking in your ear then this point is particularly important.

It is also indicated for the earliest stages of ghostly attack when it feels as if there are ghosts that are 'trying to enter the body' but have not yet managed it.

Gui Xin (鬼信) (Lu 11) ghost purity: This point was used for hysterical behaviour, disorientation and 'possessed walking' during both the day and night. If the ghost was causing a distinct draining of essence then this point was indicated.

Other indications include feeling as though there are ghosts trying to climb into your ears, eyes and throat.

Gui Lei (鬼壘) (Sp 1) ghost heap: This point was indicated for ghosts causing a person to 'shout and rave in the street' as well as ghosts that stopped them sleeping and demons that caused manic thought patterns. Psychoses with anger and rage were also indicated here.

Other indications include feeling as if the ghosts are distorting your vision and causing you visual hallucinations.

Gui Xin (鬼心) (Pc 7) ghost in the Heart Mind: Ghosts that lead to madness, hysteria and random laughter and crying are treated with this point. If the laughter becomes insane and 'distant' then the ghost is deep within the system and must be cleared with this point.

Other indications include feeling as if the ghost is taking you over and making your desires run rampant. If the ghost is 'leading' you in this way then Gui Xin can be used to help clear the effects.

Gui Lu (鬼路) (Bl 62) ghost road: Ghosts that lead to epileptic-type behaviour are treated with this point. These often come with feelings of heat and of random energies moving through the body that lead to sickness and depression.

If the ghost is causing you to strike yourself or others against your will then this point should be used.

Gui Zhen (鬼枕) (Du 16) ghost pillow: This point is for ghosts that have ridden on the Wind to enter the body. In classical thought, strong winds carried evil spirits and the potential for possession was stronger. In these cases, early treatment of invading spirits was carried out with Gui Zhen.

Gui Chuang (鬼床) (St 6) ghost bed: Ghosts that 'possess the mind' and prevent clear thinking and speech are treated with this point. It is also a general point for ghosts that cause contortion of the facial muscles. It was classically thought that strong ghosts could make their own faces be known through the face of their victims and that this was one such point for clearing these nasty critters.

Gui Shi (鬼市) (CV 24) ghost market: This point is for ghosts that cause depression, melancholic behaviour and suicidal thoughts. If there is deviation of the face and in particular the mouth then this point is indicated.

Gui Ku (鬼窟) (Pc 8) ghost hideout: If the ghost is causing convulsions and spasms that are with a full sense of awareness then this is the point to use. If there is no mental awareness during the convulsions then Gui Lu should be used instead.

Gui Tang (鬼堂) (Du 23) ghost hall: Ghosts that cause headaches, splitting pain in the middle of the brain, watering of the eyes and strong mood swings are treated with this point.

Gui Cang (鬼藏) (CV 1) ghost preserve: Ghosts that are sapping a person's consciousness are treated with this point. It is also indicated for waking somebody up from a coma. In the case of women there was a particularly awful kind of spirit that was said to come during the night and sexually assault their victims. This point was used to disrupt these spirits' connection to the victim.

Gui Chen (鬼臣) (LI 11) ghost official: This is the general point for ghosts that are causing the Shen to become disturbed and the personality to slowly begin shifting. It was also the point for ghosts coming from rituals and the actions of cult-like groups.

Gui Feng (鬼風) (Extra Point) wind ghost: This most unpleasant point to have needled was the master point for the exorcism of very strong spirits. It is located in the mouth, beneath the tongue; for this reason, we don't actually use this point.

Selection of Ghost Points

Ghost points always had a very distinct way of being used. First, they were never used in conjunction with 'non-ghost points', and second, they were always coupled with the patient's 'inherent ghost point', which is the point that has the strongest resonance with the spirit world. We shall look at what this point is for individual patients below. Essentially, this means any ghost point treatment should involve either two or three needles: two needles if there is simply the 'inherent' point and a unilateral point, and three needles in the case of bilaterally located points.

Locating the patient's inherent ghost point is dependent upon their year of birth. This is because the twelve earthly branches of time-based energy dictate which point was open at the time of conception. Each year a different acupuncture point has a stronger connection to the spirit realm. Table A2 shows the branches in the left column and the ten 'stems of Heaven' in the top bar. To select the inherent ghost point of a patient we only need the earthly branch from the left column. Find your patient's year of birth (remembering that in Chinese calendrical sciences the new year starts in February) and the name of the branch will be shown in the left column.

Table A2: Chart of the Stems and Branches for Year of Birth

Branches	Stems of Heaven									
	Jia	**Yi**	**Bing**	**Ding**	**Wu**	**Ji**	**Geng**	**Xin**	**Ren**	**Gui**
Zi	1924 1984 2044		1936 1996 2056		1948 2008 2068		1960 2020 2080		1972 2032 2092	
Chou		1925 1985 2045		1937 1997 2057		1949 2009 2069		1961 2021 2081		1973 2033 2093
Yin	1974 2034 2094		1926 1986 2046		1938 1998 2058		1950 2010 2070		1962 2022 2082	
Mao		1975 2035 2095		1927 1987 2047		1939 1999 2059		1951 2011 2071		1963 2023 2083
Chen	1964 2024 2084		1976 2036 2096		1928 1988 2048		1940 2000 2060		1952 2012 2072	
Si		1965 2025 2085		1977 2037 2097		1929 1989 2049		1941 2001 2061		1953 2013 2073
Wu	1954 2014 2074		1966 2026 2086		1978 2038 2098		1930 1990 2050		1942 2002 2062	
Wei		1955 2015 2075		1967 2027 2087		1979 2039 2099		1931 1991 2051		1943 2003 2063

Shen	1944 2004 2064		1956 2016 2076		1968 2028 2088		1980 2040 2100		1932 1992 2052	
You		1945 2005 2065		1957 2017 2077		1969 2029 2089		1981 2041 2101		1933 1993 2053
Xu	1934 1994 2054		1946 2006 2066		1958 2018 2078		1970 2030 2090		1982 2042 2102	
Hai		1935 1995 2055		1947 2007 2067		1959 2019 2079		1971 2031 2091		1983 2043 2103

Though Chinese New Year falls on a different date each year, for the purposes of selecting stems and branches of the year we generally use the start of February as our start date.

Once you have the branch of the year you will be able to select the inherent ghost point because each one is attached to an earthly branch. Below are the branches of the ghost points:

- Gui Gong (鬼宮) = Yin
- Gui Xin (鬼信) = Wu
- Gui Lei (鬼壘) = Hai
- Gui Xin (鬼心) = Shen
- Gui Lu (鬼路) = Xu
- Gui Zhen (鬼枕) = Chou
- Gui Chuang (鬼床) = Chen
- Gui Shi (鬼市) = Mao
- Gui Ku (鬼窟) = Wei
- Gui Tang (鬼堂) = Zi
- Gui Cang (鬼藏) = never the inherent ghost point
- Gui Chen (鬼臣) = You
- Gui Feng (鬼風) = Si (if this is the case, Gui Gong is used instead)

So, your treatment for expelling ghosts will then include the inherent ghost point which is needled neutrally (no tonifying nor reducing techniques) and the other point or points which you have selected for the treatment according to the symptoms presented by the patient.

Needles are retained until there is a clear 'relaxation' of the mind and associated symptoms. Failing this, there needs to be clear change present in the pulses of the patient. In my personal experience, it generally takes around thirty minutes or so for the needles to have their full influence.

In Conclusion

As stated at the start of this appendix, I don't wish to scare anybody off Nei Gong training. The chances of developing these kinds of conditions are very slight. But at the same time, the risks should be acknowledged, or else we are simply burying our heads in the sand. I also wanted to give a clear description of some of the major imbalances and how they may be tackled through Chinese medical treatments. Obviously, these kinds of suggestions are always too prescriptive. You need a full and individual diagnostic process for every patient who comes into a Chinese medicine clinic, but these suggested protocols can help you to start looking in the right direction. There is often a lack of awareness of Qi Gong sicknesses, what they are and how they manifest within a person, and this is a problem. Qi Gong and similar internal practices are going through a surge in popularity here in the West, but we are often still lacking in the associated theory and safety information.

Glossary of Pinyin Terms

This is a glossary of Chinese words in Pinyin along with their original characters. These terms are taken from this book as well as previous titles by Damo Mitchell.

Ba Chu (八觸) **Eight touches** These are eight ways in which Qi phenomena can be tangibly felt within the body during Qi Gong practice.

Ba Gua (八卦) Eight trigrams These are eight symbols that form the basis of Yi Jing (I Ching) theory. They represent the eight key forms of Qi that may manifest and transform during any singular point in the unfolding of Ming.

Ba Zi (八字) Eight pillars reading A form of astrological reading based in the four key pillars of time (year, month, day and hour) and how they interact with the stems and branches. A Ba Zi reading gives a great deal of information on a person's astrological makeup.

Bai Hui (百會) Hundred meetings An important acupuncture point that sits on the crown of the head. It is the meeting point of many channels of the body and a major point that is used in Nei Gong practice. It is the energetic Yang 'pole' of the body.

Bai Shi (拜師) Ceremony This is a ceremony of initiation used by teachers of the internal arts to accept a student as a close disciple. The student is said to be 'inside the door' once the ceremony has been completed and, as such, goes deeper into the tradition than other students.

Ban Yun (搬運) Telekinesis The ability to move matter using Qi or Shen in the Daoist internal arts. It is a sign of attainment that arises in some Nei Gong masters when they have reached a very high level.

Bi Yan Hu (碧眼胡) Blue-eyed foreigner A name for Bodhidharma, the patriarch of Chan Buddhism within China, the mythological founder of the sinew-changing and marrow-washing teachings who resided at the Shaolin monastery for many years. He also appears on the Nei Jing Tu, an important alchemical chart within northern sects of Daoism.

Bodhidharma (菩提達摩) Indian monk See *Bi Yan Hu*

Bu (補) Nourish One of the key ways in which Qi should be regulated through Qi Gong practice. If an art lacks any kind of nourishment then it is considered to be imbalanced.

Cai Qi Gong (采氣) Gathering Qi This is the practice of collecting energy from the environment. This energy is then used to either supplement or cleanse the practitioner's own Qi.

Can Tong Qi (參同契) Triplex unity The earliest alchemical textbook to come out of China. It is an important part of any alchemical Daoist's study.

Chan (禪) Chinese Buddhism The form that Buddhism took when it made its way to China. It is closely linked to the Shaolin monastery and has many crossovers with Daoism.

Chen (沈) Feeling of sinking One of the common ways that Qi can be somatically experienced through Qi Gong practice. It is generally linked to an increase in Yin Qi movement.

Chen Tuan (陳摶) Daoist sage An important sage who lived around the start of the Song dynasty. He is credited with the formation of the martial art Liu He Ba Fa as well as various alchemical methods.

Cheng Jiu (成就) Siddhi The various supernatural abilities that can arise out of Nei Gong and meditation practice. Rather than a goal of the training, they are considered a signpost of attainment. They can be based in cultivation of Qi, Shen and Ling.

Da Zhou Tian (大周天) Large heavenly orbit An extension of Qi that circulates out of the body into the surrounding environment when a practitioner reaches a certain stage of development in their practice.

Dan (丹) Elixir The Dan is the 'elixir' which is sought out through alchemical training within the Daoist tradition. Often depicted as red and likened to the ore of cinnabar.

Dan Tian (丹田) Elixir field Usually refers to the lowest of the three 'elixir fields', though there are three main Dan Tian within the body. The primary function of the lower Dan Tian is the conversion of Jing to Qi as well as the moving of Qi throughout the channel system.

Dan Tian Hu Xi (丹田呼吸) Dan Tian breathing The absorption and emission of Qi from the lower Dan Tian. This should evolve naturally out of your practice and is a mechanism involved in the storage of Qi within the Dan Tian.

Dan Tian Xi Qi (丹田吸氣) Dan Tian inhales the Qi A reference to the 'drawing in' process of Qi into the lower Dan Tian that takes place when Yin and Yang have been cultivated to a certain degree.

Dan Yuan (丹元) Field of Qi The extension of Qi into the space around your body once full radiation of Qi begins to occur. It is an aspect of the auric field.

Dao (道) Dao The nameless and formless origin of the universe. Daoism is the study of this obscure concept, and all internal arts are a way of experientially understanding the nature of Dao.

Dao De Jing (道德經) The Virtue of Following the Way Scripture The classical text of Daoism attributed to the great sage, Laozi. Also written as Tao Te Ching. Often mistaken for a book of philosophy or political commentary, it is primarily a meditative text.

Dao Wai Cai Yao (道外採藥) Picking herbs to use as an external way to Dao This is a branch of the Daoist tradition that uses herbal formulae and pills as a way to develop the body and mind towards Dao. It is derived from the 'external alchemy' tradition.

Dao Yin (導引) Guiding and pulling exercises These are the ancient exercises developed by the shamanic Wu people to purge the energy body of pathogenic energies. They are generally very stretched out and physical in comparison to Qi Gong training.

Dao Yin Tu (導引圖) Guiding and Pulling Chart An ancient chart showing Dao Yin principles dated to around 168 BCE. The chart is known as the oldest known record of moving energetic exercises.

Dao Zang (道藏) Daoist canon The Dao Zang is the Daoist canon of classical writings which includes over 1,400 pieces of scripture. It is a compendium of alchemical and medicinal writings that are collected from various Daoist lineages.

De (德) Virtue The congenital manifestation of the transient emotions. De is born from deep within the true human consciousness which is usually buried beneath the various layers of the acquired mind.

Di Qi (地氣) Earth Qi The name for the Qi of the Earth that manifests as fields of energy. It is the Qi utilised in the early stages of Nei Gong training in order to awaken the body's Qi.

Diao (掉) Shaking A common phenomenon that can occur in Qi Gong and Nei Gong training. It can be an internal form of vibration or, sometimes, can manifest into the muscles of the body.

Ding (鼎) Cauldron The 'cauldron' of Daoist Nei Dan. This is a location within the energy body where two energetic substances are being combined. Named after the Ding which sits within most Daoist temples.

Ding (定) Stabilise A quality of the mind that is both developed and required for certain stages of Nei Gong training.

Du Huo Gong Xin (毒火攻心) Poison fire tainting the heart An affliction of the mind and body that can arise as a result of unsafe or incorrect Qi Gong practice. It is particularly prevalent amongst those who practise sexual-based Qi Gong methods in an incorrect fashion.

Dui (兌) Dui trigram One of the eight trigrams of Daoist Ba Gua theory. Its energetic manifestation is metaphorically likened to a lake.

Er Ting (耳聽) Listening with ears A metaphor for the earliest stages of using the awareness to interact with a bodily process. The use of the term 'ears' means that you are listening in a very superficial manner as if you were using your physical sense organs.

Fa (法) Method The earliest stages of practising an exercise or element of the Chinese arts. When studying according to Fa you are closely following the instructions and have not yet attained expertise.

Fa Lun (法輪) Wheel of law The name for the radiant wheel of light that circulates within the microcosmic orbit as a reaction to the movement of Shen. It is so named because it is said to cleanse the spirit of Karmic debris according to some esoteric Buddhist sects.

Fa Qi (發氣) Emit Qi The ability to emit energy out of the body, generally through the hands and fingers. It is generally used as a medical tool as well as a way of teaching. There are many different strengths and qualities of Fa Qi depending on the cultivation of the practitioner and the system of practice.

Feng Shui (風水) Wind and water geomancy This is the Daoist study of environmental energies and the influence of the macrocosm upon the human energy system and consciousness.

Fu (符) Talismanic transmission The magical talismanic drawings of the ancient Daoists. The skilled practitioner of magical Daoism could draw Fu to heal sickness, curse people or perform countless other functions. An almost extinct art in modern times.

Fu (浮) Feeling light A common sensory experience within Qi Gong practice. It can result from the movement of Qi or the extension of the Huang.

Gan Ying (感應) Sensory echoes The ability to tangibly feel the quality of another's energetic or physical health. This can be done through energetic palpation, extension of the mind or harmonisation of the energetic field with the subjects.

Gan Zhi (感知) Sensory knowing The ability to cognitively 'know' and understand the quality of another's energetic or physical health. At very high levels it can also be used to know the thoughts of another.

Gen (艮) Gen trigram One of the eight trigrams of Daoist Ba Gua theory. Its energetic manifestation is likened to that of a mountain.

Gong (功) Skill or quality The attainment of a high-level skill within any art. It can be likened to reaching the state of transforming your practice into an inherent 'quality' that is a part of your being. There are 'lesser Gong', which are small sections of a wider art form, and 'higher Gong', which is the achievement of mastery of an art. Higher Gong can take a lifetime of diligent practice to reach.

Gu (固) Firm A quality of the mind that is both developed and required for certain stages of internal development.

Gua (卦) Trigram These are the eight sacred symbols which make up Daoist Ba Gua theory. They are a way to conceptualise the various vibrational frequencies of the energetic realm and how they interact. They are the mainstay of Yi Jing (I Ching) theory.

Guan Chan (觀禪) Realised perception method This was a specific branch of Daoist practice aimed at enabling a person to attain a full understanding of the nature of reality. To Daoists who followed this school of thought, enlightenment was to be found through realisation of the nature of manifested phenomena as opposed to a reconvergence of Yin and Yang.

Hou Tian (後天) Acquired The 'post-Heaven' state which humankind exists within according to Daoist thought. Hou Tian exists as a state within both the mind and energetic matrix.

Hu Lu (葫蘆) Gourd The Calabash or 'gourd' is an important symbol within Daoist artwork and practice. It shows the shape of the Huang as it needs to be formed in advanced Nei Gong practice. It is also a container for the 'immortal fluids' of the Daoist deities.

Huan (緩) Slow and gradual A core quality of the breath that was classically advised within Daoist practice. It should develop out of the practice of regulating the breathing. This will then transfer into the mind and body on various levels.

Huang (肓) Membranes Generally translated as 'membranes', these are the soft tissues that fill the spaces of the body, surrounding and enwrapping the organs. It is through the Huang that the deeper aspects of the channel system are formed.

Hui Yin (會陰) Meeting of Yin An important acupuncture point located at the perineum. It is named after the fact that it is situated within the most Yin region of the human body. It is the 'Yin pole' of the body's Qi.

Hun (魂) Yang soul The ethereal soul which continues to exist after our death. It is usually housed within the Liver. The Hun is an important element of the mind when in an acquired state and is classically said to be divided into three parts.

Hundun (混沌) Original chaos A term generally translated as 'original chaos'. Within Daoist philosophy it refers to a state which lay dormant within the centre of human consciousness as well as an aspect of the process of creation.

Ji Ben Qi Gong (基本氣功) Fundamental Qi Gong The primary foundation-level exercises taught within the Lotus Nei Gong School of Daoist Arts. The set comprises eight movements that are designed to help a student understand the principles of correct and efficient practice.

Jian (堅) Feeling tight A common somatic experience that can be felt in the channels or Huang of the body as a result of an increased movement of Qi. It should be noted that the tightness of Jian is not the same as habitual tension, which is a quality we need to shed through our practice.

Jin Dan Da Dao (金丹大道) Great path of the golden elixir This is the overriding name for the alchemical traditions of Daoism. This was the path of working systematically with the substances of Jing, Qi and Shen in order to develop the 'elixir' of Daoism.

Jing (精) Essence The lowest vibrational frequency of the three main energetic substances of humans. Usually translated as 'essence' and often misunderstood as being human sexual fluids. It is one of the three 'internal treasures' of humanity according to Daoism.

Jing (靜) Quiet A quality of the mind that will arise out of correct practice of Nei Gong and regulation of mental activities.

Jing Ding (靜定) Stillness leads to stability A two-word causation chain of instruction that essentially shows how making the mind still will result in a stabilisation of the mind's form.

Jing Jin (經筋) Sinew channels Lines of connective tissue that run throughout the body. These lines serve as 'riverbeds' for the flow of Qi that runs through the channel system. These are the lines of tissue that run near to the surface of the body; they encase the outermost aspect of the channel system.

Jing Luo (經絡) Channel system The human channel system which is made up of numerous energetic pathways that regulate the body and transport Qi to and from our organs and tissues. It comprises major and minor channel pathways through which Qi and the accompanied substance of blood flow.

Kan (坎) Kan trigram One of the eight trigrams of Daoist Ba Gua theory, which is usually likened to the energetic manifestation of water. It is a symbol often attributed to the quality of Qi within the lower abdomen and kidney region.

Kan Qi (看氣) Qi vision The ability to perceive Qi within the visual spectrum. This is an ability that commonly arises out of Nei Gong development. It often arises as a result of the opening of the 'spiritual eye'.

Kua (胯) Inguinal crease An area of the body that needs training in order for the regulation of the body stage of practice to be completed. It can be likened to the 'bikini line' if students are confused as to its location.

Kun (坤) Kun trigram One of the eight trigrams of Daoist Ba Gua theory. Its energetic manifestation is usually likened to that of the planet.

Kun Lun Shan (崑崙山) The Kun Lun Mountains A mythical mountain within Daoist legend that was said to reach up into the Heavens. Though there are actual mountains with this name in China, the Daoists generally refer to the mythical Kun Lun Mountains in their teachings.

Lao Gong (勞宮) Palace of toil An acupuncture point situated in the centre of the palm. Its name means 'palace of toil' due to it being on the human hand which carries out a lot of physical work. Within Daoism this point is also known to be very important in venting heat from the heart and so it is rarely at rest. It is a very important point in Qi Gong practice as it regulates the internal temperature and also allows us to emit Qi in practices such as external Qi therapy.

Laozi (老子) The Great Sage The 'original Daoist' who is purported to have written the Dao De Jing. Supposedly he left this text with a border watchman when he retreated into hermitage in the western mountains of China.

Leng (冷) Feeling cold A common somatic experience to be had from Qi Gong practice. It is generally the result of increased Qi movement or else can be the result of a blockage that needs to be cleared.

Li (理) Regulate One of the key principles of Qi Gong practice. It concerns harmonising Yi and Yang as well as the overall quality of the body's Qi.

Li (離) Li trigram One of the eight trigrams of Daoist Ba Gua theory. Its energetic manifestation is usually likened to fire.

Liang Yi (兩儀) Twin poles The collective name for Yin and Yang when they are in a state of inter-relationship.

Ling (靈) Magical spirit The evolved state of the Shen when it is still manifest within the earthly realm. The Ling is the basis of higher levels of perception as well as many of the mind-based Siddhi that may develop out of Nei Gong training.

Ling Bao (靈寶) Spiritual Treasure Sect An alchemical sect of Daoism that uses a number of meditation methods as well as environmental methods of regulating Yin and Yang. It was developed in the Jin dynasty as a merger of Daoist and Buddhist teachings.

Ling Zi (靈子) Magical particles This is the name for the spiritual energy that holds together even the tiniest particles of existence in Daoism. It is through the action of the Ling Zi that Dao is expressed into the manifested realm.

Liu Yi Ming (劉一明) Daoist sage Liu Yi Ming was a high-level Daoist master born in 1734. He was a major figure within the northern Daoist traditions who left behind many writings and commentaries on the alchemical arts.

Liu Zi Jue (六字訣) Six healing sounds A commonly practised Qi Gong system that involves making six different sounds, each used to nourish one of the key organs of the body. The system is based upon six internally generated sounds that can manifest as a result of increased Qi movement.

Long Dao Yin (龍導引) Dragon Dao Yin A set of four short sequences based upon the preliminary training methods from the martial style of Baguazhang. They twist the spine and open the joints to assist with the energetic purging process.

Long Mai (龍脈) Dragon lines Somewhat akin to the Western concept of ley lines, these are regions of the Earth through which flow strong lines of natural Qi. These lines are often sought out by Qi Gong practitioners as beneficial places to practise their arts. Many temples were classically built upon Long Mai and shrines were often set up at 'node points' along these lines.

Long Men (龍門) Dragon Gate Sect A northern alchemical sect of Daoism based in meditative practices and purification methods. They are the most widely spread of the Daoist traditions and have many branches around the world.

Lu (爐) The furnace This is the place within the body where expansion is created, which generates Heat. This Heat is then usually added to the Ding in order to create alchemical change. The Lu is situated at the perineum region of the body.

Mian (綿) Cotton soft One of the key qualities that we wish to seek out in our breathing. When the breath is regulated according to this principle it will start to transfer the quality into your energy system and body.

Ming (命) Life path Your life path; a mix of concepts such as fate, destiny, purpose and also the series of events that unfold throughout your life. There are three levels of Ming: the Ming of Heaven, the Ming of Earth and the Ming of humanity.

Ming Huo (命火) Ming fire An expansion of Qi that sits near to the Kidneys on your lower back. This region of the body serves as a catalyst for the actions of Qi that take place within your Governing channel as well as initiating the actions of the Jing.

Ming Men (命門) Door to your life path An acupuncture point in the lower back which is very important in Nei Gong practice. It is connected to the several very important aspects of training including your Kidney health, the quality of your Jing and the strength of the body's Yang.

Nei Dan (內丹) Internal alchemy The Daoist form of alchemical meditation usually associated with the northern sects of Daoism. Through working with various energetic and spiritual substances within the body, the practitioner seeks states of transcendence and, ultimately, immortality.

Nei Gong (內功) Internal development The process of internal change and development which a person may go through if they practise the internal arts to a high level. The Nei Gong process takes the form of a (mostly) sequential series of developmental stages. Different traditions will interpret the Nei Gong process in different ways.

Nei Guan (內觀) Inner looking The process of 'turning around the light', or placing your conscious awareness inside of the body rather than allowing it to look outwards into the external world.

Nei Jing Tu (內經圖) Chart of the Inner Landscape One of two important alchemical charts carved into a courtyard wall of the White Cloud Monastery in Beijing. It shows the theory behind many alchemical processes, Nei Gong and the microcosmic orbit.

Nu Dan (女丹) Female alchemy Women-specific alchemical practices that take into account the inherent individuality of the female energetic system. Generally, most of these traditions can be traced back to the Daoist sage Sun Bu Er.

Ping Heng Gong (平衡功) Balancing and harmonising practice This is the overriding name for using the Qi and energetic fields of the environment to harmonise the body's own Qi. This can include work with rivers, crystals, mountains, elemental energies and, most famously, trees. Many people would understand the term Ping Heng Gong to refer specifically to work with trees.

Po (魄) The Yin soul The 'Yin soul', which dies with the human body. Largely connected to our physical senses, the Po resides in the Lungs. Classically there are said to be seven Po, each of which forms the basis for one of our key emotional attachments.

Pu (樸) Simplicity Often likened to an uncarved block. The ideal state of mind according to the Daoist tradition. This has much to do with shedding the layers of the acquired self which pull you away from existing in a 'simple' state.

Qi (氣) Energy A term that is often difficult to translate into English. In Nei Gong theory it is an energetic vibration which transports information through the energy system. It can exist in various forms, including a more electrical-type form that passes through the channel system in a very linear fashion, or a more magnetic type of energy that forms fields in and around the body.

Qi Chen Dan Tian (氣沈丹田) Submerge the Qi in the Dan Tian A key principle of advanced Nei Gong whereby the Qi that is developed through practice is then sunk and submerged into the field of the lower Dan Tian.

Qi Gong (氣功) Energy exercises Usually gentle exercises which combine rhythmic movements with breathing exercises to shift Qi through the body. The term means 'energy exercises', although it is sometimes translated as 'breathing exercises'. Within the system I teach, Qi Gong exercises are used as a tool to move along the Nei Gong process.

Qi Gong Chu Pian (氣功出偏) Qi Gong deviation An error in Qi Gong practice whereby the Qi is sent the wrong way within the channel system or else there are blockages that are leading to the development of disharmony. In the majority of cases, this will require treatment from a skilled teacher or Chinese medical practitioner.

Qi Hai (氣海) Sea of Qi An acupuncture point which sits in front of the lower Dan Tian. Its name in English is 'Sea of Qi' as it is the point from where Qi is generated and where it flows from. Like water returning to the sea in rivers and streams, Qi returns to the lower Dan Tian when it has circulated through the microcosmic orbit.

Qi Ting (氣聽) Listening with the Qi A stage of absorbing the awareness into the body and becoming aware of the subtly shifting phenomena that take place as a result of the actions of Qi.

Qian (乾) Qian trigram One of the eight trigrams of Daoist Ba Gua theory. Its energetic manifestation is usually likened to the movements of Heaven.

Re (熱) Heat One of the key somatic experiences to be had through Qi Gong training. This Heat can come from an increased flow of Qi and Blood, consolidation of the Jing or internal resistance to the movement of Qi.

Ren (人) Humanity Within Daoism, Ren is 'humanity'. Humanity sits between Heaven and Earth and is a reflection of their fluctuations and movements. Ren is nourished by Earth and stimulated to development through the actions of Heaven.

Ren Ming (人命) Will of humanity The personal life path of humankind. This is the aspect of Ming that we are most influenced by on a daily basis and the branch of Ming that we have the most control over.

San Bao (三寶) Three treasures A collective name for the three key aspects of various levels of existence. On the level of Earth, the San Bao are water, wind and fire; on the level of humanity, the San Bao are Jing, Qi and Shen; on the level of Heaven, the San Bao are sun, moon and stars. Within the realm of virtue, the San Bao are wisdom, compassion and humility. Generally, unless otherwise specified, the term 'San Bao' is used in the context of humanity and the Jing–Qi–Shen axis.

San Gong (散功) Dispersal of skill An error in your development that can come from incorrect practice. Most of these errors involve forceful use of will or tightening of muscles. The result is that, at a certain point, your Qi will disperse and your health start to break down. It is a key error that can result from not following the principles of the Sinew-Changing Classic.

Shaolin (少林) Small Forest Monastery An important place for the development of Buddhism in China. Famous for its fighting monks and as the place where Bodhidharma is said to have created the Sinew-Changing Classic and the Marrow-Washing Classic.

Shen (神) Spirit The energy of consciousness. Vibrates at a frequency close to that of Heaven. You should be cautious with this term as it can be used in many ways to refer to many different aspects of mind, consciousness and spirit. When studying Shen, look closely at how the term is being used by the author or teacher.

Shen Gong (神功) Spirit skill This is the arcane skill of working with the substance of consciousness. Within Daoism it is said that a skilled Shen Gong practitioner can manipulate the very energy of the environment. It is the basis of Siddhi and another name for the use of the Ling.

Shen Ming (神明) Spiritual divinity The state of hitting profound awareness of the nature of reality. It is often heralded with the convergence of Yuan Shen and a brilliant white light that is all-consuming.

Shen Qi Xiang He (神氣相合) Shen and Qi harmonise with one another The stage of the spirit and the energetic matrix becoming one. This is a natural development that will arise out of your practice once you hit a certain stage.

Shen Xian (神仙) Heavenly immortal A full realisation of the possibility of spiritual immortality which is the final goal of Daoist Nei Dan. It should be noted that not many practitioners are said to have achieved this level of attainment!

Sheng Ren (聖人) Sage A level of attainment in the Daoist arts that is the equivalent of a wise and virtuous person. It indicates a high level of spiritual development and generally an eradication of attachment to the self.

Shou Yin (手印) Hand shape The Chinese name for mudra. Various patterns and uses of the hands that serve to adjust the quality of Qi and Shen. The Daoist tradition is said to have over 800 Shou Yin, though many of them are produced internally.

Shu Liao Fa (樹療法) Tree therapy The act of practising Qi exchange and harmonisation with trees. This is a specific branch of Qi Gong utilised by almost all traditional systems of Daoist practice.

Shuang Xiu (雙修) Paired cultivation tradition A branch of Daoism that was concerned primarily with paired Qi Gong practice. This could take the form of massage, projection of Qi or even sexual practices. Though a part of many Daoist traditions, it was never seen as one of the major paths to Dao.

Shun (順) Unconscious path along Ming The name for the form of energy that pulls us unconsciously through life along the path of Ming. There is a stage in Nei Gong training whereby you generally become aware of Shun and how it can speed up or slow down according to your mindset.

Song (松) Letting go One of the key qualities that should be developed within all of the internal arts that came out of China. Often mistaken for a form of passive relaxation, Song is actually quite different. It is the process of shedding habitual physical and mental tensions through the use of posture, inner change and (within Nei Gong) breathing.

Sun (巽) Sun trigram One of the eight trigrams of Daoist Ba Gua theory. Its energetic manifestation is usually likened to that of the wind.

Sun Wu Kong (孫悟空) Monkey king The main character of the Chinese classic *Journey to the West*. Sun Wu Kong is a representation of the transformation that a mind will go through on its journey towards spiritual enlightenment.

Taiji (太極) The great limit A Daoist concept that is literally translated as the 'great limit' but in fact would be better translated as the 'motive force of creation'. It is manifest into life as a spiralling force that causes the various inter-relations of Yin and Yang.

Taiji Tu (太極圖) Chart of Taiji The classical name for the image we commonly refer to as the Yin Yang symbol.

Taijiquan (太極拳) Internal martial art An internal martial art based upon the actions of Taiji, Yin, Yang and the process of Song.

Taiyi (太一) The great pole Within Daoist philosophy, this is the single point of union which moves out of stillness. It is also the name of a standing posture utilised in advanced female-specific Nei Gong training.

Tao Hong Jing (陶弘景) Daoist A Daoist sage credited with the formation of the Shang Qing sect of Daoism. Tao Hong Jing was a famous herbalist and astrologer as well as an alchemical practitioner.

Tian (天) Heaven Not to be mistaken with the Christian concept of Heaven; this refers to the vibrational frequency of the macrocosm. Within the microcosm of the body Heaven is used to metaphorically refer to human consciousness. Alchemical Daoism uses it as a reference to the movement of the stars and planets.

Tian Gan (天干) Heavenly stems This is a model of the Yin and Yang divisions which take place within the Wu Xing when they exist as a part of the heavenly realm. It is used extensively in astrology, Feng Shui and some forms of Chinese medicine.

Tian Gui (天癸) Heavenly water An energetic component involved in the formation of menstrual Blood in women. It is a direct conversion of the Jing that takes place according to the lunar cycles.

Tian Tu (天突) Heavenly crevice An important acupuncture point that sits in the suprasternal notch. It is the key point that is sunk downwards in order to empty the chest of tensions and sink the Qi within the torso.

Tiao Ying Wei (調營衛) To adjust the nourishment and protective functions A medical phrase for the changes that need to take place within the channel system if we wish them to function efficiently. It suggests a change to the way that our Qi nourishes the body and strengthens the protective layer of energy that surrounds our body.

Ting (聽) Listening Within the Daoist arts this is the key descriptive term for the quality of your awareness that should be present when you practise. It is a deliberately passive form of mental intention that discourages active visual experiences.

Tou Shi (透視) X-ray vision An advanced skill that can arise within very high-level Nei Gong or alchemical practitioners. It literally gives them the ability to look through your outer layers and view the state of your physical organs.

Wai Dan (外丹) External alchemy An almost (but not entirely) extinct practice based upon the development of external pills that may lead a person to spiritual elevation and Dao. These pills comprised herbs and various metals as well as the Qi of the pills' creator. In some traditions, these pills were created in a similar vein to modern Chinese herbal medicine, whilst in others, vast furnaces and bellows were used to create the pills.

Wai Qi Liao Fa (外氣療法) Qi Gong healing A form of medical treatment based upon the emission of Yin, Yang or neutral Qi. The therapist can use their own Qi either to 'give' energy or to adjust the quality of your own internal state. It is an advanced form of Qi Gong practice that needs many years of practice if it is ever to move beyond the most basic levels.

Wan Wu (萬物) Ten thousand things A name for the various phenomena and entities that arise as a result of the actions of Dao, Heaven and Earth. Within the world of manifestation, it means all of the physical objects and life forms. Within the microcosm of the human mind it refers to our thought processes.

Wei Lu (尾櫚) Tail palm-leaf A classical name for the sacrum and coccyx. This is an important part of the body for the opening of the Governing channel.

Wu (悟) Awakening A term referring to the stage of inner development whereby you fully realise the false nature of 'self' and thus shed all attachments to its actions.

Wu (巫) Chinese shaman The shamanic Wu were the historical ancestors of the Daoists. They served as medicine men, bringers of rain and general mystics to the ancient tribes of China. Many Daoist sects absorbed many of the Wu people's practices but then shunned other shamanic aspects of their practice. The logic behind this was that the shamanic path was a path too attached to the realm of Earth; this meant that progression into the realm of Heaven would be limited.

Wu Ai Bu Ai (五愛不愛) The five biases The name for the way in which the five spirits start to form the conditioning of the acquired mind. It quite literally means 'the five loves and not-loves'; this shows that the idea of good and bad is a key reason why our conditioned thinking begins to develop.

Wu Ai Zhi (五愛執) The five attachments The five key attachments of the spirits are key mental distortions that affect the way in which our acquired mind develops. The shedding of attachments within Daoism is essentially concerned with regulating the nature of these five spirits.

Wu Dao Yin (五導引) Five Dao Yin A series of five purging energetic exercises used within the Lotus Nei Gong school to help clear Xie Qi from the body. They are a simple enough series of movements that open the joints and move the Qi in a powerful fashion.

Wu Du (五毒) The five poisons A somewhat overly dramatic name for the five key emotions. They are known as 'poisons' due to the detrimental effect that they may have upon the state of your mind.

Wu Ji (無極) Without projection The Daoist concept of non-existence. The blank canvas upon which reality is projected and an important part of Daoist creation philosophy. It is also the name used for the main standing practice in the majority of Qi Gong systems.

Wu Qi (五氣) The five Qi This is a reference to the way that the five spirits can begin to affect the quality of our body's internal Qi. These five energies are then categorised according to the five elemental movements.

Wu Qi Chao Yuan (五氣朝元) Return the five Qi to their origin A term used within Qi Gong practice to show that we need to harmonise the elemental qualities of our inner state. This is generally achieved through regulation of the body's Qi, via the channel system, as well as through harmonising the five spirits. This principle is understood to be the basis for good health, longevity and mental balance.

Wu Shen (五神) The five spirits The collective name for the Shen, Hun, Yi, Zhi and Po. Many practitioners of Qi Gong will see the five spirits as models of higher consciousness and spiritual development; in fact, they are a model of the acquired state of thinking and they come into existence as a refraction of original spirit.

Wu Shen Chao Yuan (五神朝元) Return the five spirits to their origin A Qi Gong and alchemical term meaning that we should aim to recombine the five spirits into their original unified state of Yuan Shen or 'original spirit'. This is a key focus of many Daoist meditation systems.

Wu Tong (五通) Five communications These are five Siddhi that can arise out of reaching a high level with your spiritual development. The five communications are communication with the past, communication with the present, communication with the future, communication with Ming and communication with Heaven.

Wu Wei (無為) Non-doing The act of 'non-governing'. An important philosophical concept within the Daoist tradition. This term is often misunderstood to mean that Daoists should 'do' nothing and thus are essentially lazy. This misunderstanding comes from missing the fact that you cannot 'non-do' until you can first 'do'.

Wu Xiang (五象) The five manifestations This is a model for the way in which the five spirits express themselves through the physical tissues, sense organs and viscera. It is a more traditional name for the five-element categorisation model that is common to all Chinese medicine traditions.

Wu Xing (五行) Five elemental movements The five elemental states which are an important part of Daoist creation theory, psychology and medicine. The model is used as a way to understand the refraction of an original state into the acquired level of manifestation as well as how interaction then takes place during an evolutionary process.

Wu Xing Qi Gong (五行氣功) Five elemental energy exercises Five simple exercises based upon the movement and interactions of the Wu Xing energies. There are many expressions of the Wu Xing Qi Gong exercises as different teachers each had their own take on the principles.

Wu Yao (五藥) The five cures These are five answers to all mental disturbance and health issues within the Daoist arts. They are: harmonious Qi, a still mind, a tranquil nature, forgetting the emotions and having the five spirits in harmony.

Wu Zei (五賊) The five thieves This is a name for the five senses of sight, hearing, smell, touch and taste. They are 'thieves' as they take away from your inner stillness. Note that, in some traditions, the five thieves were listed as the emotions and not the senses. In the tradition taught within this book, the thieves are the senses whilst the emotions are known as the poisons.

Xi Sui Jing (洗髓經) Marrow-Washing Classic An important series of classical teachings traditionally attributed to Bodhidharma. These teachings concern higher-level internal development and as such were absorbed into advanced Qi Gong, Nei Gong and alchemical systems.

Xi Wang Mu (西王母) The Holy Mother of the West A Daoist immortal and deity associated with the power of the western Heavens, prosperity and immortality. She is often the patron deity of many female Daoist practitioners. She is associated with the seven-star constellation.

Xian Tian (先天) Congenital The 'before Heaven' congenital state which is all important within Nei Dan training. It is here that diligent practitioners of the Daoist arts are seeking to return.

Xian Yao (仙藥) Immortal medicine Another name for the Wu Yao. These are five answers to all mental disturbance and health issues within the Daoist arts. They are: harmonious Qi, a still mind, a tranquil nature, forgetting the emotions and having the five spirits in harmony.

Xiao Dao (消導) Guide out and expel A Chinese medical principle referring to the process involved in clearing stagnant and pathogenic energies from the channel system. It is a large part of Dao Yin practice as well as a process that can take place on the level of consciousness once a practitioner reaches a certain level of internal cultivation.

Xiao Zhou Tian (小周天) Microcosmic orbit The various processes involved in circulating Qi and other components of the San Bao through the two key channels of the back and front of the body. It serves as a safety mechanism, a recycling orbit for the energies of the body and a pathway through which Qi and Shen may nourish the brain.

Xie (泄) Purge One of the key ways in which Qi should be regulated through Qi Gong practice. If an art lacks any kind of purging then it is considered to be imbalanced.

Xie Qi (邪氣) Demonic Qi A somewhat overly dramatic name for the pathogenic forms of energy that can stick within the channel system. Its name heralds back to a time when all sicknesses were believed to originate in demonic possession or invasion of the body by ghosts. In contemporary practice, we could instead translate the term as 'sick Qi'.

Xin (心) Heart Mind This is the framework with which we attempt to understand the various aspects of human consciousness. Originally a Buddhist concept, it was absorbed into Daoist teachings.

Xin Fen Xi (心分析) Mind analysis A practical method used within Nei Gong training to help understand and unfold the various layers of the mind.

Xin Ling Li (心靈力) Psychic ability development A system of Daoist practice whereby the practitioner uses specific exercises and practices with the sole aim of developing Siddhi and psychic abilities. It should be noted that this is a very risky path to follow and many of the Daoist sects viewed this as a deviant system.

Xin Ting (心聽) Listening with the mind A stage of development that your awareness will move through during internal practice. Here, the mind begins to contemplate what is happening inside the body and mind. It is not an 'incorrect' stage but is a stage we should move past through continued training.

Xin Yin (心印) Mind stamp A name for the way in which an initiated teacher will pass on psychic information to their students. Each transmission of this kind carries with it the personal imprint of the teacher, much like a personalised 'chop' or 'stamp'.

Xin Zhai (心齋) Heart Mind fasting A principle of meditation within the Daoist tradition whereby the Heart Mind is starved of stimuli from the sense faculties. In some lineages, it is a set of specific training methods, whereas in others it is a guiding principle.

Xing (性) Your nature This is the expression of the various energetic and spiritual components of consciousness. It is one of the core concerns for Daoist alchemical practitioners who seek to harmonise the Xing, along with the Ming.

Xiu Zhen Tu (修真圖) The Chart of Cultivating Perfection A highly influential chart within the Daoist alchemical tradition. It is often paired with the Nei Jing Tu and shows many of the theories and views associated with the viscera and their functions.

Xu (虛) Emptiness A state of no thought and no mental action that is attained through meditation practice. It is understood to be a precursor for the arrival of Shen Ming.

Xuan Men (玄門) Mysterious pass The passageway through which the true spirit may arise. Rather than being a physical place in the body, it manifests when the body and mind are in harmonious states.

Yang (陽) The active Daoist philosophical extreme of movement, masculinity and action. One of the two great points which is required to manifest existence.

Yang Ming (陽命) Will of Heaven The way that Heaven influences the Ming of all people. This is the level of Ming that we have the least governance over. All concepts of higher purpose are linked to the influence of Yang Ming.

Yang Qi (陽氣) Yang energy An electrical type of energy that flows within the channel system, generally near to the surface of the body. It is linked to consciousness and the realm of mind. Within Daoist cosmology, it is the primal energy that sparked the creation of reality.

Yang Sheng Fa (養生法) Healthy living Literally 'life-nourishing principles'. This is the Daoist practice of living healthily which should be studied alongside all internal arts. No matter how good your practice, if you smoke, drink and eat a load of rubbish, your health will suffer the consequences.

Ye (業) Cause and effect The Daoist rule that is the nearest equivalent to Karma. It is the basis for how all actions unfold within the realm of manifestation.

Yi (意) Intention The aspect of our mind that is able to focus and have intention behind it. Within Daoist theory, it is also the aspect of our mind that is subject to mental movements.

Yi Jin Jing (易筋經) Sinew-Changing Classic An important series of classical teachings traditionally attributed to Bodhidharma. These teachings concern how to develop the body according to an effective series of internal processes as well as how to open the channel system.

Yi Jing (易經) Change Classic An ancient Daoist text which is based upon Ba Gua theory. Commonly written as I Ching. It is a model of how Ming and associated energies interact with one another and transform at any given moment. It is used to inform almost all Daoist practice, though in modern times, it is commonly known as a purely divinational text.

Yi Shou Dan Tian (意守丹田) Guard the mind within the Dan Tian An important Qi Gong principle that governs the way in which the awareness should reside within the lower Dan Tian during the phase of leading Qi there.

Yin (陰) The receptive The Daoist philosophical pole of stillness, femininity and quietude. One of the two poles required in order for existence to come into being.

Yin Ming (陰命) The 'lower' will of Heaven This can be likened to the idea of fate. It suggests a certain degree of pre-ordained potential but not necessarily a 'higher' purpose.

Yin Qi (陰氣) Yin energy Our internal energy that serves to shape the body and form the basis of the organs' function. Can also be used within alchemical theory to describe the movement of Wuji as it coalesces around the condensed energy of Yang Qi.

Yong Quan (涌泉) Surging spring An acupuncture point on the base of the foot. This is the main point through which Earth energy is drawn into the body.

Yu Ye (玉液) Jade fluid The special form of saliva that arises as a result of the congenital actions of the microcosmic orbit. It is a sweet-tasting substance that signifies the production of more Jing within the body.

Yuan Jing (元精) Original essence The original essence which exists prior to the beginning of the movement of the acquired Jing; it is said to reside in the space between the Kidneys.

Yuan Qi (元氣) Original energy The original state of Qi prior to its movement into the acquired realm.

Yuan Shen (元神) Original spirit The original state of the human psyche prior to the movement from the congenital to the acquired. It exists as a brilliant white light within the space of the human Heart Mind.

Yuan Xi (元息) Original breath The 'breath of life' which is passed down into existence from Dao. Yuan Xi is an expression of the movement of Yuan Qi.

Zang Fu (臟腑) Internal organs The collective name for the Yin and Yang organs of the body. Whilst some functions of these organs are the same as within Western biological thought, ancient Chinese models of the organs are more concerned with the energetic and spiritual properties that they pertain to.

Zhan Zhuang (站樁) Standing stake practice A common name for the practice of static postures that are held by Qi Gong practitioners for long periods of time. Often known as standing meditation, this is not quite true. Zhan Zhuang actually initiates a very active process within the body, quite different from the aim of inner stillness that is the basis for the majority of meditation systems.

Zhen (震) Zhen trigram One of the eight trigrams of Daoist Ba Gua theory. Its energetic manifestation is often likened to thunder.

Zhen Ren (真人) True person The 'true person' of Daoism is a high-level state of attainment possible through alchemical cultivation of the inner state. Many fantastical tales and supernatural skills are attributed to the Zhen Ren in Daoist lore.

Zheng Yi (正一) Orthodox Unity Sect The Daoist lineage founded during the Tang dynasty. It is a tradition with a mix of meditation practices, rituals and magical training.

Zhi (志) Willpower An element of human consciousness which is directly linked to the state of our Kidneys. The nearest translation in English is 'willpower'.

Zhu Chu Shi Men (逐出師門) Thrown out of door The act of removing somebody from a lineage that they have previously been initiated into. This can, in some cases, be a simple excommunication of the person, whilst in other cases it can involve energetic rituals to sever a person's connection to the frequency of that tradition.

Zhuang Zi (莊子) Daoist sage An important sage within the Daoist tradition. Zhuang Zi was known for his humour and the fact that he poked fun at almost every aspect of life. The teachings of Zhuang Zi are an indication of one of the key qualities of Daoism – light heartedness.

Zi Fa Gong (自發功) Self-expression practice The process of releasing spontaneous energetic movements through the body. This happens as stagnant energetic pathogens are released and the body begins to return to some kind of order. In this instance, the 'self' being expressed is the distorted quality of the acquired energetic system. The resultant reaction is often known as 'spontaneous Qi movement' in the West.

Ziran (自然) Harmonisation with nature The Daoist philosophical concept of acting in harmony with nature and returning to an original state.

Zou Huo Ru Mo (走火入魔) Entering the fire to invite demons A kind of sickness that can arise out of unsafe or incorrect Qi Gong practice. In this case, the build-up of pathogenic Heat within the body leads to psychiatric or emotional disorders. In these cases, all practice should immediately be ended and treatment sought from a skilled Chinese medical practitioner.

Zuo Wang (坐忘) Sitting and forgetting An important Daoist principle of meditation and Nei Gong whereby the mind is allowed to fade into the background so that stillness can arise. Within some traditions there are actual methods associated with Zuo Wang, whilst others use the term as an overriding principle that should be applied to all practice.

About the Author

Damo Mitchell was born into a family of martial artists and so began his studies at the age of four with martial arts. Since this time, he has continued to explore and practise the arts of Asia following the classical evolution of martial studies through into medicine and spiritual practice. Damo's studies have taken him into China, Taiwan and South-East Asia where he has spent many years travelling and researching these arts within several different traditions. Though his studies have included lengthy periods of time in Buddhist temples, it is the tradition of Daoism that has fully absorbed Damo and, in particular, the arts of Nei Gong and alchemical meditation.

Damo is the head of the Lotus Nei Gong International School of Daoist Arts, which has branches around Europe and the USA, as well as being one of the heads of the Xian Tian College of Chinese Medicine.

For more information on Damo, his background and his teachings, please visit his main website at www.lotusneigong.com

Index